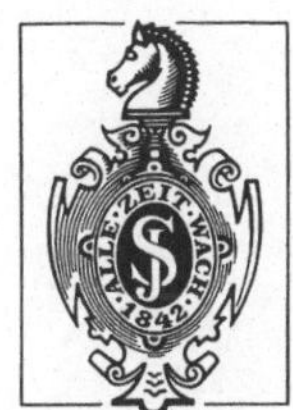

International Symposium, Mainz, Germany
October 1 and 2, 1979

International Boehringer Mannheim Symposia

Hypertension: Mechanisms and Management

Edited by
Th. Philipp and A. Distler

With 72 Figures and 17 Tables

Springer-Verlag Berlin Heidelberg New York 1980

Professor Dr. med. Thomas Philipp
Professor Dr. med. Armin Distler
Johannes-Gutenberg-Universität Mainz
I. Medizinische Klinik und Poliklinik
D-6500 Mainz, Langenbeckstraße 1

ISBN-13: 978-3-540-10171-0   e-ISBN-13: 978-3-642-67712-0
DOI: 10.1007/978-3-642-67712-0

Library of Congress Cataloging in Publication Data. Main entry under title:

Hypertension, mechanisms and management. (International Boehringer
Mannheim symposia) International symposium held Oct. 1–2, 1979, in Mainz at
the Akademie der Wissenschaften, and organized by the 1st Medical Dept. of
the University of Mainz. Bibliography: p. Includes index. 1. Hypertension-
Congresses. I. Philipp, Thomas, 1942 – II. Distler, Armin. III. Mainz. Universität.
Erste Medizinische Klinik und Poliklinik. IV. Series. [DNLM: 1. Hypertension-
Congresses. WG340 H9955 1979] RC685.H8H79 616.1'32 80-21560

Table of Contents

List of Contributors

Amann, F.W., Dr. med.
Division of Cardiology, Department of Medicine, University of Basel,
4031 Basel, Switzerland

Arlart, I., Dr. med.
Ulm University Medical Center, Steinhövelstraße 9, D-7900 Ulm,
Federal Republic of Germany

Bahlmann, J., Prof. Dr. med.
Department of Medicine, Medical School, Hannover, D-3000 Hannover,
Federal Republic of Germany

Beretta-Piccoli, C., Dr. med.
Medizinische Universitätspoliklinik, Freiburger Str. 3, 3010 Bern, Switzerland

Bertel, O., Dr. med.
Division of Cardiology, Department of Medicine, University of Basel,
Switzerland

Birkenhäger, W.H., Prof. Dr. med.
Department of Internal Medicine, Zuiderziekenhuis, Rotterdam,
The Netherlands

Bock, K.D., Prof. Dr. med.
Abteilung für Nieren- und Hochdruckkrankheiten, Medizinische Klinik der
Universität Essen, Hufelandstr. 55, D-4300 Essen, Federal Republic of Germany

Bönner, G., Dr. med.
Pharmakologisches Institut der Universität, Im Neuenheimer Feld 360,
D-6900 Heidelberg, Federal Republic of Germany

Bolli, P., Dr. med.
Division of Cardiology, Department of Medicine, University of Basel,
4031 Basel, Switzerland

Bouma, B.N., Dr. med.
Department of Haematology, University of Utrecht, The Netherlands

Brod, J., Prof. Dr. med.
Department of Medicine, Medical School, Hannover, D-3000 Hannover,
Federal Republic of Germany

van Brummelen, P., Dr. med.
Division of Cardiology, Department of Medicine, University of Basel,
4031 Basel, Switzerland

Brunner, H.R., Prof. Dr. med.
Centre Hospitalier Universitaire Vaudois, Department of Medicine,
1011 Lausanne, Switzerland

de Bruyn, J.H.B., Dr. med.
Department of Internal Medicine I, University Hospital Dijkzigt,
Erasmus University, Rotterdam, The Netherlands

Bühler, F.R., Prof. Dr. med.
Division of Cardiology, Department of Medicine, University of Basel,
4031 Basel, Switzerland

Carretero, O.A., M.D.
Department of Medicine, Henry Ford Hospital, Detroit, Michigan, 48202, USA

Cordes, U., Prof. Dr. med.
Abt. für Endokrinologie, II. Med. Klinik, Universitätskliniken, Langenbeckstr. 1,
6500 Mainz, W.-Germany

DeQuattro, V., M.D., Professor of Medicine
Department of Medicine, University of Southern California, Los Angeles,
California, 90033, USA

Derkx, F.H.M., Dr. med.
Department of Internal Medicine I, University Hospital Dijkzigt,
Erasmus University, Rotterdam, The Netherlands

Distler, A., Prof. Dr. med.
I. Medizinische Klinik, Universitätskliniken, Langenbeckstr. 1, D-6500 Mainz,
Federal Republic of Germany

Doyle, A.E., M.D., Professor of Medicine
University of Melbourne, Department of Medicine, Austin Hospital,
Heidelberg, Victoria 3084, Australia

Fuchs-Hammoser, R., Dr. med.
Division of Endocrinology, Department of Medicine, Klinikum Steglitz,
Freie Universität Berlin, D-1000 Berlin, Germany

Ganten, D., Prof. Dr. med.
Pharmakologisches Institut der Universität, Im Neuenheimer Feld 360,
D-6900 Heidelberg, Federal Republic of Germany

Glück, Z., Dr. med.
Medizinische Universitätspoliklinik, Freiburger Str. 3, 3010 Bern, Switzerland

Gordon, D., M.D.
Academic Surgical Unit, St. Mary's Hospital, London, W.2., Great Britain

Grimm, M. Dr. med.
Medizinische Universitätspoliklinik, Freiburger Str. 3, 3010 Bern, Switzerland

Grobecker, H., Prof. Dr. med.
Fachbereich Chemie und Pharmazie, Pharmakolog. Institut, Universität
Regensburg, D-8400 Regensburg, Federal Republic of Germany

Gross, F., Prof. Dr. med.
Pharmakolog. Institut der Universität, Im Neuenheimer Feld 360,
D-6900 Heidelberg, Federal Republic of Germany

Gutzwiller, F., Dr. med.
National Research Program 1, Kantonspital, 4031 Basel, Switzerland

Haehn, K.D., Prof. Dr. med.
Lehrstuhl für Allgemeinmedizin, Medizinische Hochschule Hannover,
D-3000 Hannover, Federal Republic of Germany

Hayduk, K., Prof. Dr. med.
Innere Abteilung des Marien-Hospitals, Rochusstr. 2, D-4000 Düsseldorf,
Federal Republic of Germany

Heck, J., Dr. med.
Medizinische Universitätspoliklinik, Wilhelmstr. 35, D-5300 Bonn,
Federal Republic of Germany

Heidland, A., Prof. Dr. med.
Nephrologische Abteilung, Medizinische Universitätsklinik, D-8700 Würzburg,
Federal Republic of Germany

Helber, A., Prof. Dr. med.
Krankenhaus Merheim, Universitäts-Poliklinik, Ostmerheimer Str. 200,
D-5000 Köln 91, Federal Republic of Germany

Henquet, J.W., Dr. med.
Rijsuniveriteit Limburg, Faculty of Medicine, P.O.Box 616, 6200 Maastricht,
The Netherlands

Hilfenhaus, M., Dr. med.
Department of Medicine, Medical School, Hannover, D-3000 Hannover,
Federal Republic of Germany

Hubrich, W., Dr. med.
Department of Medicine, Medical School, Hannover, D-3000 Hannover,
Federal Republic of Germany

Hummerich, W., Dr. med.
Krankenhaus Merheim, Universitäts-Poliklinik, Ostmerheimer Str. 200,
D-5000 Köln 91, Federal Republic of Germany

Jäger, H., Dr. med.
Ulm University Medical Center, Steinhövelstr. 9, D-7900 Ulm,
Federal Republic of Germany

Jahnecke, J., Prof. Dr. med.
St. Johannis-Hospital, Kölnstr. 54, D-5300 Bonn, Federal Republic of Germany

Johnston, W., M.D.
Department of Medicine, University of Southern California, Los Angeles,
California, 90033, USA

Kaufmann, W., Prof. Dr. med.
Krankenhaus Merheim, Medizinische Universitäts-Poliklinik, Ostmerheimer
Str. 200, D-5000 Köln 91, Federal Republic of Germany

Keusch, G., Dr. med.
Medizinische Universitätspoliklinik, Freiburger Str. 3, 3010 Bern, Switzerland

Kho, T., Dr. med.
Rijsuniversiteit Limburg, Faculty of Medicine, P.O.Box 616, 6200 Maastricht,
The Netherlands

Kiowski, W., Dr. med.
Division of Cardiology, Department of Medicine, University of Basel,
4031 Basel, Switzerland

Kobayashi, K., M.D.
Department of Medicine, University of Southern California, Los Angeles,
California, 90033, USA

Kolloch, R., Dr. med.
Medizinische Universitäts-Poliklinik, Wilhelmstr. 35, D-5300 Bonn,
Federal Republic of Germany

Krück, F., Prof. Dr. med.
Medizinische Universitäts-Poliklinik, Wilhelmstr. 35, D-5300 Bonn,
Federal Republic of Germany

Kühnert, M., Dr. med.
Medizinische Universitäts-Poliklinik, Wilhelmstr. 35, D-5300 Bonn,
Federal Republic of Germany

Laaser, U., Dr. med.
DIHB, Postfach 101409, D-6900 Heidelberg, Federal Republic of Germany

Landmann, R., Dr. med.
Division of Cardiology, Department of Medicine, University of Basel,
4031 Basel, Switzerland

Laragh, J.H., M.D.
Professor of Medicine, New York Hospital, Cornell University Med. Center,
525 E 68th Street, New York, 10021, USA

De Leeuw, P.W., Dr. med.
Department of Internal Medicine, Zuiderziekenhuis, Rotterdam, The Netherlands

Lever, A.F., M.D.
Medical Research Council, Blood Pressure Research Unit, Western Infirmary,
Glasgow G11 9NT, Great Britain

Liebau, H., Prof. Dr. med.
Department of Medicine, Medical School Hannover, D-3000 Hannover,
Federal Republic of Germany

Losse, H., Prof. Dr. med.
Med. Univ.-Poliklinik, Westring 3, D-4400 Münster, Federal Republic of Germany

Lüth, J.B., Dr. med.
I. Medizinische Klinik, Universitätsklinken, Langenbeckstr. 1, D-6500 Mainz,
Federal Republic of Germany

Man in t'Veld, A.J., Dr. med.
Department of Haematology, University of Utrecht, The Netherlands

Marin-Grez, M., Dr. med.
Pharmakologisches Institut der Universität, Im Neuenheimer Feld 360,
D-6900 Heidelberg, Federal Republic of Germany

Mariss, P., Dr. med.
Department of Medicine, Medical School Hannover, D-3000 Hannover,
Federal Republic of Germany

Meier, A., Dr. med.
Medizinische Universitätspoliklinik, Freiburger Str. 3, 3010 Bern, Switzerland

Meurer, K.A., Prof. Dr. med.
Krankenhaus Merheim, Universitäts-Poliklinik, Ostmerheimer Str. 200,
D-5000 Köln 91, Federal Republic of Germany

Miano, L., M.D.
Department of Medicine, University of Southern California, Los Angeles,
California, 90033, USA

Minder, I., Dr. med.
Medizinische Universitätspoliklinik, Freiburger Str. 3, 3010 Bern, Switzerland

Möhring, J. (†), Prof. Dr. med.
Merell Research Center, 16, rue d' Ankara, 67084 Strasbourg, France

Muscholl, E., Prof. Dr. med.
Pharmakolog. Institut der Universität, Obere Zahlbacher Str. 67,
D-6500 Mainz, Federal Republic of Germany

Oelkers, W., Prof. Dr. med.
Division of Endocrinology, Department of Medicine, Klinikum Steglitz,
Freie Universität Berlin, D-1000 Berlin, Germany

Overlack, A., Dr. med.
Medizinische Universitätspoliklinik, Wilhelmstr. 35, D-5300 Bonn,
Federal Republic of Germany

Philipp, Th., Prof. Dr. med.
I. Medizinische Klinik, Universitätskliniken, Langenbeckstr. 1, D-6500 Mainz,
Federal Republic of Germany

Pretschner, P., Dr. med.
Department of Medicine, Medical School Hannover, D-3000 Hannover,
Federal Republic of Germany

Rahn, K.H., Prof. Dr. med.
Rijsuniversiteit Limburg, Faculty of Medicine, P.O.Box 616, 6200 Maastricht,
The Netherlands

Rascher, W., Dr. med.
Pharmakologisches Institut der Universität, Im Neuenheimer Feld 360,
D-6900 Heidelberg, Federal Republic of Germany

Rastetter, B., Dr. med.
Pharmakologisches Institut der Universität, Im Neuenheimer Feld 360,
D-6900 Heidelberg, Federal Republic of Germany

Reid, J.L., M.D.
Department of Materia Medica, Stobhill General Hospital, Glasgow,
G21 3UW, Great Britain

Ressel, C.
Medizinische Universitätspoliklinik, Wilhelmstr. 35, D-5300 Bonn,
Federal Republic of Germany

Rockhold, R.W.
Pharmakologisches Institut der Universität, Im Neuenheimer Feld 360,
D-6900 Heidelberg, Federal Republic of Germany

Röckel, A., Prof. Dr. med.
Nephrologische Abteilung, Medizinische Universitätsklinik, D-8700 Würzburg,
Federal Republic of Germany

Rosenthal, J., Priv.Doz., Dr. med.
University Medical Center, Steinhövelstr. 9, D-7900 Ulm, Federal Republic
of Germany

Schalekamp, M.A.D.H., Dr. med.
Department of Internal Medicine I, University Hospital Dijkzigt, Erasmus
University, Rotterdam, The Netherlands

Schalekamp, M.P., Dr. med.
Department of Internal Medicine I, University Hospital Dijkzigt, Erasmus
University, Rotterdam, The Netherlands

Schmid, G., Dr. med.
Nephrologische Abteilung, Medizinische Universitätsklinik, D-8700 Würzburg,
Federal Republic of Germany

Schober, O., Dr. med.
Department of Medicine, Medical School Hannover, D-3000 Hannover,
Federal Republic of Germany

Schölkens, B., Dr. med.
Hoechst AG, Abt. für Pharmakologie, D-6230 Frankfurt-Hoechst,
Federal Republic of Germany

Schöneshöfer, M., Dr. med.
Division of Endocrinology, Department of Medicine, Klinikum Steglitz,
Freie Universität Berlin, D-1000 Berlin, Germany

Schols, M., Dr. med.
Rijsuniversiteit Limburg, Faculty of Medicine, P.O.Box 616, 6200 Maastricht,
The Netherlands

Schultze, G., Dr. med.
Division of Endocrinology, Department of Medicine, Klinikum Steglitz,
Freie Universität Berlin, D-1000 Berlin, Germany

Schwartz, F.W., Dr. med.
Zentralinstitut für die kassenärztliche Versorgung, Haedenkampstr. 5,
D-5000 Köln 91, Federal Republic of Germany

Scicli, A.G., M.D.
Department of Medicine, Henry Ford Hospital, Detroit, Michigan, 48202, USA

Seldin, D.W., M.D., Professor of Medicine
Department Int. Med., University of Texas, South Western Medical School,
Dallas, Texas 75235, USA

Sever, P., M.D.
Academic Surgical Unit, St. Mary's Hospital, London, W.2., Great Britain

Speck, G., Dr. med.
Pharmakologisches Institut der Universität, Im Neuenheimer Feld 360,
D-6900 Heidelberg, Federal Republic of Germany

Stürmer, G., Dr. med.
Nephrologische Abteilung, Medizinische Universitätsklinik, D-8700 Würzburg,
Federal Republic of Germany

Stumpe, K.O., Prof. Dr. med.
Medizinische Universitätspoliklinik, Wilhelmstr. 35, D-5300 Bonn, Federal
Republic of Germany

Tan-Tjong, H.L., Dr. med.
Department of Internal Medicine I, University Hospital Dijkzigt, Erasmus
University, Rotterdam, The Netherlands

Thijssen, H., Dr. med.
Rijsuniversiteit Limburg, Faculty of Medicine, P.O.Box 616, 6200 Maastricht,
The Netherlands

Unger, Th., Dr. med.
Pharmakologisches Institut der Universität, Im Neuenheimer Feld 360,
D-6900 Heidelberg, Federal Republic of Germany

Vecht, R.J., M.D.
Academic Surgical Unit, St. Mary's Hospital, London W.2., Great Britain

Venema, F., Dr. med.
Division of Endocrinology, Department of Medicine, Klinikum Steglitz,
Freie Universität Berlin, D-1000 Berlin, Germany

Wambach, G., Dr. med.
Krankenhaus Merheim, Universitäts-Poliklinik, Ostmerheimer Str. 200,
D-5000 Köln 91, Federal Republic of Germany

Ward, G.W., M.P.H.
National Heart, Lung, and Blood Institute, National Institutes of Health,
Bethesda, Maryland, 20205, USA

Weidmann, P., Prof. Dr. med.
Medizinische Universitätspoliklinik, Freiburger Str. 3, 3010 Bern, Switzerland

Wenting, G.J., Dr. med.
Department of Internal Medicine I, University Hospital Dijkzigt, Erasmus
University, Rotterdam, The Netherlands

Wester, A., Dr. med.
Department of Internal Medicine, Zuiderziekenhuis, Rotterdam,
The Netherlands

Willemse, P.J., Dr. med.
Department of Internal Medicine, Zuiderziekenhuis, Rotterdam, The Netherlands

Wolff, H.P., Prof. Dr. med.
I. Medizinische Klinik, Universitätskliniken, Langenbeckstr. 1, D-6500 Mainz,
Federal Republic of Germany

Preface

This volume presents the proceedings of the Symposium on "Hypertension., Mechanisms and Management" held at the "Akademie der Wissenschaften" in Mainz on the 1st and 2nd October, 1979. The Symposion has been dedicated to Professor Hanns-Peter Wolff, who has been the Chairman of the First Department of Internal Medicine at the University of Mainz since 1968, on the occasion of his 65th birthday.

The conference was mainly devoted to pathophysiological aspects of high blood pressure. A first series of papers discussed the possible role of the sympathetic nervous system in the pathogenesis of arterial hypertension. Despite considerable methodological progress made in the measurement of circulating catecholamines it is still unclear whether catecholamines are raised in essential hypertension, and if so, whether this is important for the pathogenesis of high blood pressure. Practically all papers of the first session were related to this question.

For several decades the renin-angiotensin system has been the central topic of any hypertension meeting. We thought that additional lectures or papers on this subject might fail to provide new aspects. We therefore asked five experts who have been working in this field for many years to discuss in a Round Table whether or not the renin-angiotensin system might play a significant role in human hypertension.

A further topic were the renal tissue hormones other than renin-angiotensin. The papers discussed in particular kallikrein and its possible role in activating renin and thereby possibly contributing to high blood pressure.

In the last session of the meeting the problem was discussed of what to do with the many persons in this country who have high blood pressure. This question is still widely unresolved in Germany and we are particularly greatful to our colleagues from abroad for reporting here on the efforts made in their countries.

We are deeply indebted to Boehringer Mannheim, particularly to Dr. H. Wenzel and Mr. E. Rühl, for their generous support and help with the organization of the meeting.

Mainz, August 1980

Armin Distler
Thomas Philipp

Sympathetic Nervous System and Hypertension

Circulatory Neurohormones in Primary Hypertension: Probes in Etiology and Treatment

V. DeQuattro, R. Kolloch, K. Kobayashi, W. Johnston,
L. Miano

Summary

Plasma noradrenaline content may be a biochemical marker of sympathetic
nerve function in man and of value in determining the pathophysiology and
therapy of primary hypertension. This paper describes our findings of the concentrations of the circulatory neurohormones, adrenaline (A), noradrenaline
(NA) and its metabolite normetanephrine (NMN) in normotensive volunteers
and patients with primary hypertension. A and NA were measured in blood
from both arterial and venous sites and NMN was determined in venous blood.
Venous plasma NA and NMN, but not A, appear to be reliable markers of net
sympathetic tone in man and are increased in young patients with primary
hypertension. These findings may indicate an enhanced central sympathetic
noradrenergic tone which is especially amenable to therapy with centrally acting alpha agonist antihypertensive drugs.

Introduction

Sympathetic nerve function is assessed in animal models with hypertension by
measuring tissue content, biosynthesis and turnover of noradrenaline [1]. Noradrenaline and adrenaline enter the venous circulation after neuronal release at
the synaptic cleft and after exocytosis from the adrenal medulla, respectively.
The contents of these catecholamines and metabolites in plasma are the net
result of their rates of entry, degradation and excretion and at steady state reflect the level of sympathetic nerve activity [2].

This paper describes our findings of the concentrations of: 1) noradrenaline,
adrenaline and normetanephrine in venous plasma of normotensives and age-
matched hypertensives during stimulation and suppression of sympathetic
nerve tone, 2) noradrenaline and adrenaline in venous and arterial plasma of
both normotensives and hypertensive patients with various illnesses before and
during postural stress and 3) noradrenaline in venous plasma of hypertensive
patients before, during and after therapy with an alpha agonist congenor of
clonidine, tiamenidine. The results suggest that plasma concentrations of NA,
A and NMN in venous plasma reflect sympathetic nerve tone and are elevated

in some hypertensives and can predict which patients are especially responsive
to drugs which suppress central sympathetic nerve function.

Methods

Subjects

Three different groups of patients were studied. Group I were young hypertensives and volunteers age twenty to forty (mean 30 ± 1); Group II were fourteen
patients with various illness age 22 to 70 (mean 52 ± 4); Group III were sixteen
patients age 23 to 61 (mean 51 ± 2) with uncomplicated primary hypertension
who were studied before, during and after therapy with tiamenidine, 3 mg per
day. Patients were classified as hypertensive if supine blood pressure on three
consecutive visits were averaged as 140/90 mm Hg or greater.

Protocol

All subjects signed informed consents approved by the institutional review
committee. Blood samples were taken after sixty minutes in the supine position. Subjects of Groups II and III then stood five and sixty minutes, respectively and another blood sample was obtained. Some normotensive subjects of
Group I had blood samples taken after ambulation and at fifteen minute intervals during one hour each of lying and standing. Simultaneous arterial samples
were obtained from Group II subjects via radial artery puncture during both
supine and upright positions.

Assays

Plasma NA and A were measured via: 1) a radioenzymatic method [3] for
Group I subjects and 2) a fluorimetric method (Renzini) in Groups II and III
[4]. NMN was measured after conversion of NMN to MN^3H with tritiated SAM
and isolation of the product on thin layer chromatography [5].

Plasma was collected in EGTA gluthathione or EDTA chilled tubes for the
enzymatic and fluorimetric assays, respectively.

Results

Group I

The postural variation of plasma concentrations of NA and NMN are shown for
three normotensive subjects during ambulation and subsequently while supine

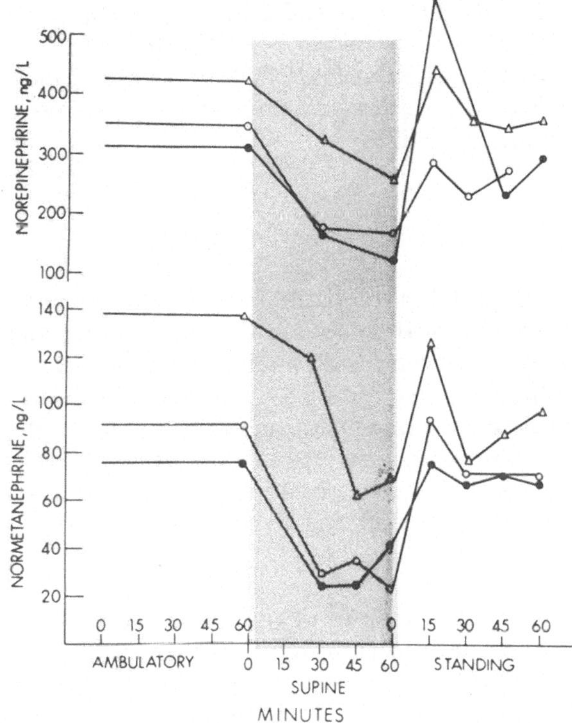

Fig. 1. The fluctuations of the concentrations of NA and NMN in plasma of normotensive volunteers during ambulation, supine rest, and standing

and standing (Fig. 1). The means of the plasma concentrations of NA, A and NMN of young normotensives and hypertensives of Group I in the supine position are given in Table 1. The values of all three substances were increased in the hypertensives, but only NA and NMN increases were significant.

Table 1. Elevated circulatory neurohormones in young hypertensives during basal conditions

	Noradrenaline	Adrenaline ng/L	Normetanephrine
Normotensives (8) (31 ± 1)	219 ± 51	26 ± 8	64 ± 11
Hypertensives (12) (30 ± 2)	348 ± 24	40 ± 5	95 ± 9
P	<.05	NS	<.02

Values (means ± SEM) in parenthesis are those of N and age in years, respectively

The mean plasma concentration of NA, A and NMN of five normotensives after one hour ambulation were: 432 ± 68, 113 ± 31 and 100 ± 15 ng/L, respectively. These values were all reduced by fifty percent (P <.01 for each) after thirty minutes in the supine position. The NA and NMN concentrations returned to ambulatory levels after fifteen minutes standing. The A levels returned to ambulatory levels after 45 min standing.

Group II

The means of arterial and venous NA and A for the patients, both supine and standing, are given in Table 2. The levels of both venous and arterial noradrenaline and those of arterial adrenaline, but not venous adrenaline were increased significantly (above two-fold) after standing five minutes compared to the supine values. There were no differences in the concentrations of NA in arterial vs. venous plasma during either the supine or standing positions. However, the plasma concentration of A in arterial plasma was increased significantly compared to venous plasma while supine and after standing five minutes.

Table 2. The responsiveness of plasma concentrations of noradrenaline and adrenaline of the arterial and venous circulations to upright posture

| | Nanograms/Liter | | Difference |
	Supine	Standing	(Su) vs. (St)
Noradrenaline			
Venous	392 ± 69	803 ± 163	< .01
Arterial	395 ± 58	637 ± 105	< .01
Difference			
(V) vs. (A)	NS	NS	
Adrenaline			
Venous	50 ± 18	83 ± 22	NS
Arterial	107 ± 33	187 ± 41	< .05
Difference			
(V) vs. (A)	< .05	< .01	

Values are Mean ± SEM.
Students "t" test for paired data was used

Group III

These hypertensive patients were divided into two additional subgroups as determined by their plasma NA concentration after one hour supine rest. Patients in subgroup I were those whose plasma NA concentrations were less than 200 ng/L. Patients in subgroup II had concentrations equal or greater than 200 ng/L. The mean values of the two subgroups while supine were 133 ± 12 and 280 ± 27 ng/L, respectively (P <.01). The mean systolic and diastolic blood pressure responses of these two subgroups both supine and standing are shown after three months therapy and 48 hours after discontinuation of therapy (Fig. 2). The eight patients with the higher mean supine plasma NA had greater and significant reductions in systolic and diastolic blood pressure in both supine and standing positions. From a systolic of 183 ± 7 and a diastolic of 109 ± 11 to 158 ± 8 and 98 ± 4 (P < .05, < .05) while supine and from systolic 177 ± 9 and diastolic 114 ± 3 to 147 ± 8 and 100 ± 4 while standing (P < .05, < .01). The other eight patients with the lower plasma NA had a diastolic blood pressure change only in the standing position from a mean of 118 ± 3 to 103 ± 6 mm Hg (P <.05).

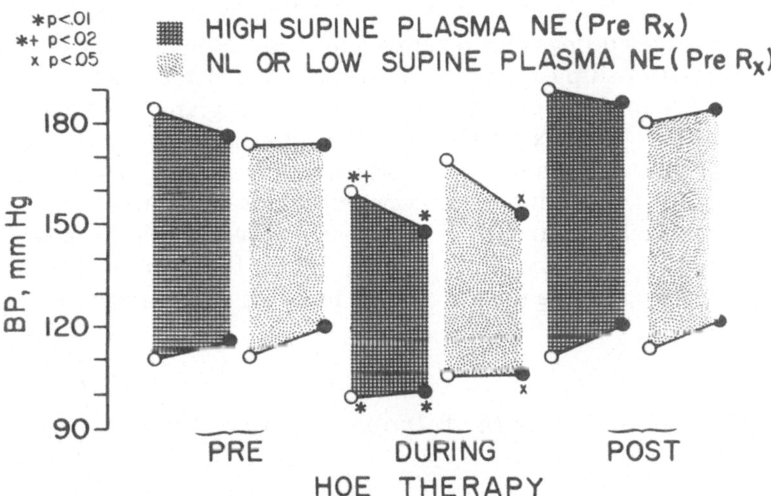

Fig. 2. Supine and standing blood pressures of hypertensive patients segregated according to basal concentrations of plasma NA before, during and after cessation of therapy with tiamenidine (HOE 440), a clonidine congenor

Discussion

Plasma Neurohormones as Biochemical Markers

Plasma noradrenaline, adrenaline and normetanephrine concentrations increased in venous blood during standing and ambulation in the range of two to three-fold as compared to values in the supine position.

These increments reflect recruitment of the sympathetic neuronal activity required to enhance venous return and offset reduced cardiac output during upright posture. These changes in the concentrations of neurohormones could also follow reduced glomerulo filtration and renal clearance. However, these renal factors apparently have a minor influence on plasma NA since postural increments have been reported in anephric patients [6].

The corresponding increases in plasma NMN concentration support the notion that the increased plasma NA reflects enhanced synthesis and release of neurotransmittor rather than diminished uptake, degradation and excretion. Kopin has demonstrated that NMN, the product of NA which increases in venous effluent from innervated organs after neuronal stimulation, is the metabolite which best reflects synthesis and release of newly formed norepinephrine [7].

Venous plasma adrenaline may not be as reliable a marker of peripheral sympathetic tone. Plasma concentrations of adrenaline measured from arterial sites in convalescing patients with various physical illnesses exceeded those from venous sites especially after the additional stress of upright posture. This finding may be interpreted as a result of clearance of adrenaline from the arterial circulation by perfused nerve endings and receptors or a consequence of not reaching a steady state relationship of venous to arterial concentrations after sixty minutes supine or five minutes of standing. The latter explanation does not seem plausible since the plasma NA level at five minutes is 75 to 80 percent of that reached at sixty minutes [8] and that steady states of plasma NA are reached in venous blood after five minutes of constant intravenous infusion of noradrenaline [9]. Higher levels of adrenaline in arterial vs. venous blood have been reported previously [10, 11]. Therefore, arterial rather than venous plasma adrenaline concentrations may be more accurate markers of sympathetic nerve tone.

Circulatory NA and NMN as Probes for the Pathophysiology of Primary Hypertension

The findings in this small group of hypertensives support those of several groups [12] studying young agematched normotensives and hypertensives. The elevated values of plasma NA and NMN are thought to reflect increased synthesis and release of transmitter into the neural cleft and subsequently the venous blood. We do not suggest that the elevated NA has a pharmacological or physiological effect on distal receptors. The evidence suggests only that some patients, perhaps 25 to 30 percent, have raised plasma NA or NMN, a reflection of increased central and peripheral sympathetic nerve activity perhaps a major cause of their elevated blood pressure [13]. Further, evidence suggests that increased noradrenergic activity as a pathogenic factor in primary hypertension is not tenable in older patients [5]. It appears likely then with aging and with the development of renal and vascular sequelae of the hypertension the enhanced neurogenic tone is buffered by secondary factors which then become prominent in maintaining the hypertension.

Basal Plasma NA as a Probe for Rational Therapy

Pari passu with the observation that some hypertensives have increased noradrenergic tone as a pathogenic factor is the expectation that the blood pressures
of these patients should be more responsive to drugs which suppress sympathetic tone. This hypothesis has been tested, and its validity supported by Louis
and Doyle with a ganglionic blocking agent [14]. In our study we found enhanced
responsiveness of arterial blood pressure of patients with raised noradrenergic
tone to long term therapy with the centrally acting inhibitor of sympathetic
nerve function, the alpha agonist congenor of clonidine, tiamenidine. Similar
findings after clondine were reported earlier by Louis and Doyle [15].

We also observed greater blood pressure lowering in the standing position of
both groups of hypertensives-indirect evidence of the enhanced noradrenergic
recruitment during upright posture. The findings with tiamenidine therapy in
this small group of hypertensives suggest that further measurements of circulating neurohormones may provide more effective and rational mono-drug
therapy for patients with primary hypertension.

Acknowledgment. We gratefully acknowledge the technical assistance of
Daantje Meijer and the preparation of the manuscript by Mrs. Nancy King.

References

1. DeQuattro V, Nagatsu T, Maronde R, Alexander L (1969) Catecholamine
   synthesis in rabbits with neurogenic hypertension. Circ Res 24:545-555
2. Popper CW, Chiueh CC, Kopin IJ (1977) Plasma catecholamine concentrations in unanesthetized rats during sleep, wakefulness, immobilization and
   after decapitation. J Pharmacol Exp Ther 202:144-148
3. Peuler JD, Johnson GA (1978) Simultaneous single isotope radioenzymatic
   assay of plasma norepinephrine, epinephrine and dopamine. Life Sciences
   21:625-636
4. Miura Y, Campese V, DeQuattro V, Meijer D (1977) Plasma catecholamines
   via an improved fluorimetric assay; comparison with an enzymatic method.
   J Lab Clin Med 89:421-427
5. Kobayashi K, Kolloch R, DeQuattro V, Miano L (1979) Increased plasma
   and urinary normetanephrine in young patients with primary hypertension. Clin Sci Mol Med, in press
6. Brecht HM, Ernst W, Koch KM (1975) Plasma noradrenaline levels in regular hemodialysis patients. Proc Eur Dial Transpl Assoc 12:281-289
7. Kopin IJ, Breese GR, Krauss KR, Weise VK (1968) Selective release of newly synthesized norepinephrine from the cat spleen during sympathetic
   nerve stimulation. J Pharmacol Exp Ther 161:271-278
8. DeQuattro V, Chan S (1972) Raised plasma-catecholamines in some patients with primary hypertension. Lancet 1:806-809
9. Cohen G, Holland B, Sha J, Goldenberg M (1959) Plasma concentrations of

epinephrine and norepinephrine during intravenous infusions in man. J Clin Invest 38:1935-1941

10. Vendsalu A (1960) Studies on adrenaline and noradrenaline in human plasma. Acta Physiol Scand (Suppl. 173) 49:1
11. Miura Y, Haneda T, Sato T, Miyazawa K, Sakuma H, Kobayashi K, Minai K, Shirato K, Honna T, Takishima T, Yoshinaga K (1976) Plasma catecholamine levels in the coronary sinus, aorta and femoral vein of subjects undergoing cardiac catheterization at rest and during exercise. Japanese Circ J 40:929-934
12. Miura Y, Kobayashi K, Sakuma H, Tomioka H, Adachi J, Yoshinaga K (1978) Plasma noradrenaline concentrations and hemodynamics in the early stage of essential hypertension. Clin Sci Mol Med 55:69s-71s
13. Eide I, Kolloch R, DeQuattro V, Miano L, Dugger R, Van der Meulen J (1979) Raised cerebrospinal fluid norepinephrine in some patients with primary hypertension. Hypertension 1:255-260
14. Louis WJ, Doyle AE, Anavekar S (1973) Plasma norepinephrine levels in essential hypertension. N Engl J Med 288:599
15. Louis WJ, Doyle AE, Anavekar SN, Johnston CI, Geffen LB, Rush R (1974) Plasma catecholamine, dopamine-beta-hydroxylase, and renin levels in essential hypertension. Circ Res Suppl I: 57-61

Plasma Catecholamine Levels and the Renin-Angiotensin-System in Subjects with Borderline Hypertension

K. H. RAHN, J. W. HENQUET, T. KHO, M. SCHOLS, H. THIJSSEN

The role of the sympathetic nervous system in the pathogenesis of essential hypertension is still controversial. Upon sympathetic nervous stimulation, noradrenaline is released from nerve endings. The majority of it is taken up again into the neurons but a small fraction reaches the systemic circulation. Thus, plasma noradrenaline concentration can be used as an index of sympathetic nervous activity. In man, most if not all adrenaline in plasma stems from the adrenal medulla.

Increased plasma catecholamine levels have been found in patients with essential hypertension at rest and during physical activity (Engelman et al., 1970; De Quattro and Chan, 1972; Louis et al., 1974; Chodakowska et al., 1975; Planz et al., 1976). In other studies, however, such differences were not detected (Pedersen and Christensen, 1975; Lake et al., 1977; Taylor et al., 1978). The discrepancies might be due to differences in the composition of the groups of subjects studied. Thus, it could be that elevated plasma catecholamine concentrations exist only in an early phase of hypertension. Furthermore, increased plasma catecholamine levels could be the consequence rather than the cause of blood pressure elevation. One would then expect catecholamine concentrations to increase with the progression of hypertension, little or no rise of plasma catecholamine concentrations in normotensives and in patients with borderline hypertension.

It seemed possible that differences in plasma catecholamine concentrations might become more evident during physical exercise, that is in a situation with increased sympathetic activity. Furthermore, the sympathetic nervous system is known to be a mediator of renin secretion by the kidney. Thus, there could be altered plasma renin activities concomitant with changes of plasma catecholamine levels. Therefore, both plasma catecholamines and plasma renin were measured at rest and during physical activity.

The study was performed in male subjects whose age ranged from 18 to 30 years. 25 of them were normotensives, that is, their blood pressure after 2 min standing was 125/85 mm Hg or less at two measurements performed with an interval of one week. The other 25 subjects were borderline hypertensives. For the purpose of this study, borderline hypertension is defined as standing blood pressure reading of 140/90 or above but less than 160/100 mm Hg at two measurements with one week's interval. In order to recruit volunteers for the study, all 18 to 30 years old men attending an outpatient clinic of the Maastricht University Hospital were asked to participate provided no diagnosis other than mild hypertension had been made. Furthermore, three general practitioners were requested to recruit volunteers in the same way. Secondary hypertension was excluded by history, physical examination, urinanalysis, determination of potassium and creatinine in serum as well as vanilmandelic acid excretion in urine and by intravenous pyelography. None of the subjects with borderline hypertension had retinal changes. None of them ever had received antihypertensive therapy.

In all subjects studied, the urinary excretion of sodium, vanilmandelic acid, noradrenaline and adrenaline was measured. Subsequently, maximum work capacity during bicycle ergometry was determined. Five to seven days thereafter, heart rate, blood pressure, plasma catecholamines, plasma renin activity and plasma renin concentration were measured after 30 min supine rest as well as at the end of a 5 min ergometry period at 50 and 75% of maximum work capacity. Noradrenaline and adrenaline in plasma were determined by means of a radioenzymatic method. Plasma renin activity and plasma renin concentration were measured by radioimmunoassay.

In the normotensives, 24 h urinary excretion averaged 186 mval for sodium, 2.2 mg for vanilmandelic acid, 59 µg for adrenaline. The values determined in subjects with borderline hypertension did not differ from these data. Maximum work capacity was in the average 210 watt in the normotensives. This value was 185 watt in the subjects with borderline hypertension. The difference is statistically significant. Both groups of subjects achieved an average heart rate of 180 beats/min at maximum work capacity.

Resting heart rate averaged 63 beats/min in the normotensives. It was 73 beats/ min in the subjects with borderline hypertension. The difference is statistically significant. In both groups of volunteers heart rate increased during physical activity corresponding to 50 and 75% of maximum work capacity. At both work levels, the heart rate was significantly higher in subjects with borderline hypertension than in normotensives. Thus, only at maximum work capacity both groups had identical heart rates.

Blood pressure at supine rest averaged 120/80 mm Hg in the normotensives. It was 150/95 mm Hg in the subjects with borderline hypertension. In both groups, systolic blood pressure rose significantly during physical activity, whereas diastolic blood pressure was higher in borderline hypertensives than in normotensives at a physical activity corresponding to 50 and 75% of maximum work capacity.

At rest, plasma noradrenaline concentration averaged 0.35 ng/ml in the normotensives studied. This parameter rose to an average of 1.25 ng/ml at physical exercise corresponding to 75% of maximum work capacity. The noradrenaline concentrations measured in the subjects with borderline hypertension did not differ from the data determined in the normotensives.

Resting adrenaline concentration was 0.09 ng/ml in normotensives. It rose to 0.21 ng/ml at 75% of maximum work capacity. Again there was no difference between normotensives and subjects with borderline hypertension.

The same is true for plasma renin activity, which corresponded to 1.2 ng angiotensin I/ml · h. This parameter rose to an average of 2 ng angiotensin I/ml · h at physical exercise corresponding to 75% of maximum work capacity.

There was also no difference between the two groups of subjects studied in plasma renin concentration at rest and during physical activity.

In the present study, there were no differences between normotensives and subjects with borderline hypertension in the plasma concentrations of noradrenaline and adrenaline as well as in plasma renin activity and plasma renin concentration. The results do not support the assumption that there is an increased activity of the sympathetic nervous system at the begin of essential hypertension. However, one has to consider that only in a minor portion of subjects with borderline hypertension blood pressure will reach definitively hypertensive levels in the course of some years. It could be that only in these subjects plasma catecholamine levels rise as compared with normotensive persons.

Recently, Robertson et al. (1979) published a study of the sympathetic nervous system in borderline hypertensives. These authors, too, found no differences in plasma noradrenaline levels at supine rest between subjects with borderline hypertension and normotensive controls. However, in their study plasma noradrenaline concentrations in borderline hypertensives were higher than in normotensives during physical activity. Several points of their paper ought to be discussed. First of all, their essential conclusions are based on a very small number of subjects, that is seven normotensives and eight to nine borderline hypertensives. There is substantial overlapping of the plasma noradrenaline levels of the two groups. Inclusion of a few more subjects could make the differences no longer statistically significant. In the second place, the authors used exercise on a treadmill without taking into account that there might be differences between the two groups of subjects studied in the maximum tolerated work load. Thus, differences in conditioning could contribute to or even cause the differences in plasma noradrenaline levels observed. Taken together, the study by Robertson et al. (1979) does not give convincing evidence of increased sympathetic nervous system activity in subjects with borderline hypertension. Our own study is limited by the fact that the volunteers were studied only at rest and during physical exercise. It seems possible that by using other stimuli to activate the sympathetic nervous system differences between normotensives and borderline hypertensive subjects become demonstrable.

References

Chodakowska J, Nazar K, Wocial B, Jarecki M, Skórka B (1975) Plasma catecholamines and renin activity in response to exercise in patients with essential hypertension. Clin Sci Mol Med 49:511-514

DeQuattro V, Chan S (1972) Raised plasma catecholamines in some patients with primary hypertension. Lancet 1:806-809

Engelman K, Portnoy B, Sjoerdsma A (1970) Plasma catecholamine concentrations in patients with essential hypertension. Circ Res Suppl 1 27:141-145

Lake CR, Ziegler MG, Coleman MD, Kopin IJ (1977) Age-adjusted plasma norepinephrine levels are similar in normotensive and hypertensive subjects. N Engl J Med 296:208-209

Louis WJ, Doyle AE, Anavekar SN, Johnston CI, Geffen LB, Rush R (1974) Plasma catecholamine, dopamine-beta-hydroxylase, and renin levels in essential hypertension. Circ Res Suppl 1 34:57-61

Pedersen EB, Christensen NJ (1975) Catecholamines in plasma and urine in patients with essential hypertension determined by double-isotope derivate techniques. Acta Med Scand 198:373-377

Planz G, Gierlichs HW, Hawlina A, Planz R, Stephany W, Rahn KH (1976) A comparison of catecholamine concentrations and dopamine-beta-hydroxylase activities in plasma from normotensive subjects and from patients with essential hypertension at rest and during exercise. Klin Wochenschr 54:561-565

Robertson D, Shand DG, Hollifield JW, Nies AS, Frölich JC, Oates J (1979) Alterations in the response of the sympathetic nervous system and renin in borderline hypertension. Hypertension 1:118-124

Taylor AA, Pool JL, Lake CR, Ziegler MG, Rosen RA, Rollins DE, Mitchell JR (1978) Plasma norepinephrine concentrations — no differences among normal volunteers and low, high or normal renin hypertensive patients. Life Sci 22.1499-1510

Sympathetic Nervous Activity, Noradrenaline Reactivity, and Blood Pressure Control

A. DISTLER, TH. PHILIPP, B. LÜTH, U. CORDES

Slightly to moderately increased plasma noradrenaline levels thought to reflect increased sympathetic tone have been observed in a proportion of patients with essential hypertension [1, 2, 3]. However, some authors have also reported on normal plasma noradrenaline levels in essential hypertension [4, 5].

We have previously shown that an inverse correlation exists between plasma noradrenaline concentration during physical exercise and reactivity to exogenous noradrenaline in normotensive subjects [6]. This relationship was invariably disturbed in age-matched patients with essential hypertension. In the patients with high plasma noradrenaline levels the pressor response to noradrenaline was not diminished appropriately, and in the patients with normal or low noradrenaline reactivity to noradrenaline was inappropriately increased. A multiple regression analysis revealed a highly significant correlation between the combination of both factors and the height of mean arterial blood pressure (Fig. 1) suggesting that sympathetic nervous activity and pressor response to noradrenaline together form an important determinant of arterial blood pressure level.

We were now interested in the *dynamic* interrelations between sympathetic nervous activity and reactivity to noradrenaline. For this purpose we studied patients who had undergone total thyroidectomy for thyroid cancer and who were in hypo- and hyperthyroid state at different times. In addition, we studied normotensive healthy volunteers who were given the synthetic mineralocorticoid fludrocortisone.

It is known from the literature that plasma noradrenaline is increased in hypothyroidism [7] and decreased in hyperthyroidism [8]. — Little is known so far about sympathetic nervous function in mineralocorticoid hypertension in man. However, previous studies in deoxycorticosterone-saline hypertensive rats conducted by de Champlain et al. [9] and by Reid et al. [10] had suggested that increased adrenergic activity might be an important factor in the development of this type of hypertension.

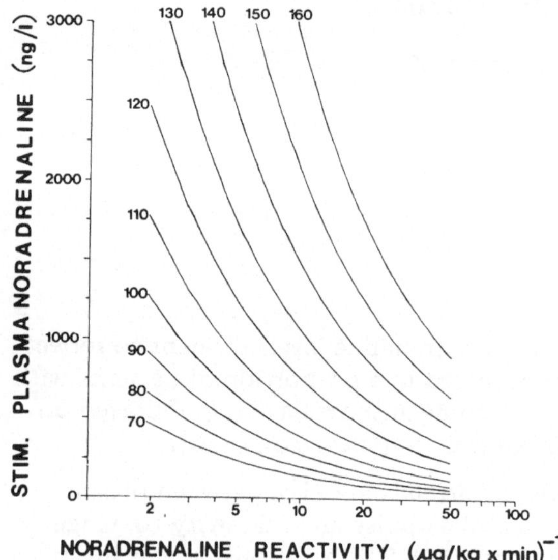

Fig. 1. Computer plot based on data from 29 normotensives and 29 patients with essential hypertension illustrating the dependency of mean arterial pressure on the combination of stimulated plasma noradrenaline concentration and reactivity to noradrenaline (from [6])

1. Studies in Hyper- and Hypothyroid State

Patients and Methods

The patients who had undergone total thyroidectomy for thyroid cancer ($n = 11$) were first studied while they were in a slightly hyperthyroid state resulting from high dose substitution therapy with 200-350 μg thyroxine/day. The high doses of thyroxine were necessary to suppress TSH release and to prevent a possible cancer spreading. — A second study of the same patients was done after substitution therapy had been withdrawn for at least four weeks. This stop was necessary to accomplish the annual total body radioiodine scan. At that time the patients were markedly hypothyroid as documented by very low plasma levels of tri-iodothyronine and thyroxine.

As an index of sympathetic nervous activity plasma noradrenaline concentration was measured at rest and after a standardized workload of 100 W for 2 min. Plasma noradrenaline was determinded by the method of Renzini et al. [11]. Reactivity to exogenous noradrenaline was estimated by determining so called "pressor doses". Reactivity is expressed in terms of reciprocal values of the pressor doses as described previously [6].

16

Results

Plasma noradrenaline was significantly higher both during recumbency and following exercise in the hypo- than in the hyperthyroid state (Fig. 2). Reactivity to noradrenaline was descreased in all patients in the hypothyroid state as compared to the hyperthyroid state (Fig. 3).

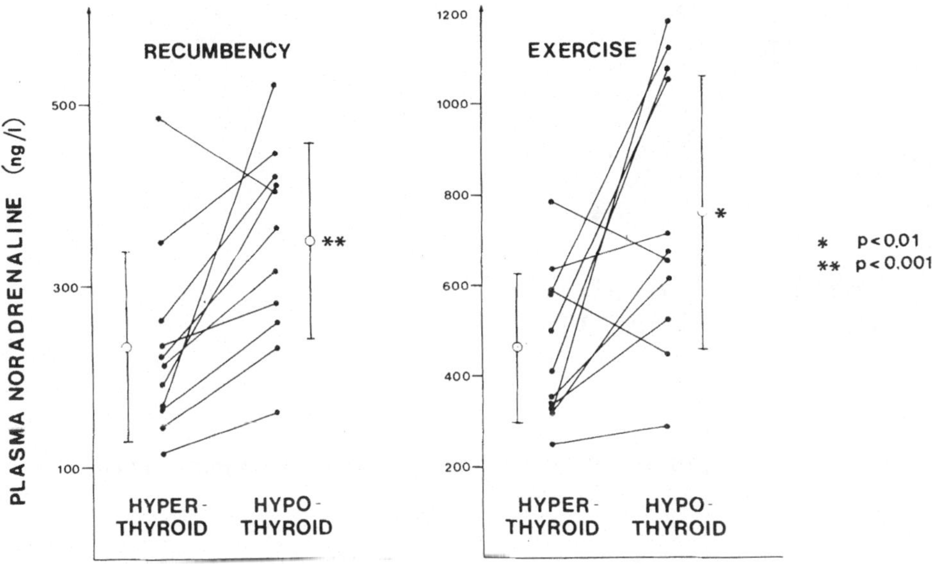

Fig. 2. Plasma noradrenaline concentration in eleven thyroidectomized patients in hyper- and hypothyroid state

Mean arterial blood pressure was slightly increased (by 6 mm Hg on the average) in the hypothyroid state as compared to the hyperthyroid state.

Discussion

These data seem to indicate again that there is an inverse relationship between plasma noradrenaline and reactivity to noradrenaline. When plasma noradrenaline increases as observed in the hypothyroid state reactivity to noradrenaline decreases. A likely explanation for this would be that the availability of noradrenaline receptors falls with increasing sympathetic nervous activity and vice versa. The inverse relationship between sympathetic tone and reactivity to noradrenaline appears to be of importance for the homoeostasis of the blood pressure. If an increased sympathetic tone were not counterbalanced by a decreased responsiveness to noradrenaline an excessive rise in blood pressure would occur.

17

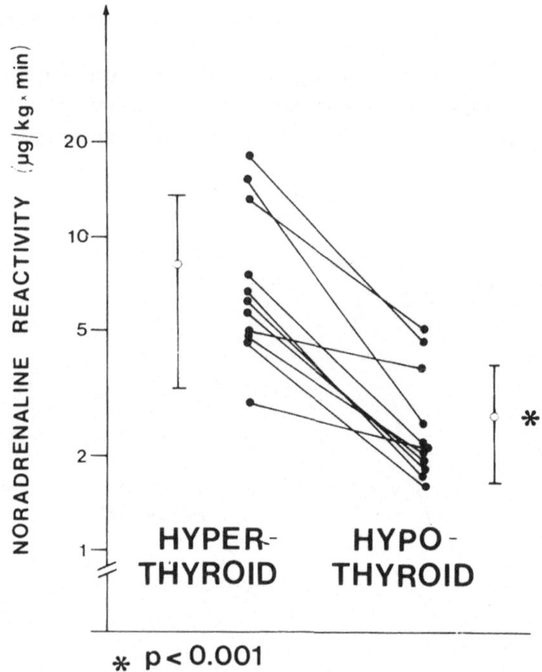

Fig. 3. Reactivity to exogenous noradrenaline in eleven thyroidectomized patients in hyper- and hypothyroid state

2. Studies During Mineralocorticoid Application

Subjects and Methods

The volunteer subjects ($n = 7$), who were between 22 and 25 years of age, were fully informed of the nature and the purpose of the study. Fludrocortisone was given orally in a daily dose of 0.8 mg for a period of six weeks. No dietary restrictions were made.

Plasma noradrenaline concentration was measured at rest and after a standardized workload of 200 W for 2 min. Plasma noradrenaline was determined by the method of da Prada and Zürcher [12]. Plasma renin activity (PRA) was determined after a 30 min resting period in recumbent position and after combined stimulation by 40 mg of furosemide i.v. and active orthostasis as described elsewhere [13]. Reactivity to exogenous noradrenaline and angiotensin II was estimated by determining so-called "pressor doses" as described in the foregoing section.

Results

Data on plasma noradrenaline and PRA are given in Table 1. Basal as well as
stimulated plasma noradrenaline levels fell within the first week of treatment
and remained depressed during the following weeks. Responsiveness to exogenous noradrenaline increased up to the third week. Thereafter responsiveness
to noradrenaline appeared to decrease once again. However, after the 6th week
of fludrocortisone administration, the responsiveness to noradrenaline was still
significantly higher (p < 0.01) than before treatment.

Table 1. Plasma noradrenaline (NA) concentration, plasma renin activity (PRA)
and reactivity to exogenous noradrenaline (pd NA^{-1}) and angiotensin II (pd ANG^{-1})
in seven normotensive subjects given 0.8 mg fludrocortisone daily for six weeks.
Studies were made before as well as after the first, third and sixth week of
steroid administration. Mean values are given ± SEM. Significance of changes
compared with control data: * P < 0.025; ** P < 0.01

	Control	Week 1	Week 3	Week 6
Plasma NA (ng/l)				
basal	299 ± 43	136 ± 24**	155 ± 21**	150 ± 34**
stimulated	898 ± 124	580 ± 116**	430 ± 91**	354 ± 25**
pd NA^{-1} (μg min^{-1} kg^{-1})	3.3 ± 0.4	6.2 ± 1.0**	8.8 ± 2.0**	5.1 ± 0.7**
PRA (ng h^{-1} kg^{-1})				
basal	3.7 ± 0.8	0.8 ± 0.1**	0.6 ± 0.1**	0 6 + 0.1**
stimulated	8.2 ± 1.9	1.3 ± 0.2**	1.4 ± 0.3**	1.1 ± 0.2**
pd ANG^{-1} (μg min^{-1} kg^{-1})	95 ± 14	163 ± 23*	301 ± 64**	222 ± 39**

Basal and stimulated PRA decreased during the first week of fludrocortisone
administration and remained depressed. Responsiveness to exogenous angiotensin II increased up to the 3rd week and declined thereafter, but was still
significantly higher (p < 0.01) than before fludrocortisone administration.

Discussion

As shown by haemodynamic studies, fludrocortisone causes a rise in blood
pressure which initially is a consequence of an increase in stroke volume and
in cardiac output. Later on, elevated blood pressure is caused by an increased
total peripheral resistance [14].

Studies in deoxycorticosterone-saline hypertensive rats [9, 10] had suggested
that increased adrenergic activity may be an important factor in the development of this type of hypertension. Our findings of a fall in plasma noradrena-

line concentration point toward a decreased rather than an increased sympathetic tone during mineralocorticoid-induced blood pressure increase in man.

The increase in reactivity to noradrenaline observed during fludrocortisone application is probably a compensatory phenomenon resulting from decreased noradrenaline-receptor occupancy due to decreased sympathetic tone, and does not appear to be the cause of the blood pressure rise. For the same reason the increase in reactivity to angiotensin II (which is probably the consequence of the fludrocortisone-induced renin suppression) does not appear to contribute to the blood pressure elevation.

Summary and Conclusions

As shown in a previous study [6], sympathetic tone (as reflected by stimulated plasma noradrenaline levels) and reactivity to noradrenaline form an important determinant of blood pressure in normotensives and in patients with essential hypertension.

To gain insight into the *dynamic* interrelations between sympathetic tone and reactivity to noradrenaline we studied eleven patients who had undergone total thyroidectomy for thyroid cancer and who were in hypo- and hyperthyroid state at different times. Plasma noradrenaline was significantly higher both during recumbency and following physical exercise in the hypo- than in the hyperthyroid state. Reactivity to exogenous noradrenaline was deccreased in all patients in the hypothyroid state as compared to the hyperthyroid state. Mean arterial pressure was slightly increased (by 6 mm Hg on the average) in the hypothyroid state as compared to the hyperthyroid state.

Plasma noradrenaline concentration during rest and following physical exercise as well as reactivity to exogenous noradrenaline were also studied in seven normotensive volunteer subjects before and during administration of the synthetic mineralocorticoid fludrocortisone (0.8 mg daily) for a period of six weeks. Plasma noradrenaline concentration decreased and reactivity to noradrenaline increased during steroid administration. The mechanism underlying the increase in blood pressure during long-term mineralocorticoid administration remains unclear. Increased sympathetic tone does not seem to be a factor since plasma noradrenaline decreased considerably. Pressor response to noradrenaline increased which was probably due to decreased sympathetic tone.

The data obtained seem to indicate that an increase in plasma noradrenaline concentration (probably reflecting increased sympathetic tone) *normally* leads to a decrease in reactivity to noradrenaline and vice versa. Therefore, when discussing the role of the sympathetic nervous system in essential hypertension, it is important to consider sympathetic tone in conjunction with its effectiveness — i.e., reactivity to noradrenaline. An increased sympathetic tone appears to contribute to high blood pressure only if reactivity to noradrenaline is *not* decreased.

References

1. Engelman K, Portnoy B (1970) A sensitive double-isotope derivative assay for norepinephrine and epinephrine: Normal resting human plasma levels. Circ Res 26: 53
2. Louis WJ, Doyle AE, Anavekar SN, Johnston CI, Geffen LB, Rush R (1974) Plasma catecholamine, dopamine-beta-hydroxylase, and renin levels in essential hypertension. Circ Res 34/35 Suppl I:57
3. Champlain J de, Farley L, Cousineau D, Ameringen M-R van (1976) Circulating catecholamine levels in human and experimental hypertension. Circ Res 38:109
4. Pedersen EB, Christensen NJ (1975) Catecholamines in plasma and urine in patients with essential hypertension determined by double-isotope derivative techniques. Acta Med Scand 198:373
5. Lake CR, Ziegler MG, Coleman MD, Kopin IJ (1977) Age-adjusted norepinephrine levels are similar in normotensive and hypertensive subjects. N Engl J Med 296:208
6. Philipp Th, Distler A, Cordes U (1978) Sympathetic nervous system and blood-pressure control in essential hypertension. Lancet 2:959
7. Christensen NJ (1972) Increased levels of plasma noradrenaline in hypothyroidism. J Clin Endocrinol Metab 35:359
8. Stoffer SS, Jiang NS, Gorman CA, Pikler GM (1973) Plasma catecholamines in hypothyroidism and hyperthyroidism. J Clin Endocrinol Metab 36:587
9. Champlain J de, Ameringen MR van (1972) Regulation of blood pressure by sympathetic nerve fibers and adrenal medulla in normotensive and hypertensive rats. Circ Res 31:617
10. Reid JL, Zivin JA, Kopin IJ (1975) Central and peripheral adrenergic mechanisms in the development of deoxycorticosterone-saline hypertension in rats. Circ Res 37:569
11. Renzini VC, Brunori CA, Valori C (1970) A sensitive and specific fluorimetric method for the determination of noradrenaline in human plasma. Clin Chim Acta 30: 587
12. DaPrada M, Zürcher G (1976) Simultaneous radioenzymatic determination of plasma and tissue adrenaline, noradrenaline and dopamine within the femtomole range. Life Sci 19:1161
13. Distler A, Keim HJ, Cordes U, Philipp Th, Wolff HP (1978) Sympathetic responsiveness and antihypertensive effect of beta-receptor blockade in essential hypertension. Am J Med 64:446
14. Distler A, Philipp Th, Lüth B, Wucherer G (1979) Studies on the mechanism of mineralocorticoid-induced blood pressure increase in man. Clin Sci 57:303s

Cardiovascular Pressor Reactivity as Related to Plasma Catecholamines: Role in the Pathogenesis of Essential Hypertension and in the Antihypertensive Mechanism of Diuretic Treatment[1]

P. WEIDMANN, M. GRIMM, A. MEIER, Z. GLÜCK, G. KEUSCH, I. MINDER, C. BERETTA-PICCOLI

Abstract

The role of the adrenergic effector-response axis in the pathogenesis of essential hypertension and in the hypotensive mechanism of diuretic treatment was evaluated by combined analysis of plasma catecholamine levels and pressor sensitivity to norepinephrine (NE).

Under placebo conditions, plasma NE, epinephrine and dopamine concentrations did not differ significantly between normal subjects and patients with borderline or established essential hypertension. The pressor dose (Δ mean blood pressure + 20 mm Hg) of infused NE correlated positively (P < 0.05) with endogenous plasma NE; however, this relationship was shifted in hypertensive patients so that NE pressor dose at any basal plasma NE level tended to be decreased. Compared to normal subjects, NE pressor dose was decreased. Compared to normal subjects, NE pressor dose was decreased slightly (P < 0.01) in borderline and markedly (P < 0.001) in established hypertension; it correlated inversely (P < 0.01) with basal blood pressure.

Adrenergic neuronal blockage with debrisoquine decreased plasma NE by 50% in all three groups; blood pressure remained largely unchanged in normal subjects, decreased only slightly (-5%) in borderline and fell significantly more in established hypertension (-21%). Thus, the ratio between debrisoquine-induced changes in blood pressure and plasma NE was greater (P < 0.001) in established hypertension than in normal or borderline hypertensive subjects.

Following six weeks of treatment with thiazidelike diuretics, basal plasma catecholamines, NE pressor dose and blood pressure remained unchanged in normal subjects. In hypertensive patients, diuretics caused a reduction (P < 0.01) in blood pressure and NE pressor reactivity, while basal plasma catecholamine levels were not significantly changed. Diuretic-induced changes in blood pressure and NE pressor dose were correlated (R = 0.40; P < 0.05).

---

1 A modified version of this paper has been presented at the Symposium of the Swiss Association against High blood pressure, June 1979, Glion, Switzerland. Therefore, it appeared with slight modifications also as a part of the proceedings of the Glion Symposium in Clin. Exp. Hypertension, 1979

These findings suggest that increased cardiovascular reactivity to NE occurs already at the borderline stage of hypertension. Borderline or established essential hypertension may be maintained, at least in part, by the inappropriate association of normal adrenergic activity with increased NE pressor reactivity. Diuretics may decrease blood pressure in essential hypertension by reducing an inappropriately high NE pressor reactivity without causing a concomitant equivalent increase in adrenergic nervous activity.

Introduction

The sympathetic nervous system is an important factor complementing the body sodium-volume state, the renin-angiotensin-aldosterone system and some other components in the regulation of blood pressure. Whether and to what extent this complex neuro-humoral axis plays a role in the pathogenesis of hypertension not associated with pheochromocytoma is still unclear. Since a direct analysis of neurotransmittor discharge under clinical conditions is not possible, measurement of norepinephrine (NE) in urine or plasma have been used as an approximate index of adrenergic activity. Several authors reported increased plasma or urinary NE or total catecholamine levels in sizeable groups of patients with essential hypertension [8, 9, 12, 13, 28, 33], but others found normal values [20, 29, 36, 38, 44].

For judging catecholamine measurements, the dietary sodium intake and the age of the patient should be considered. In normal adult man, plasma and urinary NE increase with aging [16, 20, 29, 33, 37, 38] and in response to marked sodium depletion [2, 31, 38]. Plasma epinephrine and dopamine concentrations are also elevated during sodium restriction [31]. In the more recent studies in which age was considered as a modulating factor, circulating NE was found to be usually normal in borderline or established essential hypertension [16, 20, 29, 38]. Nevertheless, there appeared to be a tendency for supernormal plasma NE in patients with established hypertension below the age of 40 to 50 years [16, 33, 38]. Blood levels of epinephrine, which may reflect the activity of the adrenomedullary effectors axis, were normal [38] or slightly increased [16], and no abnormality in circulating dopamine was noted [16]. Although mild hypercatecholeminemia may occur in some patients, it appears probable that the maintenance of essential hypertension cannot usually be explaned by such alterations in the circulating levels of catecholamines *per se*. Other important pressor factors or correlates such as plasma aldosterone, body sodium, extracellular fluid volume, blood volume and circulating renin levels are also normal, or the two latter sometimes even low, in most patients with benign essential hypertension [21, 22, 32, 36, 38].

Analyses of pressor factors alone allow only limited insight in the overall blood pressure control. Thus, the pressor effects of NE, angiotensin II or sodium may be modulated by variations in cardiovascular responsiveness. It has been known for many years that patients with essential hypertension tend to have an increased pressor responsiveness to both exogenous NE [11, 27] and angiotensin

II [19]. It was felt that the tendency for increased angiotensin-reactivity may be a physiologic adaptation to low endogenous plasma renin levels [19, 34].

However, studies of the relationship between plasma NE and its pressor action, based on simultaneous evaluation of these two parameters, were performed only recently by our own [39-41] and another group [30]. It became now apparent, that NE pressor sensitivity tends to be increased or inappropriately high relative to the concomitant level of circulating NE in established essential hypertension [30, 39, 40] as well as in mild to moderate hypertension associated with diabetes mellitus [41]. This report combines some of our previous findings [39, 40] with a presentation of more recent studies of cardiovascular pressor reactivity as related to plasma catecholamines in untreated and diuretic-treated normal subjects and patients with borderline or established essential hypertension.

Subjects and Methods

Studies With Norepinephrine Inhibition

Our initial approach to the problem under study was designed to investigate blood pressure-dependence on endogenous NE. Pharmacological inhibition of sympathetic nerve endings by the adrenergic neuron blocking agent, debrisoquine, provided a model to evaluate this. Normal subjects and patients with borderline (141/91 to 160/100 mm Hg) or established essential hypertension (> 160/100 mm Hg) were studied. In these studies and those described below, secondary forms of hypertension were excluded, serum creatinine was always normal (< 1.3 mg/100 ml), antihypertensive drugs were discontinued at least two to four weeks before the study and replaced by placebo tablets; and all subjects were instructed not to add salt to their food, starting at least five days before the first test [37, 38].

Blood pressure and plasma NE and epinephrine levels were obtained between 08.00 and 11.00 h under placebo conditions and again after two to six weeks of treatment with debrisoquine. Indwelling plastic needles were inserted in an antecubital vein at least 30 min before blood sampling. 24-hour urinary sodium and potassium excretions were comparable between the normal and borderline or established hypertensive subjects on the study days. Debrisoquine was administered orally; the starting dose of 15 mg/day was increased weekly until side effects developed or blood pressure in hypertensive subjects decreased to normal. These studies have already been reported in detail previously [39, 40].

Studies With Norepinephrine Infusion

Increases in circulating NE were induced by intravenous infusion in 25 normal subjects and 35 patients with borderline (141/91-159/94 mm and sometimes below) [18] or established essential hypertension ($\geq$160/95 mm Hg). Mean age was comparable in the normal and hypertensive subjects (42 ± 17 (± SD) vs.

40 ± 16 yr); it was 33 ± 12 yr in the 18 patients with borderline hypertension and 48 ± 12 yr in the 17 with established hypertension. Studies were performed under placebo conditions, after discontinuation of any antihypertensive drugs for at least two to four weeks, and with the dietary instructions specified above. 24 hr urinary sodium and potassium excretions were comparable between normal and borderline or established hypertensive subjects on the study day. Following a one-hour stabilization period with intravenous infusion of 5% dextrose (6-12 ml/hr by infusion pump) in the supine position, NE was infused at stepwise increasing rates. Each rate was maintained for at least 10 min; three to five different dose rates were given. At least five measurements of blood pressure were obtained when the blood pressure had stabilized before and at each norepinephrine infusion rate. Blood for determination of plasma catecholamines was collected immediately before the start of norepinephrine infusion and at two dose rates, that is when increases in mean blood pressure of 5-15 and 17-35 mm Hg, respectively, were achieved.

In order to evaluate the role of plasma catecholamines and cardiovascular reactivity in the antihypertensive mechanism of diuretic treatment, the study was continued following these procedures in 19 normal subjects and 29 patients with borderline (N = 14) or established (N = 15) essential hypertension. The placebo tablet was replaced by one tablet of a thiazide-like diuretic acting at the cortical diluting segment of the distal renal tubules, chlorthalidone, 100 mg/day, or indapamide, 2.5 mg/day [42]. Determinations performed under placebo conditions were repeated after six weeks of diuretic treatment.

Analytical Procedures

Blood pressure was measured using standard cuff and sphygmomanometer; each recorded blood pressure was the mean of three measurements. For determination of the cardiovascular pressor responsiveness, blood pressure was registered with the automatic blood pressure recorder, Physiometrics SR 2. Mean blood pressure was calculated as the sum of the diastolic (disappearance of sounds) and one third of the pulse pressure. Plasma catecholamines (NE, epinephrine, dopamine) were measured by a radioenzymatic method [7] as reported previously from this laboratory [38, 40, 41].

Dose-response curves for the relationship between infused NE and changes in blood pressure were plotted on semilogarithmic paper and further analyzed as follows. A regression line was constructed based on two to three data points below and above the level of a NE-induced increase in mean arterial pressure of 20 mm Hg; the steepest part of the dose-response curve was chosen for this regression line, because it represents most closely the linear part. Each regression line was used to calculate a) the steepness (slope) of this line, b) the NE pressor dose, i.e. the dose increasing mean arterial pressure by 20 mm Hg; and c) the NE threshold dose as obtained by the extrapolated dose causing zero change in mean arterial pressure.

For t-tests and regression analysis, the natural logarithm transformation of
plasma catecholamine levels and of NE pressor and threshold doses was used.

Results

Studies With Norepinephrine Inhibition

Before adrenergic neuronal blockage with debrisoquine, normal subjects and
patients with borderline or established essential hypertension did not differ
significantly in their mean upright plasma NE (35 ± 7, 51 ± 10 and 37 ± 4 (±
SEM) ng/100 ml, respectively) or epinephrine levels. Mean blood pressure averaged 85 ± 4, 114 ± 3 and 154 ± 6 mm Hg, respectively.

Adrenergic blockage with debrisoquine caused similar reductions in plasma NE
($P < 0.005$) in normal subjects and patients with borderline or established hypertension ($-46 ± 2, -50 ± 6$ and $-49 ± 5\%$, respectively). In contrast, the
decrease in blood pressure was statistically not significant in normal subjects
($-3 ± 3\%$), slight but significant ($P < 0.05$) in borderline hypertension ($-5 ±
2\%$), and significantly ($P < 0.005$) more marked in established hypertension
($-21 ± 4\%$). The corresponding ratios between debrisoquine-induced changes
in blood pressure and plasma NE in the three groups averaged 0.14 ± 0.27,
0.43 ± 0.13 and 2.86 ± 0.58, respectively (Fig. 1). Thus, the fall in blood pressure for any given NE reduction did not differ significantly between normal
and borderline hypertensive subjects, but was significantly ($P < 0.001$) greater
in established essential hypertension. Mean plasma epinephrine levels remained
unchanged after debrisoquine. These findings have been reported in detail
previously [39, 40].

Studies With Norepinephrine Infusion

a) In the Untreated State (Placebo Conditions)

Plasma NE was increased up to 1200 ng/100 ml during infusion, that is 55-
fold above the mean preinfusion level of about 22 ng/100 ml. There was an
excellent positive correlation between NE infusion rate and plasma NE measured during infusion ($P < 0.001$); this relationship was similar in normal and
hypertensive subjects.

The slopes of the NE dose-blood pressure response curves were comparable
in the normal and hypertensive subjects (Fig. 2). However, dose-response curves in the hypertensive patients were in the average shifted to the left, with a
significant ($P < 0.001$) decrease in threshold dose (20 ± 10 as compared to
43 ± 26 (± SD) ng/kg · min in normal subjects). The threshold dose was decreased slightly in borderline (25 ± 12 mg/kg · min; $P < 0.02$) and markedly
in established hypertension (16 ± 6 ng/kg · min; $P < 0.001$).

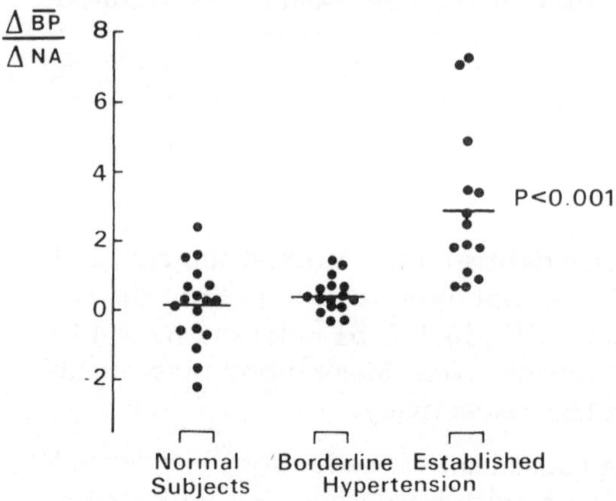

Fig. 1. Ratio between changes in blood pressure and plasma norepinephrine following adrenergic neuronal blockage. P < 0.001 denotes a statistically significant difference between patients with established hypertension compared to normal or borderline hypertensive subjects. From P. Weidmann et al. [40] by permission of J Clin Endocrinol Metab

The mean NE pressor dose was also significantly (P < 0.01) lower in hypertensive as compared to normal subjects (86 ± 42 vs. 140 ± 71 ng/kg · min) (Fig. 3). The NE pressor dose was decreased slightly in borderline (97 ± 31 ng/kg · min; P < 0.01) and markedly in established hypertension (75 ± 47 ng/kg · min; P < 0.001). In contrast, normal subjects and patients with borderline or established essential hypertension did not differ significantly in their mean pre-infusion levels of plasma NE (Fig. 3), epinephrine (3.3 ± 2.1, 4.5 ± 3.0 and 4.1 ± 2.6 ng/100 ml) and dopamine (5.2 ± 2.8, 7.2 ± 2.3 and 7.5 ± 2.2 ng/100 ml).

The NE pressor dose correlated positively with basal plasma NE in both normal (P < 0.01) or hypertensive subjects (P < 0.05). However, the NE pressor dose at any given basal plasma NE level tended to be increased in hypertensive patients. Moreover, analyzing all subjects together there was a significant (P < 0.01) inverse relationship between NE pressor dose and basal (pre-infusion) mean arterial pressure (r = 0.41; P < 0.01). A similar inverse relationship was found between NE threshold dose and basal blood pressure.

b) Effect of Diuretic Treatment

Findings under placebo conditions before diuretic therapy were comparable to those in the slightly larger study groups described above. In normal subjects blood pressure as well as mean NE pressor dose (Fig. 4) and plasma NE (Fig. 5) remained unchanged following diuretic treatment. In the hypertensive patients, blood pressure was decreased by an average of 11%

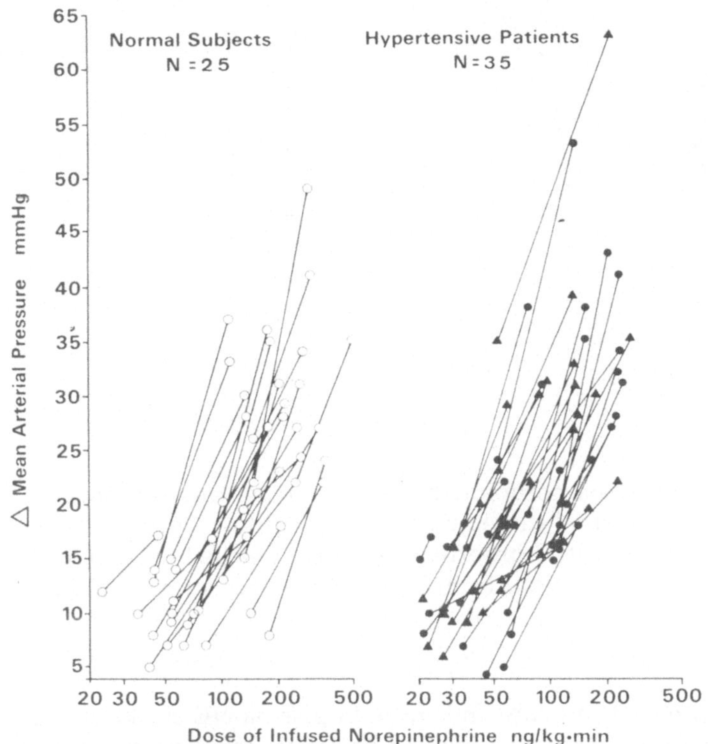

Fig. 2. Relationship between dose of infused norepinephrine and changes in
mean arterial pressure in normal subjects and patients with borderline (●) or
established (▲) essential hypertension

($P < 0.01$), NE pressor dose rose from the initially low levels into the normal
range (Fig. 4), while plasma NE levels were again not significantly changed
(Fig. 5). Analyzing all subjects together, diuretic-induced changes in blood
pressure correlated inversely with changes in NE pressor dose ($r = 0.40$; P
< 0.05).

Discussion

Pharmacologic reduction of neurotransmittor discharge by the adrenergic neuron blocking drug, debrisoquine, provided us with a model to estimate the actual blood pressure dependence on endogenous sympathetic activity [39, 40].
Except for depleting NE in sympathetic nerve endings and in the circulation
[14, 40] this agent has no known direct effects on other blood pressure-regu-
lating mechanisms and, in particular, does not alter the sensitivity of blood
vessels to NE or angiotensin II [6, 17]. Therefore, the ratio between debriso-

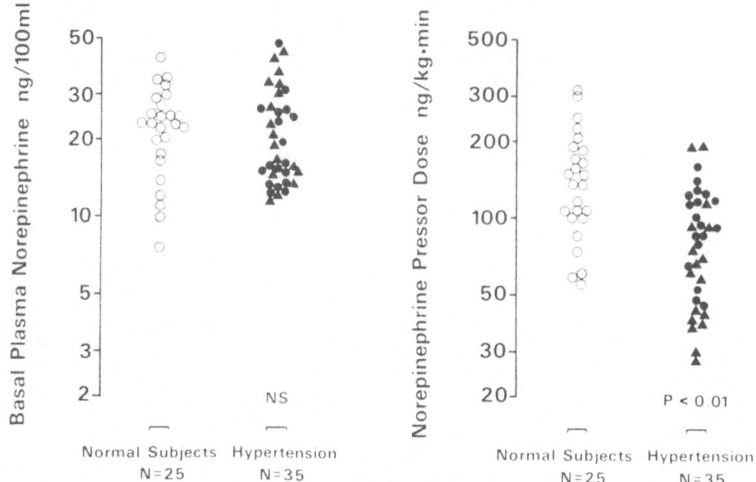

Fig. 3. Basal (pre-infusion) plasma norepinephrine concentrations and norepinephrine pressor doses in normal subjects and norepinephrine pressor doses in normal subjects and patients with borderline (●) or established (▲) essential hypertension. P < 0.001 denotes a significant difference between normal subjects and all hypertensive patients analyzed together

quine-induced changes in blood pressure and those in plasma NE could be considered as an index of cardiovascular reactivity to the adrenergic input. In these earlier studies [39, 40] from which parts have been incorporated in the present report, the depressor response to sympathetic inhibition and, hence, the pressor sensitivity to NE were found to be exaggerated in established essential hypertension. Thus, the ratio between desbrisoquine-induced percentile changes in blood pressure and circulating NE was significantly (P < 0.001) increased in established hypertension as compared to borderline hypertensive or normal subjects (Fig. 1). Although debrisoquine reduced mean plasma NE evenly by almost 50% in all three groups, the blood pressure was not changed significantly in normal subjects (−3%) was decreased by only 5% (P < 0.05) in patients with borderline hypertension, and fell significantly more (P < 0.005), namely by 21% in those with established hypertension. Pre-treatment plasma NE and epinephrine concentrations, on the other hand, did not differ significantly between the three groups [39, 40]. This combination of findings suggested that established essential hypertension may be maintained, at least in part, by the inappropriate association of normal, or in some patients even supernormal [33, 38] adrenergic activity with increased NE pressor reactivity.

An essentially similar conclusion was reached when the blood pressure-NE relationship was studied by an alternative approach, namely by simultaneous analysis of endogenous plasma NE and the pressor response to intravenously infused NE [30]. However, the latter report differs somewhat from our ex-

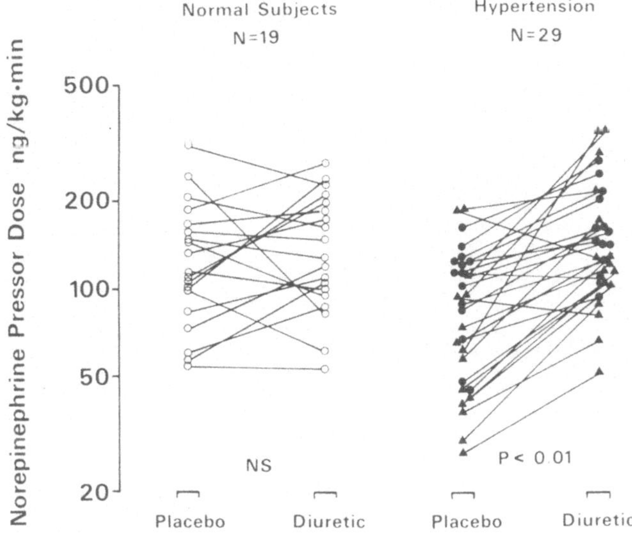

Fig. 4. Influence of diuretic treatment on norepinephrine pressor dose in normal subjects and patients with borderline (●) or established (▲) essential hypertension

perience and that of others [16, 20, 29, 38, 40], since high plasma NE levels were noted commonly in patients with established essential hypertension; moreover, no patients with borderline hypertension were evaluated [30].

The NE infusion studies performed in our laboratory included 25 normal subjects, 18 patients with borderline hypertension and 17 with established essential hypertension. The method was validated by the demonstration of an excellent positive correlation between NE infusion rate and plasma NE measured during infusion (P < 0.001). The findings from this investigation indicate that cardiovascular reactivity to an acute elevation in circulating NE may be increased already at the borderline stage of hypertension. Compared to our normal control subjects, mean NE pressor dose (e.g. the infusion rate increasing mean arterial pressure by 20 mm Hg) was decreased slightly (P < 0.01) in borderline and markedly (P < 0.001) in established hypertension (140 ± 71 vs. 97 ± 31 vs. 75 ± 47 (± SD) ng/kg · min), respectively (Fig. 3). NE pressor dose correlated inversely with basal (pre-infusion) mean blood pressure (r = 0.41; P < 0.01) which ranged from 73 to 143 mm Hg. NE pressor dose correlated positively with endogenous plasma NE in our normal subjects and those of others [30], pointing to a physiologic regulatory mechanism. Such a relationship existed also in hypertension (P < 0.05), but it was shifted so that NE reactivity at a given basal plasma NE level tended to be higher. Therefore, consid-

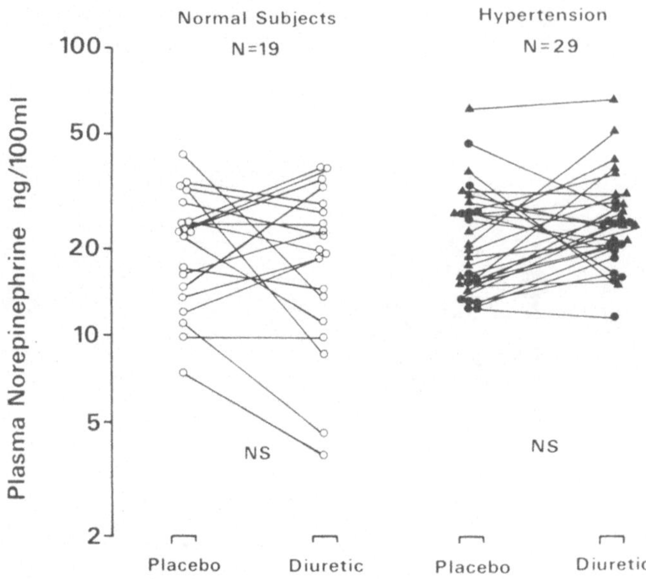

Fig. 5. Effect of diuretic treatment on basal (pre-infusion) plasma norepinephrine levels in normal subjects and patients with borderline (●) or established
(▲) essential hypertension

ering their normal plasma NE levels, the NE reactivity in our borderline or established hypertensive patients appeared to be inappropriately high. Nevertheless we noted a considerable overlap rather than a clear separation [30] of
values between normal and hypertensive subjects. This suggests that factors
other than cardiovascular NE reactivity and adrenergic nervous activity contribute also to the development and/or maintenance of borderline or established
essential hypertension. In fact, observations in our laboratory indicate that
cardiovascular reactivity to angiotensin II, as related to circulating plasma renin
activity tends also to be increased in borderline hypertension [24a].

Mechanisms which may influence cardiovascular reactivity include pressor factors such as the renin-angiotensin-system [23] or the body sodium-volume state
[3], baroreflex activity [11], humoral depressor agents such as prostaglandins
or bradykinin [24], sensitivity of alpha and beta-adrenergic receptors, and hy-
pertrophic alterations of the blood vessel walls [15]. Since mean plasma renin
levels, plasma and blood volumes and exchangeable body sodium did not differ
significantly between our normal and hypertensive subjects [42, 43], these factors did not appear to contribute to increased NE or angiotensin II [24a, 43]
pressor sensitivity in borderline or essential hypertension. The hyperreactivity
could probably not be explained by altered baroreflex function [30] or as an
unspecific consequence of an elevated systemic blood pressure and vascular

resistance [27, 11a]. The observed pattern is also not consistent with altered
beta receptor sensitivity; moreover, the responsiveness of cardiac beta receptors
tends to be decreased rather than increased with progressive hypertension [5].
The possibility that exaggerated sensitivity of vascular alpha and angiotensin
II receptors or a lack in vasodepressor substances could contribute to increased
NE and angiotensin II reactivity is presently speculative, but deserves further
consideration; in fact, urinary excretion of prostaglandin E was found to be
decreased in essential hypertension [1]. High blood pressure-induced hyper-
trophic changes of the blood vessel walls [15] may be yet another participating factor; its relevance has been disputed [27, 30], and it could probably not
account for the observed NE hyperreactivity in normotensive sons of hypertensive parents [11a]. The demonstration of a decreased pressor threshold to NE
and a normal slope of the NE dose-pressor response curve in our hypertensive
patients (Fig. 2) might appear to favor a mechanism related to increased vascular sensitivity [27] rather than secondary structural vascular changes [15]. Nevertheless, this observation does not allow a definite conclusion, since the whole
cardiovascular system and not the peripheral arteriolar vasculature alone was
tested by intravenous NE infusion. Whatever the exact underlying cause, and
regardless whether increased vascular reactivity is a primary pathogenic event
[27] or a consequence [15] of pre-existing hypertension, it is evident that an
exaggerated pressor responsiveness to sympathetic stimuli or angiotensin II
[24a, 43] in patients who already have an elevated blood pressure should act at
least as an aggravating factor.

In contrast to the altered cardiovascular reactivity, we found no abnormalities
in the kinetics of circulating norepinephrine in essential hypertension. This is
supported by two observations. First, during norepinephrine infusion the regression lines for the relationship between norepinephrine infusion rate and
plasma norepinephrine concentration were nearly identical in our normal and
hypertensive subjects. Second and more importantly, a recent study in our laboratory revealed that total plasma clearances of norepinephrine measured under
steady state infusion conditions were in the average similar in normal subjects
and patients with essential hypertension (5.3 vs. 5.2 liter/min) [16a]. The con-
stellation of normal endogenous plasma concentrations and a normal elimination rate of norepinephrine from the vascular compartment implies that the
overflow of neurotransmittor was also unaltered in our hypertensive patients.
Moreover, the normal plasma norepinephrine clearance [16a] upgrades the validity of plasma norepinephrine concentrations as an approximate index of adrenergic nervous activity in essential hypertension.

Diuretics have been used for many years as the major antihypertensive drugs,
but the mechanism underlying their blood pressure-lowering action has remained incompletely understood. Our observation suggests that thiazide-like diuretics may lower the blood pressure in essential hypertension by reducing an
inappropriately high NE pressor reactivity without causing a concomitant equivalent increase in adrenergic nervous activity. This concept is supported by a)
the absence of significant changes in NE pressor reactivity, plasma catecholamines and blood pressure following six weeks of diuretic treatment when the

cardiovascular system is normal, that is in our normal subjects; b) the parallel reduction in blood pressure and cardiovascular NE sensitivity towards normal values, without a significant change in endogenous catecholamine levels, in diuretic-treated patients with borderline or established hypertension; and c) the finding of a significant correlation between diuretic-induced changes in NE pressor dose and blood pressure (r = —0.40; P < 0.05). Although a decrease in vascular reactivity to NE following diuretic therapy was noted previously [25, 26], no simultaneous catecholamine determinations have been available, leaving the role of the adrenergic effector-response axis in the hypotensive mechanism of diuretic drugs unclear. It is evident that a reduction in cardiovascular pressor sensitivity will result in a net depressor effect only if it is not accompanied by an equivalent rise in the endogenous level of the specific pressor factor. The findings in our hypertensive patients correspond with the latter pattern. Compared to this mechanism, the role of extracellular sodium and fluid volume depletion in the maintenance of the blood pressure-lowering effect of thiazide-like diuretics would appear to be of lesser importance, since echangeable sodium following six weeks of diuretic treatment in our normal or hypertensive subjects [42, 43].

The tendency for the disturbance in cardiovascular NE reactivity and its relationship to circulating NE to be more pronounced with progressive blood pressure elevation is also of general pharmacotherapeutic interest. This mechanism may help to explain the observation that the blood pressure-lowering effect of both diuretic and sympathicolytic drugs is generally more pronounced in severe than in mild essential hypertension, and minimal or absent in normal subjects [4, 10, 14, 35]. Our findings may also provide a rational basis for the treatment of essential hypertension with diuretics to decrease an abnormal cardiovascular NE reactivity, and with adrenergic inhibitory agents to reduce an inappropriately normal sympathetic nervous activity.

Acknowledgements. This work was supported by Swiss National Science Foundation.

We thank Miss I. Bollinger, Mrs. J. Bürki, Mrs. G. Haueter, Miss U. Litschi and Miss R. Mosimann for skilled technical and Mrs. C. Weder for secretarial assistance.

References

1. Abe K, Yasujima M, Irokawa N, Seino M, Chiba S, Sakurai Y, Sato M, Imai J, Saito K, Haruyama T, Otsika Y, Yoshinaga K (1978) Proceedings of the Vth Scientific Meeting of the International Society of Hypertension. Paris p 7
2. Alexander RW, Gill Jr JR, Yamabe H, Lovenberg W, Keiser HR (1974) J Clin Invest 54: 194
3. Ames RP, Borkowski AJ, Sicinski AM, Laragh JH (1965) J Clin Invest 44 : 1171

4. Beretta-Piccoli C, Weidmann P, DeChâtel R, Hirsch D, Reubi FC (1977) Schweiz Med Wochenschr 107:104
5. Bertel O, Bühler FR, Kiowski W (1978) In: Circulating catecholamines and blood pressure. Birkenhäger WH, Falke HE (eds) Bunge, Utrecht, p 50
6. Cavero I, Gerold M, Saner A, Haeusler G (1978) J Pharmacol Exp Ther 206 : 123
7. DaPrada M, Zürcher G, (1976) Life Sci 19 : 1161
8. DeChamplain J, Farley L, Cousineau D, Ameringen M van (1976) Circ Res 38 : 109
9. DeQuattro V, Miura Y, Lurvey A, Cosgrove M, Mendez R (1975) Circ Res 36 : 118
10. Doyle AE, Smirk FH (1955) Circulation 12 : 543
11. Doyle AE, Fraser JRE (1961) Circ Res 9 : 755
11a. Doyle AE, Fraser JRE (1961) Lancet 2 : 509
12. Engelman K, Portnoy B, Sjoerdsma A (1970) Circ Res Suppl I 27 : 141
13. Esler M, Julius S, Zweifler A, Randall O, Harburg E, Gardiner H, DeQuattro V (1977) N Engl J Med 296 : 405
14. Flammer J, Weidmann P, Ziegler WH, Glück Z, Reubi FC (1979) Am J Med 66 : 34
15. Folkow B (1971) Clin Sci 41 : 1
16. Franco-Morselli R, Elghozi JL, Joly E, DiGiulio S, Meyer P (1977) Br Med J 2: 1251
16a. Grimm M, Weidmann P, Keusch G, Meier A, Glück Z, unpublished data
17. Haeusler G, Lorez HP, Bratholini G, Kettler R, Tranzer JP (1974) Pharmacol Exp Ther 189 : 646
18. Julius S (1977) Med Clin North Am 61 : 495
19. Kaplan NM, Silah JG (1964) J Clin Invest 43 : 659
20. Lake CR, Ziegler MG, Coleman MD, Kopin IJ (1977) N Engl J Med 296 : 208
21. Laragh JH (1973) Am J Med 55 : 261
22. Lebel M, Schalekamp MA, Beevers DG, Brown JJ, Davies DL, Fraser R, Kremer D, Lever AF, Morton JJ, Robertson JIS, Tree M, Wilson A (1974) Lancet 2 : 308
23. Malik KU, Nasjletti A (1976) Circ Res 38 : 26
24. McGiff JC (1977) Ann Int Med 87 : 369
24a. Meier A, Weidmann P, Grimm M, Keusch G, Glück Z, Minder I, Ziegler WH, unpublished data
25. Mendlowitz M, Naftchi N, Gitlow SE, Wolf RL (1960) Ann NY Acad Sci 88 : 964
26. Mendlowitz M, Naftchi N, Gitlow SE, Wolf RL (1968) Am Heart J 76 : 795
27. Mendlowitz M (1973) Am Heart J 85 : 252
28. Nestel PJ, Esler MD (1970) Circ Res Suppl II Circ Res 26/27 : 75
29. Pedersen EB, Christensen NJ (1975) Acta Med Scand 198 : 373
30. Philipp T, Distler A, Cordes U (1978) Lancet 2 : 959
31. Romoff MS, Keusch G, Wang M, Friedler RM, Weidmann P, Massry SG (1979) J Clin Endocrinol Metab 48 : 26

32. Schalekamp MA, Lebel M, Beevers DH, Fraser R, Kolsters G, Birkenhäger WH (1974) Lancet 2 : 310
33. Sever PS, Birch M, Osikowska B, Tunbridge RDG (1977) Lancet 1 : 1078
34. Weidmann P, Endres P, Siegenthaler W (1968) Br Med J 3 : 154
35. Weidmann P, Hirsch D, Maxwell MH, Okun R, Schroth P (1974) Am J Cardiol 34 : 671
36. Weidmann P, Hirsch D, Beretta-Piccoli C, Reubi FC (1977) Am J Med 62 : 209
37. Weidmann P, DeChâtel R, Schiffmann A, Bachmann E, Beretta-Piccoli C, Reubi FC, Ziegler WH, Vetter W (1977) Klin Wochenschr 55 : 725
38. Weidmann P, Beretta-Piccoli C, Ziegler WH, Keusch G, Glück Z, Reubi FC (1978) Kidney Int 14 : 619
39. Weidmann P, Keusch G, Flammer J, Ziegler WH, Reubi FC (1978) Schweiz Med Wochenschr 108 : 1974
40. Weidmann P, Keusch G, Flammer J, Ziegler WH, Reubi FC (1979) J Clin Endocrinol Metab 48 : 727
41. Weidmann P, Beretta-Piccoli C, Keusch G, Glück Z, Mujagic M, Meier A, Ziegler WH (1979) Am J Med   :
42. Weidmann P, Keusch G, Meier A, Glück Z, Grimm M, Beretta-Piccoli C (1979) Excerpta Med   :
43. Weidmann P, Meier A, Grimm M, Keusch G, Glück Z unpublished data
44. Wolf RL, Mendlowitz M, Roboz J, Gitlow SE (1965) N Engl J Med 273 : 1459

Blunting of Beta-Adrenoceptor-Mediated Cardiovascular Responses and Increasing Alpha-Receptor-Mediated Vasoconstriction: An Age-Dependent Transformation of Essential Hypertension

F. R. Bühler, W. Kiowski, F. W. Amann, P. Bolli, O. Bertel,
P. van Brummelen, R. Landmann

Summary

The role of the sympathetic nervous system in cardiac, renal and peripheral vascular adrenoceptor-mediated responses was investigated in patients with essential hypertension and age-matched normotensive subjects. Regardless of age, plasma adrenaline was significantly higher in hypertensive when compared with normotensive subjects. This suggests a sympatho-adrenal factor in essential hypertension. Plasma noradrenaline tended to increase with age but its similarity between normotensive and hypertensive subjects points to similar postganglionic neural activity and/or similar overflow of noradrenaline into the circulation. On the other hand, beta-adrenoceptor-mediated tachycardia in response to exercise and intravenous isoproterenol as well as the forearm vasodilator response to intraarterial isoproterenol decreased in normal subjects with older age. In hypertensives this age-dependent beta-receptor-related effect tends to be enhanced as judged from the greater reduction of cardiac isoproterenol sensitivity and the blunted renin response to exercise stimulation.

The dilator response to alpha-adrenoceptor blockade with phentolamine was not different in both groups. Therefore a qualitative rather than quantitative derangement of sympathetic control of vascular resistance — in which beta-dilator effects are reduced and alpha-constrictor mechanisms prevail — may contribute to the maintenance of established hypertension.

Introduction

Clinical investigation into the role of the sympathetic nervous system in the pathophysiology of essential hypertension thus far revealed controversial results which in part may be due to the methodology employed. A direct measurement of the activity of the sympathetic nerves proved to be difficult. Over the last years, as an alternative approach specific and sensitive radioenzymatic assays have been developed [13] and applied [37] to the measurement of the catecholamines adrenaline and noradrenaline in human plasma. At present plasma noradrenaline is considered to be an index of sympatho-neural activity which reflects in the rate of release at postganglionic nerve endings. On the other hand, plasma adrenaline is considered a marker of preganglionic sympatho-adrenal activity and acts as neuro-hormone on adrenoceptors, particularly those of the beta type.

The response of an organ to sympathetic stimulation, however, is not only determined by the activity of the sympathetic nervous system but it also depends on the response mediated by postjunctional adrenoceptors. In sympathetic cardiovascular control adrenoceptors play a pivotal role since heart rate and cardiac output as well as the renin-angiotensin system are to a large degree regulated via beta-adrenoceptors. Peripheral vascular tone, in addition to the renin-angiotensin vasoconstrictor axis — is modulated by the balance of an alpha-adrenoceptor-mediated vasoconstrictor and beta-adrenoceptor-mediated vasodilator force.

In order to obtain a more comprehensive view of the involvement of the sympathetic nervous system in circulatory regulation and of its interaction with adrenoceptor-mediated cardiovascular functions, a series of experiments were designed for simultaneous assessment of plasma catecholamines and different beta- or alphaadrenoceptors-mediated cardiovascular responses. To this end, heart rate, plasma renin activity, and blood pressure were measured and related to plasma catecholamine concentrations in age-matched groups of normotensive and hypertensive subjects. In addition to physiological stimulation by change of posture and by ergometry isoproterenol was used to test the beta-adrenoceptor-mediated response of heart rate and forearm blood flow. Phentolamine was administered to quantify its inhibitory effect on the alpha-adrenoceptor-mediated neurogenic vasoconstrictor tone.

Plasma Adrenaline — not Noradrenaline — is Elevated in Hypertension

In the past, measurements of plasma noradrenaline concentrations revealed differing results and conclusions. In some studies, subgroups of patients with supranormal levels were described [15, 39, 14, 43] whereas in others no difference between normotensive and hypertensive subjects was found [31, 26, 3]. These discrepancies might largely be explained on the basis of different methodology. Since plasma noradrenaline is influenced among others by physical and psychological stress, postural effects and by diurnal variations of the sympathetic nervous system all these factors must be taken into account in the study procedures. Also, one has to consider a certain degree of familiarity with laboratory procedures if normal control subjects are recruited from hospital staff [26]. With due recognition of these 'provisos' the following picture emerges from plasma noradrenaline measurements in our and other groups' studies. There is no overall differences in plasma noradrenaline concentrations between normotensive and hypertensive subjects [3, 26, 31]. Age is an important factor since noradrenaline levels tend to be higher in the older subjects [3, 31, 39, 43]. Among the patients with essential hypertension about one third of the population, those below the age of 45 years, exhibit supranormal values [3, 14, 15] most of them belonging to the high renin category [28]. It

still remains to be shown as to whether this young age pattern' in these patients bears some relationship with supranormal noradrenaline values found
in other groups of patients with borderline and mild hypertension [14, 18] or
in offsprings of hypertensive parents [21].

In contrast to noradrenaline much less is known with respect to plasma adrenaline levels in humans. To learn more about this problem we studied 86 patients with established essential hypertension with a diastolic blood pressure
$\geq$ 100 mg Hg and 38 agematched normotensive volunteers using the assay technique by Da Prada and Zürcher [13] which enables the precise and selective
measurement of noradrenaline and adrenaline. In all subjects the investigations
started between 8 and 10 a.m. with the insertion of an indwelling cannula into
an antecubital vein. After resting in a recumbent position for 30', blood for
plasma catecholamine estimation was drawn.

The plasma adrenaline results obtained at rest are shown in Figure 1. Although
there is a great overlap in the plasma adrenaline concentrations between normotensive and hypertensive subjects, the hypertensive patients exhibit significant-

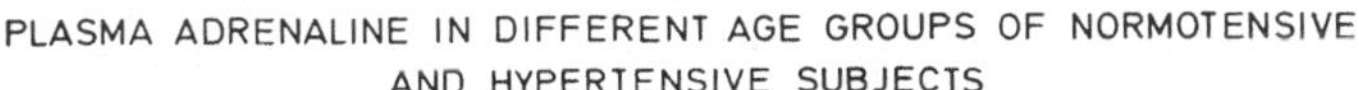

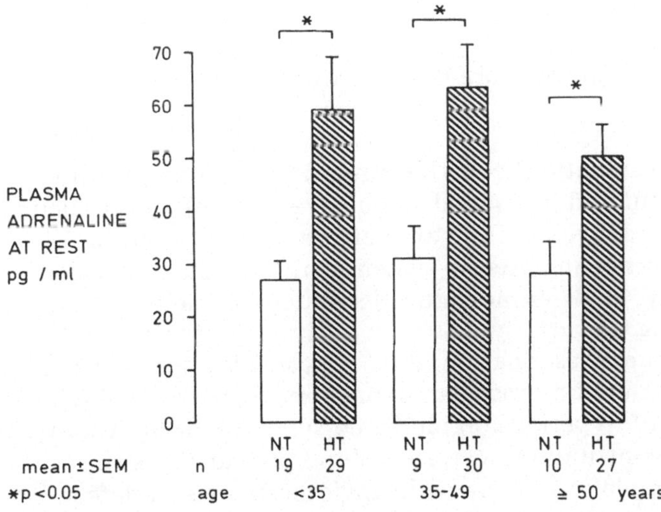

Fig. 1. Plasma adrenaline concentration measured 30 min after resting in a
supine position between 8-10 a.m. in different age groups. 86 hypertensive and
38 normotensive subjects of similar age were studied

ly higher values. This still holds true when different subgroups matched for age
were compared. Plasma adrenaline concentrations did not change with age

which contrasts the observations on noradrenaline. Thus, these data are in accord with those of other investigators [23]. Moreover, in our studies not only resting adrenaline levels but also those obtained during exercise stimulation were significantly higher which provided further support for enhanced preganglionic sympathetic activity. According to our results of elevated adrenaline levels in older hypertensives increased adrenergic activity participated not only in the development of hypertension [24] but also substantially contributes to the later maintenance of high blood pressure.

Because one might expect a more parallel change in both adrenaline and noradrenaline, the observed 'normal' noradrenaline but elevated adrenaline concentrations in hypertensive patients deserve some comments. There could be a disturbance of the noradrenaline reuptake at the nerve ending or in the vicinity of it or, alternatively, there could be an altered metabolism but all these possible explanations do not appear to hold true [19]. Furthermore, one could envisage the possibility that prejunctional betareceptors, which have been regarded to enhance noradrenaline release [1], could be hyporeactive to sympathetic stimulation and thereby reduce this facilitatory prejunctional noradrenaline release. It is tempting to speculate that the elevated plasma adrenaline concentrations over time might be the expression of an adaptive desensitization process of beta-adrenoceptors. Such a process might be promoted by adrenaline being taken up and subsequently released at postganglionic nerve endings [41].

Beta-Adrenoceptor-Mediated Functions are Blunted with Increasing Age and Pressure

Increased sympathetic nerve activity affects the regulation of blood pressure (the product of cardiac output and peripheral vascular resistance) by producing beta-adrenoceptor-mediated tachycardia and an increase in cardiac output as well as a stimulation of the renin-angiotensin-system which results in vasoconstriction and, simultaneously, aldosterone-induced sodium-volume retention with increased vascular filling. In turn, sympathetic activation of peripheral vascular beta-receptors produces vasodilation, thus opposing the sympathetic vasoconstrictor response mediated by vascular alpha-adrenoceptors. In the initial developmental phase of hypertension increased sympathetic activation of beta-adrenoceptors may contribute to elevated blood pressure by a rise in cardiac output and/or stimulation of the renin-angiotensin axis. A defect in the beta-adrenoceptor transmission would conceivably result in a reduced cardiac output, a lesser responsive renin system as well as in a diminution of a peripheral vasodilator force. Thus, on the theoretical grounds, the transition from a high output/high renin state to a high resistance form of hypertension might be linked to a defect in beta-adrenoceptor-mediated functions whereby cardiac output would tend to return to normal and peripheral vascular resistance tend to increase. In keeping with this view are findings of an agerelated decrease in exercise tachycardia [2, 3], a reduction in isoproterenol sensitivity

[3, 4, 34, 35] and a reduced heart rate response to acute beta-adrenoceptor
blockade [12]. Furthermore, with older age a low and hyporeactive renin secretion [10] and a blunted production of cAMP [36] have been observed. As a
practical consequence such age-related changes in beta-adrenoceptor-mediated
functions may have a bearing on chronic beta-blocker therapy of hypertensive
patients in whom the antihypertensive response to beta-blocker monotherapy
was found to decrease with older age and a lower renin [6, 7, 10]. With this
concept in mind, cardiac, renal and peripheral vascular beta-adrenoceptor mediated responses were tested in the following three studies.

Heart rate responses were tested by determining the chronotropic dose of intravenous isoproterenol to increase heart rate by 25 beats per minute (CD25)
using a protocol [3] which was adapted from a standard procedure [4, 11].
These pharmacological tests were also compared in the same individual with the
physiological response of plasma noradrenaline, renin activity and blood pressure during ergometric exercise [3]. As summarized in Figure 2 isoproterenol
sensitivity decreases with older age, as indicated by the higher CD25 of isoproterenol, an effect which is more pronounced in the hypertensive patients. Moreover, the reduction in isoproterenol sensitivity was paralleled by a decreased
exercise tachycardia and the isoproterenol sensitivity correlated inversely with
plasma noradrenaline concentrations and blood pressure measured during exercise stimulation [3].

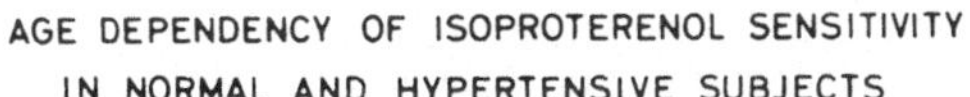
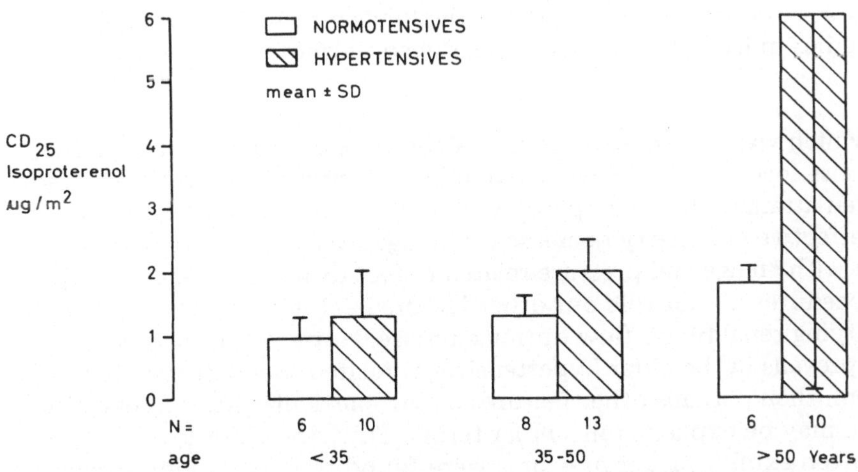

Fig. 2. Chronotropic dose 25 of isoproterenol (the dose, assessed from a dose-
response curve, to increase heart rate by 25 beats per minute corrected for
body surface in different age groups of hypertensive and normotensive subjects)

Plasma renin responses, presented in Figure 3, are based on the results from similar test procedures outlined above. In addition, for this investigation, the subjects were seated and subsequently underwent bicycle ergometry with graded work load of 25%, 50% and 75% of their maximal physical work capacity

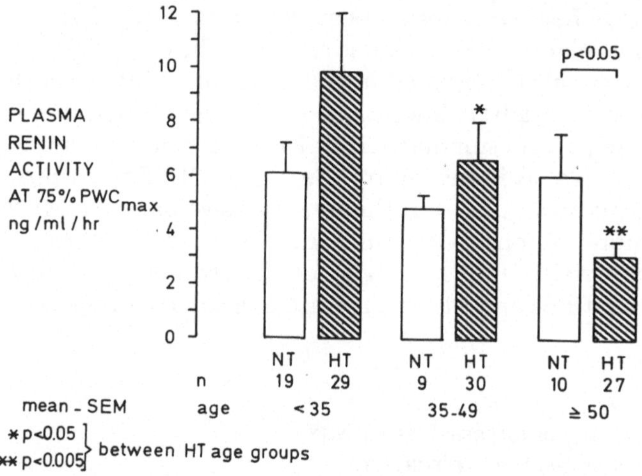

Fig. 3. Plasma renin activity as measured during steady state upright bicycle ergometry at a work load of 75% of the individual's maximal physical work capacity. Studies in hypertensive and agematched normotensive subjects

(PWCmax) which was determined on one of the days prior to the study. The level of exercise load was increased at five minutes' intervals after a new steady state had been attained. In the hypertensive patients plasma renin activity during equieffective ergometry decreased with age. Although these data would be in accord with an age and pressure-related defect of renal beta-adrenoceptors, our procedures do not rule out other factors i.e. the effect on renin release of a varying renal blood flow during exercise. However, if the low renin state which prevails in the older hypertensives is related to a defective beta-receptor system, then perhaps other features of this particular form of essential hypertension may be explained in similar terms. Thus, the older low renin patients who often exhibit higher pressures were found to have a reduced renal blood flow and an increased filtration fraction [42] which results in increased proximal sodium reabsorption [17]. Moreover, low renin patients were shown to have a slightly higher aldosterone secretion [8] which promotes distal tubular sodium reabsorption. Such a possible endogenous defect in beta-adrenoceptor-mediated postglomerular vascular tone, and perhaps in aldosterone secretion have implicit pharmacological corollaries since chronic beta-blockade was found to increase renal filtration fraction [38] and, in some patients, to retard the fall in aldosterone which usually follows renin suppression [9].

Peripheral vascular responses to isoproterenol infusions were investigated in a recent study in old and young normotensive subjects (Fig. 4). Forearm blood flow was measured using mercury in silastic strain gauge plethysmography [29] before and after a brachial artery infusion of incremental doses of isoproterenol.

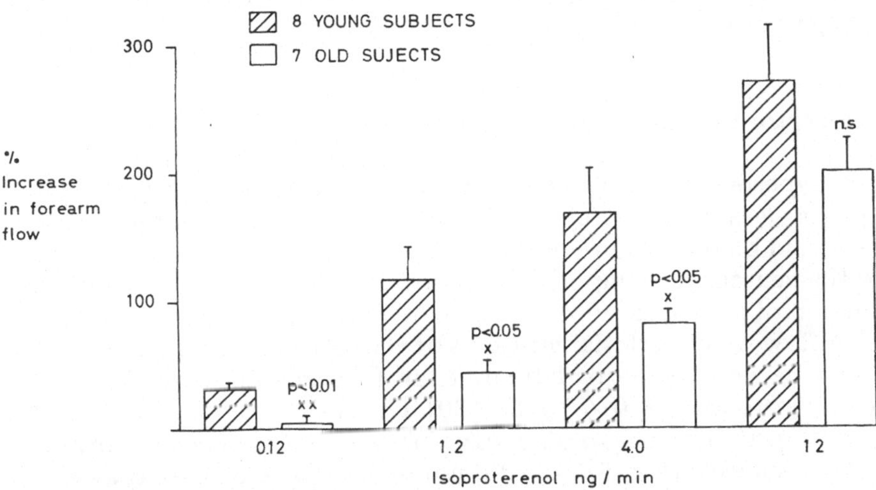

Fig. 4. Increases in forearm blood flow following beta-adrenoceptor stimulation with intraarterial infusions of isoproterenol in young and old normal subjects

Young subjects exhibited a greater vasodilator response to isoproterenol than the old subjects. In this study, too, the increments in flow correlated with the chronotropic dose (CD25) of isoproterenol as well as with the resting plasma renin acitivity.

This new information on an age-related decrease in peripheral vascular beta-adrenoceptor-mediated responses tallies with the observation of a parallel defect in cardiac and renal beta-adrenoceptor responsiveness.

The physiological and pharmacological observations of blunted beta-receptor-mediated responses in different segments of the circulation raise the question as to whether this could be accounted for by a different number or function of the individual's beta-adrenoceptors. In the last five years, receptor binding techniques with radioactively labelled beta-adrenoceptor blocking drugs were developed [33] which can be combined with procedures to activate and quantify by a beta-receptor agonist the membrane-bound enzyme adenylate cyclase and subsequent generation of the second messenger cyclic AMP. In clinical research a possibly promising approach at the moment related to the presence of adrenergic receptors on circulatory blood cells. In normotensive man, using direct binding studies with (-)H3-dihydroalprenolol it was found by one group that beta-blocker binding decreases with older age [44]. Applying the radio-receptor assay to the measurement of sofar unknown high affinity binding sites for (—)H3-dihydroalprenolol on mononuclear leucocytes with great sensitivity, we were unable to confirm an age-related decrease in binding [32]. This agrees with a most recent study [27] in which neither age nor pressure were associated with differences in beta-blocker binding. Further research in this area will clarify to whether circulating blood cells are suitable models for studying the adrenergic control of receptor-effector mechanisms in patients with different stages of essential hypertension.

Alpha-Adrenoceptor Blockade and Peripheral Blood Flow

In established hypertension — in which total peripheral resistance rather than cardiac output is elevated — the relationship between plasma noradrenaline concentrations and blood pressure observed in some studies [5, 29, 35] could be linked to the neurogenic component of vascular resistance which is predominantly a function of alpha-adrenoceptor-mediated vasoconstriction. Changes in forearm blood flow to intraarterial infusions of the alpha-adrenergic blocking drug phentolamine were therefore determined in 14 normotensive and 12 hypertensive subjects aged 18 to 70 years [30]. On the average, the increase in forearm blood flow in response to phentolamine was similar in normotensive and hypertensive subjects (Fig. 5). Age did not appear to be of importance since the responses to phentolamine were similar in young and old subjects. Because systemic blood pressure was not affected by the intraarterial infusion of phentolamine the observed increases in forearm blood flow directly reflected decreases in forearm vascular resistance dependent upon removal of alpha-adrenoceptor-mediated vasoconstriction. The possibility that there might be qualitative rather than quantitative differences is suggested by the direct relationship found between the effect of phentolamine on forearm flow and plasma noradrenaline concentration, as well as the height of blood pressure found in the hypertensive patients only [30]. This particular observation in hypertensive patients may have different explanations. Structural changes in the resistance vessels [22] and increased responses to pressure stimuli [16, 25, 40] could well be of relevance. Alternatively, in hypertension, beta-adrenoceptor-mediated effects might be inversely related to the level of sympathetic activity [3]. This could render the response to sympathetic stimulation the more dependent upon alpha-adrenoceptor-mediated mechanisms the higher sympathetic activity is. Thus, our view regarding a transformation from an initial state of intact beta-adrenoceptor-mediated cardiovascular control to a subsequent state of blunted beta-adrenoceptor but sustained alpha-adrenoceptor-mediated responses

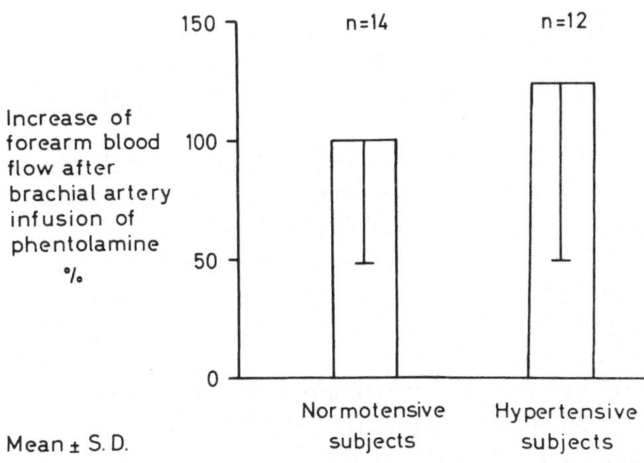

Fig. 5. Increases in forearm blood flow following alpha-adrenoceptor blockade with intraarterial infusion of phentolamine in hypertensive and age-matched normotensive subjects

is consistent with the finding that young hypertensive patients display a relatively higher cardiac output which decreases later on in association with an attendant rise in arteriolar resistance [20].

Acknowledgement. This work was supported by grants of the Swiss National Fund No. 3.894.77

References

1. Adler-Grashinsky E, Langer SZ (1975) Possible role of a beta-adrenoceptor in the regulation of noradrenaline release by nerve stimulation through a positive feed-back mechanism. Br J Pharmacol 53 : 43
2. Åstrand PO, Rodahl K (1970) Textbook of work physiology. McGraw Hill, New York
3. Bertel O, Bühler FR, Kiowski W, Lütold BE (in press) Decreased beta-adrenoreceptor responsiveness as related to age, blood pressure and plasma catecholamines in patients with essential hypertension. Hypertension
4. Bertel O, Bühler FR, Kiowski W (1978) Isoproterenol sensitivity testing in different age and renin groups of essential hypertension. In: Birkenhäger WH, Galke HE (eds), Circulating catecholamines and blood pressure. Bunge, Utrecht, p 50
5. Brecht HM, Schoeppe W (1978) Relation of plasma noradrenaline to blood pressure, age, sex and sodium balance in patients with essential hypertension and in normotensive subjects. Clin Sci 55 : 81s
6. Bühler FR, Bertel O, Lütold BE (1978) Simplified and stratified antihypertensive therapy based on betablockers. Cardiovasc Med 3 : 135

7. Bühler FR, Laragh HG, Baer L, Vaughan Jr ED, Brunner HR (1977) Propranolol inhibition of renin secretion. A specific approach to diagnosis and treatment of renin-dependent hypertensive diseases. N Engl J Med 287 : 1209

8. Bühler FR, Laragh JH, Sealey JE, Brunner HR (1973) Plasma aldosterone-renin interrelationships in various forms of essential hypertension: studies using a rapid assay of plasma aldosterone. Am J Cardiol 32 : 554

9. Bühler FR, Burkart F, Lütold BE, Küng M, Marbet G, Pfisterer M (1975) Antihypertensive beta-blocking action as related to renin and age: a pharmacological tool to identify pathogenetic mechanisms in essential hypertension. Am J Cardiol 36 : 633

10. Bühler FR (1978) Age and renin as predictors of the antihypertensive response to betablockers, In: Meyer P, Schmitt H (eds), Central nervous system and hypertension. Flammarion, Paris, p 471

11. Cleaveland CR, Rangno RE, Shand DG (1972) A standardized isoproterenol sensitivity test. The effects of sinus arrhythmia, atropine, and propranolol. Arch Intern Med 130 : 47

12. Conway J (1970) Effect of age on the response to propranolol. Int J Clin Pharmacol 4 : 148

13. Da Prada M, Zürcher G (1976) Simultaneous radioenzymatic determination of plasma and tissue adrenaline, noradrenaline and dopamine within the femtomole range. Life Sci 19 : 1161

14. De Champlain J, Farley L, Cousineau D, Van Ameringen MR (1976) Circulating catecholamine levels in human and experimental hypertension. Circ Res 38 : 109

15. DeQuattro V, Chan S (1972) Raised plasma catecholamines in some patients with primary hypertension. Lancet 1 : 806

16. Doyle AE, Fraser JRE, Marshall RJ (1959) Reactivity of forearm vessels to vasoconstrictor substances in hypertensive and normotensive subjects. Clin Sci 18 : 441

17. Early LE, Dangharty TM (1969) Sodium metabolism. N Engl J Med 281 : 72

18. Esler M, Julius S, Zweifler A, Randall O, Harburgh E, Gardiner H, DeQuattro V (1977) Mild high-renin hypertension: neurogenic human hypertension? N Engl J Med 296 : 405

19. Esler M, Korner P, Jennings G, Bobitz A, Kelleher D (1978) Rate of removal of noradrenaline from plasma in man. Abstracts of the Fifth Scientific Meeting of the International Society of Hypertension, Paris p 76

20. Fagard R, Amery A, Reybrouck T, Lijnen P, Billiet L, Joossens JV (1977) Plasma renin levels and systemic hemodynamics in essential hypertension. Clin Sci 52 : 591

21. Falkner B, Onesti G, Angelakos ET, Fernandes M, Langman C (1979) Cardiovascular response to mental stress in normal adolescents with hypertensive parents. Hypertension 1 : 1

22. Folkow B (1971) The hemodynamic consequences of adaptative structural changes of the resistance vessels in hypertension. Clin Sci 41 : 1

23. Franco-Morselli R, Elghozi JL, Joly E, Diginilio S, Meyer P (1977) Increased plasma adrenaline concentrations in benign essential hypertension. Br Med J 2 : 1251
24. Frohlich ED, Kozul VJ, Tarazi RC, Dustan HP (1970) Physiological comparison of labile and essential hypertension. Circ Res 27 : 55
25. Gombos EA, Hulet WH, Bopp P, Golding W, Baldwin DS, Casis H (1968) Reactivity of renal and systemic circulations to vasoconstrictor agents in normotensive and hypertensive subjects. J Clin Invest 41 : 203
26. Jones DH, Hamilton CA, Reid JL (1979) Choice of control groups in the appraisal of sympathetic nervous activity in essential hypertension. Clin Sci 57 : 339
27. Kafka MS, Lake R, Gullner HG, Tallmann JF, Bartter FC, Fujika T (1979) Adrenergic receptor function is different in male and female patients with essential hypertension. Clin Exp Hypertension 1 : 613
28. Kiowski W, Bertel O, Bühler FR (1979) The renin type of essential hypertension and the relationships between catecholamines, renin and age. In: Meyer P, Schmitt H (eds) Nervous system and hypertension. Flammarion, Paris, p 318
29. Kiowski W, Brummelen P van, Amann FW, Bühler FR (1979) Abnahme von kardialen, peripher vaskulären und renalen Beta-Adrenozeptor-vermittelten Funktionen im Alter. Therapiewoche 29 : 7703
30. Kiowski W, Brummelen P van, Bühler FR, Amann FW (in press) Plasma noradrenaline correlates with blood pressure and alpha adrenoceptor-mediated vasoconstriction in essential hypertension. Clin Sci
31. Lake CR, Ziegler NG, Coleman MD, Kopin IJ (1977) Age-adjusted plasma norepinephrine levels are similar in normotensive and hypertensive subjects. N Engl J Med 296 : 208
32. Landmann R, Bittinger H, Bühler FR, Dukor O (1980) High affinity beta-adrenoceptor binding sites in human mononuclear leucocytes. Abstract Book, European Society for Clinical Investigation, Annual Meeting
33. Lefkowitz RJ (1979) Direct binding studies of adrenergic receptors: biochemical, physiologic and clinical implications. Ann Int Med 91 : 450
34. London GM, Safar ME, Weiss YA, Milliez PL (1976) Isoproterenol sensitivity and total body clearance of propranolol in hypertensive patients. J Clin Pharmacol 16 : 174
35. Louis WJ, Doyle AE, Anavekar SN (1973) Plasma norepinephrine levels in essential hypertension. N Engl J Med 296 : 599
36. Lowder SC, Hamet P, Liddle GW (1976) Contrasting effects of hypoglycemia on plasma renin activity and cyclic adenosine 3', 5'-monophosphate (cyclic AMP) in low renin and normal renin essential hypertension. Circ Res 48 : 105
37. Lütold BE, Bühler FR, DaPrada M (1976) Dynamik von Plasmakatecholaminen und Beta-Adrenozeptor-Funktionen. Anwendung einer neuen radioenzymatischen Mikromethode. Schweiz Wochenschr 106 : 1735
38. Niess AA, McNiel JS, Schrier RW (1971) Mechanism of increased sodium reabsorption during propranolol administration. Circulation 44 : 596

38. Niess AA, McNiel JS, Schrier RW (1971) Mechanism of increased sodium reabsorption during propranolol administration. Circulation 44 : 596
39. Pedersen EB, Christensen NJ (1975) Catecholamines in plasma and urine in patients with essential hypertension determined by double-isotope derivative techniques. Acta Med Scand 198 : 373
40. Philipp T, Distler A, Cordes U (1978) Sympathetic nervous system and blood pressure control in essential hypertension. Lancet 2 : 959
41. Rand MJ, Majewski H, McCulloch HW, Story DF (1978) An adrenaline-mediated positive feedback loop in sympathetic transmission and its possible role in hypertension. Proceedings of the IUPHAR Satellite Symposium on 'Presynaptic Receptors', Paris, 22-23 July
42. Schalekamp MADH, Schalekamp-Kuyken MPA, Birkenhäger WH (1970) Abnormal renin haemodynamics and renal suppression in hypertensive patients. Clin Sci 38 : 101
43. Sever PS, Owikowska B, Birch M, Turnbridge RDG (1977) Plasma noradrenaline in essential hypertension. Lancet 1 : 1078
44. Schocken DD, Roth GS (1977) Reduced beta-adrenergic receptor concentrations in ageing man. Nature 267 : 856
45. Vestal RE, Wood AJJ, Shand DG (1979) Reduced beta-adrenoceptor sensitivity in the elderly. Clin Pharmacol Ther 25 : 181

Patterns of Noradrenaline and Renin in Essential Hypertension – Effects of Stress and Therapy

P. W. De Leeuw, A. Wester, P. J. Willemse, W. H. Birkenhäger

Introduction

Essential hypertension is characterized by an increased vascular resistance, which is at least in part functional [1, 2]. The mechanisms of this haemodynamic abnormality are unknown. Although a relative deficiency of vasodilator substances may be involved, it seems more practical to investigate whether there is increased activity of vasopressor systems. Although the renin-angiotension system and the adrenergic system compete for this role, both systems are closely interrelated [3, 4]. Therefore, it seems worthwhile to attempt to dissociate the two functions by designing a variety of challenge studies.

Patients and Methods

The study was divided in three parts. In the first, basal levels of noradrenaline and renin were determined in 20 normotensives and 60 essential hypertensives.

The normotensive group consisted of hospitalized patients who had been admitted for diagnostic tests or were in the reconvalescent phase of a minor illness. Their age ranged from 20-68 (average 41) years and mean blood pressure from 75-100 (average 95) mm Hg.

The hypertensives were 21-73 (average 45) years old and mean blood pressure ranged from 85-170 (average 120) mm Hg at the time of the study. The diagnosis of essential hypertension was based on routine exclusion of known causes of high blood pressure. Antihypertensive treatment was withdrawn at least three weeks prior to the study.

All subjects were studied under metabolic ward conditions, sodium intake being fixed at 55 mmoles a day.

Blood samples for determination of noradrenaline and active plasma renin concentration were drawn in the morning after an overnight fast and with the patient in the supine position. Assay methods have been published before [2, 5].

In the hypertensives we also measured cardiac output (impedance cardiography), total peripheral vascular resistance, renal plasma flow (^{125} J-hippuran), renal

vascular resistance and plasma volume (^{131}J-albumin) as described previously
[2]. In addition, intrarenal haemodynamics were assessed in 15 of the hypertensive patients by means of the Xe-washout technique [6].

In the second part of the study the possibility of a dynamic relationship
between noradrenaline and renin was investigated in several of the hypertensive
patients. Methods to activate the sympathetic system included 45° head-up
tilt (ten patients), isometric exercise by voluntary handgrip (15 patients) and a
standardized acoustical stress test [7] (15 patients). Blood samples for noradrenaline and renin were drawn prior to and three and five minutes after initiation
of the various tests. Blood pressure was measured simultaneously by Arterio-
sonde.

In the third part of the study we investigated the endocrine response to treatment with a pure vasodilator (L 6150) or with prazosin, which interferes with
post-synaptic alpha-adrenergic function. Fifteen of the hypertensive patients
were treated with L 6150 and twelve with prazosin. Noradrenaline and renin
levels were determined before therapy and after two weeks of treatment.
Throughout the treatment period patients remained hospitalized and salt intake
was kept at 55 mmoles a day.

Results

I. Basal Levels of Noradrenaline and Renin

Basal levels of noradrenaline and active renin were not different between
normotensives and hypertensives. Neither hormone was related to blood
pressure, cardiac output, total peripheral vascular resistance, or plasma volume. Likewise, there was no relationship between these hormones and renal
plasma flow (as measured by hippuran-clearance) or renal vascular resistance. However, renal cortical blood flow (assessed by Xenonwashout)
appeared to be inversely related to noradrenaline ($r = -0.75$; $p < 0.001$).

While there was a direct relationship between noradrenaline and renin in
the normotensives ($r = 0.75$, $p < 0.001$), no such relation was found in the
hypertensives. However, when the hypertensive subjects, who at the time
of the actual investigation had a mean blood pressure (<110 mm Hg were
considered separately, a positive relationship between noradrenaline and
renin was again found ($n = 14$; $r = 0.65$; $p < 0.01$). In patients with mean
blood pressure > 110 mm Hg this relation was virtually absent.

II. Stimulated Levels of Noradrenaline and Renin

During all three "stress' procedures levels of noradrenaline and renin rose,
although individual responses exhibited a wide variation. During tilting

50

both noradrenaline and renin rose by 50-100% and there was a significant relationship between changes in noradrenaline and those in renin (r = 0.72; p < 0.01). Blood pressure remained essentially unchanged under these conditions.

Both isometric exercise and acoustical stress produced a significant increase in blood pressure and in noradrenaline (Fig. 1). Although renin levels rose significantly, the change from base-line values amounted only to 10%. Noradrenaline levels, on the other hand, increased by at least 50%.

While there was a direct relationship between changes in noradrenaline and those in blood pressure (r = 0.65; p < 0.05), there was no relationship between the changes in noradrenaline and renin.

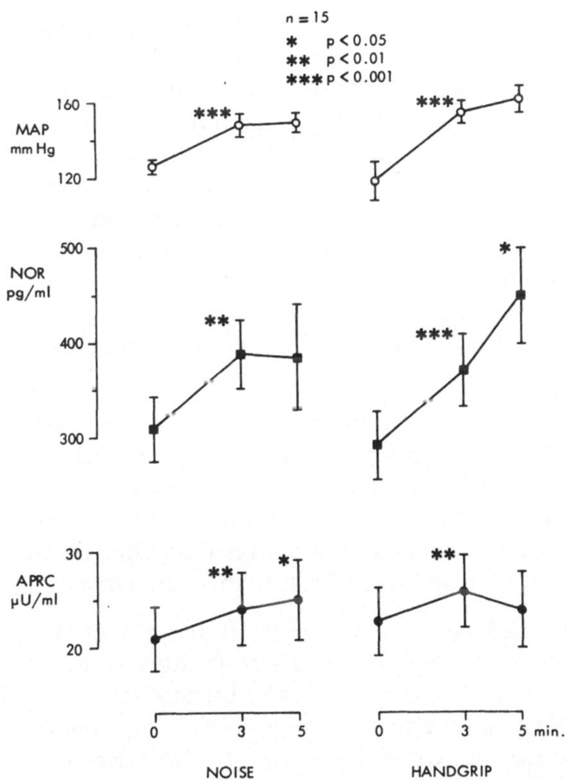

Fig. 1. Time course of changes in mean arterial pressure (MAP), and concentrations of noradrenaline (NOR) and active renin (APRC) during acoustical stress (left panel) and isometric exercise (right panel)

III. Effect of L 6150 and Prazosin on Noradrenaline and Renin

Both L 6150 and prazosin caused a two- to threefold rise in plasma noradrenaline when these drugs were given for two weeks. In the case of
L 6150 renin levels rose by about 25%. Prazosin, however, had no effect
on renin levels.

Both drugs produced a comparable fall in blood pressure and starting pressures were the same in both groups. During treatment with L 6150 there
was a weak direct relationship between changes in noradrenaline and those
in renin, but this failed to reach significance.

Discussion

It is well established that total peripheral vascular resistance is increased in essential hypertension [1, 2]. Both the renin-angiotensin system and the adrenergic system are involved in the regulation of vascular tone and blood pressure
and increased activity of either one of these systems could account for the
development of essential hypertension. Thus far, only Miura has shown a correlation of vascular resistance with noradrenaline [8]. In our own series we failed to find such a relationship. Neither did we find a relationship of noradrenaline with renal vascular resistance. However, blood flow through the outer cortex of the kidney was inversely related to noradrenaline. Assuming that a low
cortical flow rate is the result of a local increase in vascular tone, this may indicate that in a selected area vascular resistance is indeed dependent on sympathetic activity.

With respect to the renin-angiotensin system the data are conflicting and renin
is even said to correlate inversely with vascular resistance [1, 2]. On the other
hand, several studies have shown that vascular reactivity to catecholamines or
angiotensin cannot be determined simply from measuring circulating hormone
levels [9, 10]. Another problem in interpreting available data is that changes in
sympathetic function may alter the circulating level of renin and vice versa.

In earlier studies it was shown that renin levels could vary both directly [11]
and inversely [12] with catecholamines. This could indicate that there is no
relation at all between the two systems. Alternatively, it may be that such a
relationship is dependent on other factors. Our results suggest that this may be
indeed the case. In 20 normotensive subjects we found a direct relationship
between noradrenaline and renin. Although this relationship was absent when
all hypertensives were considered together, it became again apparent in those
patients who were normotensive at the time of the actual investigation. It could
be therefore, that a rise in blood pressure counteracts the stimulation of renin
secretion either directly or by tuning down beta-receptor sensitivity. Indeed,
reduced beta-receptor function has been described in essential hypertension
and this is particularly evident in older patients, who also have the highest
blood pressure [13].

Tilting, by decreasing venous return, induces reflex stimulation of sympathetic activity, which was accompanied by a rise in plasma noradrenaline. Renin levels rose in proportion to the increase in noradrenaline, yet blood pressure did not change significantly. Since in the absence of sympathetic function blood pressure would fall [14], it can be inferred that the sympathetic nervous system is necessary to maintain blood pressure. In this case the adrenergic system tries to prevent hypotension rather than to cause hypertension and thus the input signal of blood pressure at the level of the juxtaglomerular apparatus may be different as compared to the basal state. This could explain why renin levels rise in proportion to the increase in sympathetic activity. Likewise, one would anticipate that when sympathetic stimulation is accompanied by a rise in blood pressure, beta-adrenoceptor mediated renin release will be less evident. This, indeed, occurred in our patients who were subjected to isometric exercise or "noise". Renin rose by only 10%, which is in sharp contrast to the 50-100% rise during tilting, despite almost identical increases in plasma noradrenaline. Based on the foregoing one would expect vasodilator treatment to be associated with hormonal changes comparable to those during tilting. While this appeared to be true for noradrenaline, renin levels changed less (L 6150) or not at all (prazosin). However, the pharmacological properties of these drugs have not yet been fully established.

In summary, our results suggest that the sympathetic nervous system is an important determinant of renin release under normotensive conditions or under circumstances where the organism tries to prevent a drop in pressure.

Apparently the beta-adrenoreceptor function is reset or turned off by an acute or chronic rise in blood pressure. Whether the latter is related to a baroreceptor mediated suppression of renin release to exaggerated vasoconstriction, or selective alpha-adrenergic stimulation, remains to be identified.

References

1. Birkenhager WH, Schalekamp MADH (1976) Control mechanisms in essential hypertension. Elsevier, Amsterdam
2. Leeuw PW de (1978) Vasoregulation and renal function in essential hypertension. Thesis, Rotterdam
3. Davis JO (1973) The control of renin release. Am J Med 55 : 333
4. Ferrario CM, Gildenberg PL, McCubbin JW (1972) Cardiovascular effects of angiotensin mediated by the central nervous system. Circ Res 30 : 257
5. Falke HE, Punt R, Birkenhager WH (1978) Radioenzymatic estimation of noradrenaline in small plasma samples without previous extraction. Clin Chim Acta 89 : 111
6. Kolsters G, Graaf CN de (1978) Renal blood flow and intrarenal blood flow distribution assessed by the ^{133}Xenon washout technique in man. Neth J Med 21 : 188
7. Turek JV, Kuy A van der, Pelgrim C, Keyzer F de, Fuhr SLHM von der, Voerman J (1977) Blood pressure response to a new standardized stress test. Neth J Med 20 : 104

8. Miura Y, Kobayashi K, Sakuma H, Tomioka H, Adachi M, Yoshinaga K (1978) Plasma noradrenaline concentrations and haemodynamics in the early stage of essential hypertension. Clin Sci Mol Med Suppl 4 55 : 69s
9. Philipp T, Distler A, Cordes U (1978) Sympathetic nervous system and blood pressure control in essential hypertension. Lancet 2 : 959
10. Riegger AJG, Tree M, Bean BL, Casals-Stenzel J, Brown JJ, Fraser R, Lever AF, Morton JJ, Robertson JIS (1979) Does angiotensin II act in two ways to raise blood pressure in renal artery stenosis. In: Bianchi G, Bazzato G (eds) The kidney in arterial hypertension. Bunge, Utrecht
11. DeQuattro V, Miura Y (1973) Neurogenic factors in human hypertension: mechanism or myth. Am J Med 55 : 362
12. Louis WJ, Doyle AE, Anavekar SN, Johnston CI, Geffen LB, Rush R (1974) Plasma catecholamine, dopamine-beta-hydroxylase and renin levels in essential hypertension. Circ Res Suppl 1 34/35 : 57
13. Bühler FR, Bertel O, Kiowski DW (1978) Plasma noradrenaline and adrenaline and beta-adrenoceptor responsiveness in renin subgroups of essential hypertension. Clin Sci Mol Med Suppl 4 55 : 57s
14. Ziegler MG, Lake CR, Kopin IJ (1977) The sympathetic nervous system defect in primary orthostatic hypotension. N Engl J Med 296 : 293

Catecholamines, Isometric Exercise and Left Ventricular Function

R. J. VECHT, D. GORDON, P. SEVER

Introduction

The use of plasma noradrenaline as a determinant of sympathetic function has been described by several authors and has resulted from a number of investigations in which acute changes in plasma noradrenaline concentration have been determined in response to a sympathetic challenge (Lake et al., 1976; Osikowska and Sever, 1976). There are, however, major difficulties in the interpretation of isolated values of noradrenaline in plasma because of widespread inter-individual variations in both basal and stimulated levels. Recent studies from Wallin and his co-workers have given encouragement to the validity of plasma noradrenaline as a determinant of sympathetic tone since they claim a positive relationship between sympathetic muscle nerve activity and noradrenaline concentration (Wallin, G., personal communication).

The evidence for a relationship between noradrenaline and blood pressure is, however, more tenuous, as is that between sympathetic muscle nerve activity and blood pressure (Sever at al., 1979, Sundlof and Wallin, 1978). It is possible that stimulated levels of noradrenaline may more accurately reflect sympathetic activity and in certain studies relationships to blood pressure have been more clearly defined after a postural stimulus or after dynamic exercise (Sever et al., 1979; Sleight et al., 1979).

In the present study we have investigated the changes in circulating noradrenaline in response to isometric exercise and attempted to relate such changes to those occurring in heart rate and blood pressure.

We have also monitored changes in plasma noradrenaline occurring at several sites throughout the circulation in an attempt to demonstrate whether or not levels recorded from a peripheral vein are representative of those from other sites in the vascular space.

Subjects and Methods

Twenty-four patients, age range 30-57, undergoing routine cardiac catheterisation, were studied. All patients gave informed consent, were fasting, in sinus

rhythm and premedicated with diazepam 10 mg and promethazine 25 mg.
Details are given in Table 1.

Table 1

---

24 Unselected patients
20 Males : 4 Females
Age range 30-57 Years (Mean 47.4)

---

16 Ischaemic Heart Disease
 4 Rheumatic Valve Disease
 1 Non-rheumatic Mitral Regurgitation
 1 Congestive Cardiomyopathy
 1 Hypertension
 1 Normal (N)

Resting heart rate and left ventricular systolic pressures were measured through
fluid filled catheters and recorded using Hewlett Packard 120 series transducers
and 350 series multichannel recording system. The zero reference point was
taken at mid-chest. Cardiac indices at rest were derived from arterial and mixed
venous samples collected simultaneously, the oxygen uptake based on Tables.
Ejection fractions at rest were calculated planimetrically from left ventricular
angiograms.

After basal measurements had been recorded, patients performed a standardized handgrip using a balloon dynamometer, to 30% of maximum effect (approximately 0.3 kg/cm^2), ensuring that no valsalva response was being obtained.
Recordings were again obtained at 1.5 and 3 min handgrip and repeated 5 and
10 min after discontinuing the isometric effort.

At time 0 and at 1.5, 3, 5 and 10 min, simultaneous blood samples were obtained from the left ventricle and pulmonary artery. In several cases additional
samples were obtained from the superior vena cava, femoral vein, inferior vena
cava, coronary sinus and antecubital veins.

Blood samples were taken into Lithium heparin tubes, immediately centrifuged
and the plasma frozen at $-20°C$ until assayed within 21 days of collection.
Plasma noradrenaline was determined radioenzymatically (Henry et al., 1975).
Data were analysed on the C.D.C. 6000 series computer at the University of
London, using the statistical package for the social sciences.

Results

During handgrip, there was a significant rise in mean heart rate from 77 to 91
beats per minute at maximum handgrip. There was also a significant rise in left

56

ventricular systolic pressure from 129 at rest to 165 mm Hg at maximum
handgrip (Fig. 1).

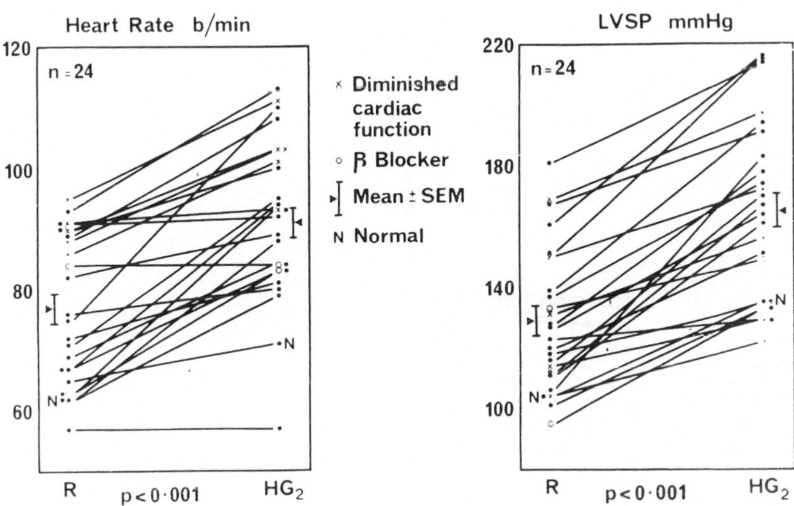

Fig. 1. Heart rate and left ventricular systolic pressure (LVSP) responses to
isometric exercise. The values given are those obtained at rest (R) and following
handgrip for three minutes (HG₂). Two patients were receiving beta-blocking
drugs at the time of the study and these individuals are identified on the slide

Resting plasma noradrenaline values showed marked variation, were similar in
pulmonary artery and left ventricle samples, and highest in those with poor
cardiac function (Fig. 2). In all individuals, plasma noradrenaline rose with
handgrip to an average of 155 pg/ml above basal values at 3 min handgrip. Expressed as a percentage this represents a 53% change at maximum handgrip
(left ventricle samples) and 43% change (pulmonary artery samples). Levels
returned to basal values after 10 min rest (Fig. 3).

An analysis of variance shows that for each individual, heart rate moves very
closely with noradrenaline during the handgrip and post-handgrip period,
(p < 0.001).

A significant inverse correlation was found between cardiac index at rest and
plasma noradrenaline concentration (Fig. 4).

In addition to the observations on cardiac index and plasma noradrenaline concentration, it can be seen from Table 2 that all other indices of left ventricular
function were inversely related to plasma noradrenaline concentration. However, so significant correlation was found between measurements of arterial pressure and plasma noradrenaline.

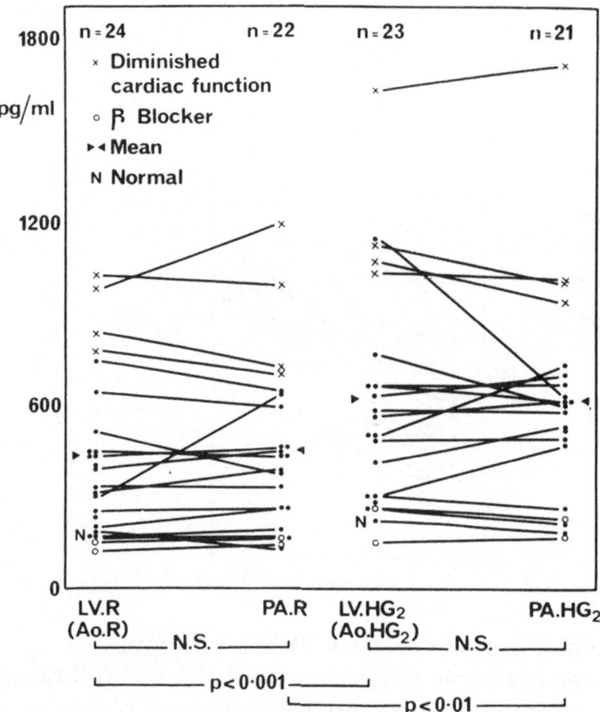

Fig. 2. Plasma noradrenaline concentrations (PNA) from left ventricle or aorta and pulmonary artery at rest (LVR, AoR, PAP) and from the same sites after three minutes of handgrip (LVHG2, AoHG2, PAHG2)

Table 3 gives details of the mean values for paired samples obtained from various sites and these have been compared using Students paired 't' test. With the exception of samples from the pulmonary artery and inferior vena cava, no significant differences were obtained, and we concluded that in general, changes occurring in plasma noradrenaline from a peripheral vein were closely paralelled by those occurring throughout the circulation. Reference to Table 3 does, however, suggest that samples obtained from the coronary sinus were also higher than those obtained from the pulmonary artery, although this difference was not siginificant.

The consistently higher plasma noradrenaline levels recorded from the inferior vena caval region below the hepatic veins when compared with the pulmonary artery concentrations (Fig. 5) strongly suggested that the liver was a major source of removal of amines from the circulation. If it is assumed that hepatic blood flow is 20 to 25% of the cardiac output, then the difference between the pulmonary artery noradrenaline concentrations and those derived from the

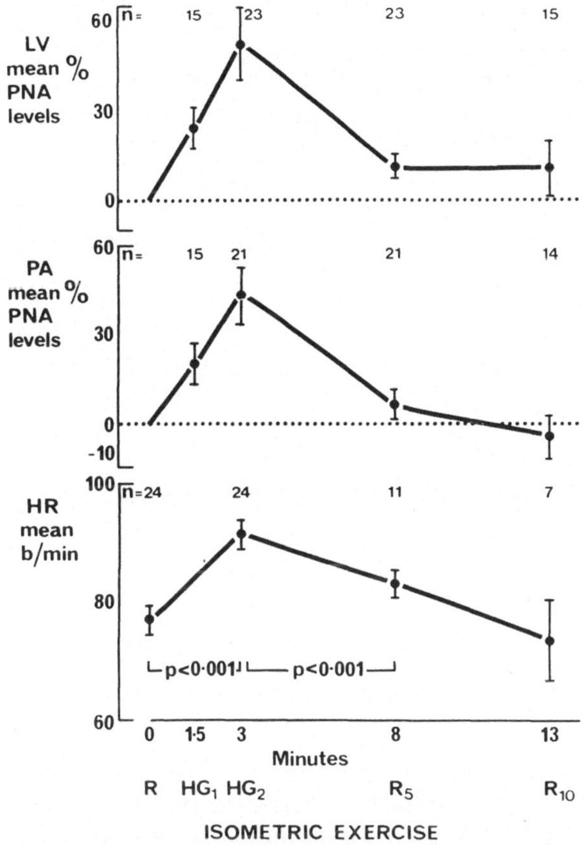

Fig. 3. Percentage changes in plasma noradrenaline concentration (PNA) following handgrip. LV = left ventricle, PA = pulmonary artery, HR = heart rate, R = Rest, HG1 = 1 1/2 min handgrip, HG2 = 3 min handgrip, R5 = 5 min rest, R10 = 10 min rest post handgrip

inferior vena cava implies between 55 and 70% extraction of noradrenaline occurs on a single pass through the liver.

Two patients were taking beta-blocking drugs at the time of the investigation. A re-analysis of the data omitting observations on these two patients does not alter the conclusions presented here.

Discussion

Isometric or static exercise exert profound haemodynamic changes. The dramatic rise in arterial pressure is considered to result from the combined effects of a modest rise in heart rate, a positive ionotropic mechanism and peripheral vasoconstriction. It is thus likely that a major part of this haemodynamic response

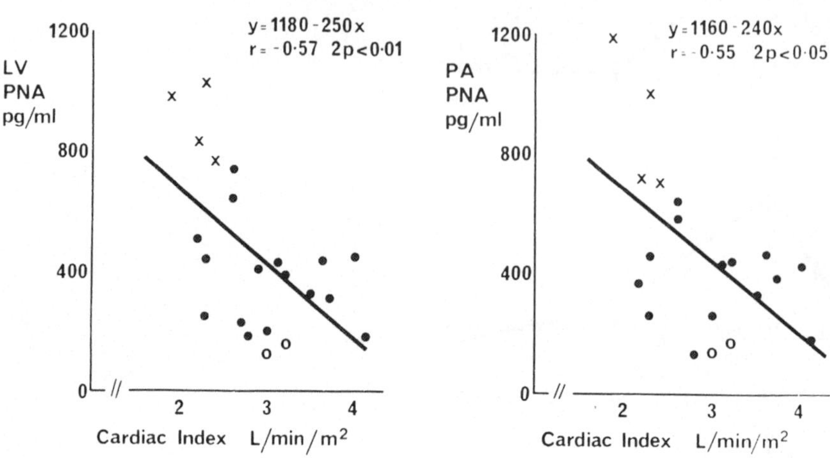

Fig. 4. Symbols as for previous figure

is mediated through their activation of the sympathetic nervous system (Vecht et al., 1978).

The results of these investigations have shown a modest rise in plasma noradrenaline in response to isometric effort. This rise is much less than that occurring in response to dynamic exercise (Sleight et al., 1979) and appears only to occur in those subjects with reduced left ventricular function. Thus, earlier reports of a rise in noradrenaline with isometric exercise must be reviewed with reference to the type of patient upon which the studies were carried out. These observations provide a further example of the necessity for careful appraisal of the type of subjects used in any study incorporating measurements of plasma catecholamines.

The high resting and stimulated levels of noradrenaline found in association with poor cardiac function could indicate increased sympathetic activity. Nevertheless, the possibility that reduced clearance could account for these findings has not been eliminated.

Resting heart rates and their response to the isometric effort were closely correlated with changes in circulating noradrenaline. However, the relationship to blood pressure was not significant.

Despite earlier reports suggesting significant clearance of catecholamines by the lungs (Sole et al., 1979), this has not been confirmed in the present study, and the only major differences found on multiple-site sampling were those between the inferior vena cava and the pulmonary artery, suggesting significant elimination of circulating noradrenaline by the liver.

Table 2. Correlations with Pulmonary Artery and Left Ventricular Plasma Noradrenaline Concentrations

	Pulmonary Artery	Left Ventricle
Age	.16 (22)	.16 (24)
Heart Rate	.52 (59)[a]	.55 (65)[a]
Left ventricular systolic pressure	.16 (59)	.19 (65)
Left ventricular end diastolic pressure	.35 (28)	.39 (31)[a]
DP/DT	-.48 (9)	-.39 (12)
Cardiac index	-.55 (20)[a]	-.57 (22)[a]
Ejection fraction	-.41 (18)	-.44 (20)[a]

[a] 2p < 0.05

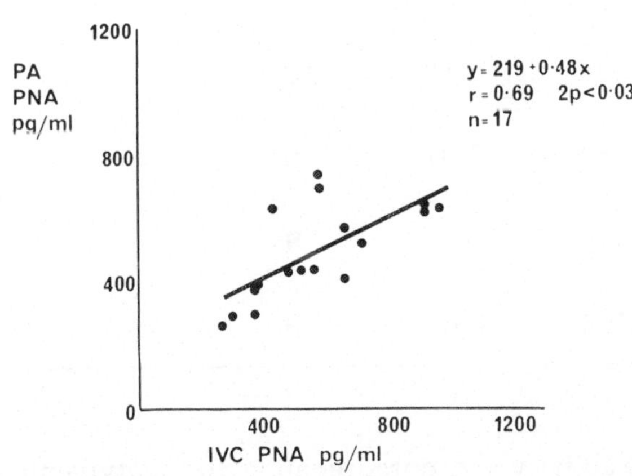

Fig. 5. IVC = inferior vena cava. Other symbols as for previous figures

The results of these studies shed little light on the mechanism underlying the pressor response to isometric exercise and it may again be pointed out that the changes in sympathetic muscle nerve activity during this manoeuvre are not as dramatic as those that are seen during postural stimulus. No comparison is

61

Table 3. Multiple-Site Sampling for Noradrenaline

Sites	Mean Values (pg/ml)		Paired 't'	Number of Pairs
	1	2	2p	
Pulmonary artery[1] and left ventricle[2]	504	504	0.99	91
Pulmonary artery[1] and superior vena cava[2]	485	491	0.76	24
Pulmonary artery[1] & femoral vein[2]	442	445	0.92	10
Pulmonary artery & inferior vena cava[2]	493	571	0.06	17
Pulmonary artery[1] & cubital sinus.[2]	504	563	0.19	10
Pulmonary artery[1] & cubital vein.[2]	476	454	0.66	9
Left ventricle[1] and superior vena cava[2]	473	497	0.23	25
Left ventricle[1] and femoral vein[2]	426	446	0.45	10
Left ventricle[1] and inferior vena cava[2]	547	561	0.68	17
Left ventricle[1] and coronary sinus[2]	403	444	0.15	15
Left ventricle[1] and cubital vein[2]	460	454	0.91	9
Superior vena cava[1] & inferior vena cava[2]	557	570	0.80	9
Femoral vein[1] and cubital vein[2]	483	454	0.67	9

available for changes in muscle nerve activity and noradrenaline during dynamic exercise. It is possible that the dramatic elevations in noradrenaline seen with change in posture and with dynamic exercise may predominantly reflect release of this amine from nerve endings in the walls of the veins or, alternatively, that these two stimuli are associated with a marked reduction in the clearance of noradrenaline from the circulation.

Acknowledgement. We are grateful to Miss May Petrie and Miss Barbara Osikowska for their technical assistance and to Miss Gery Bartlett for typing the manuscript.

This work was partly supported by a grant from the Wellcome Trust.

References

Lake CR, Ziegler MG, Kopin IJ (1976) Use of plasma norepinephrine for evaluation of sympathetic neuronal function in man. Life Sci 18 : 1315

Sever PS, Peart WS, Davies IB, Tunbridge RDG, Gordon D (in press) Ethnic differences in blood pressure with observations on noradrenaline and renin. 2. An hospital hypertensive population. Clin Exp Hypertension

Sundlof G, Wallin BG (1978) Human muscle nerve sympathetic activity at rest. Relationship to blood pressure and age. J Physiol 274 : 621-637

Sleight P, Floras JS, Hassan MO, Jones JV, Osikowska BA, Sever PS, Turner KL (in press) Baroreflex control of blood pressure and plasma noradrenaline during exercise in essential hypertension. Cli Sci Mol Med

Henry DP, Starman BJ, Johnson DG, Williams RH (1975) A sensitive radio-enzymatic assay for norepinephrine in tissues and plasma. Life Sci 16 : 375

Sole MJ, Drobac M, Schwartz L, Hussain MN, Vaughan-Neil EF (1979) The extraction of circulating catecholamines by the lungs in normal man and in patients with pulmonary hypertension. Circulation 60 : 160-163

Vecht RJ, Graham GWS, Sever PS (1978) Plasma noradrenaline concentrations during isometric exercise. Br Heart J 40 : 1216-1220

Plasma Noradrenaline as an Index of Sympathetic Activity

J. L. Reid

Plasma noradrenaline represents the small fraction of neurotransmitter noradrenaline released from peripheral sympathetic nerve endings which is not taken up into neuronal or extraneuronal tissue or metabolised by methylation or deamination and which overflows into the circulation. Plasma adrenaline in contrast is derived from the adrenal medulla and exerts its action as a blood borne hormone on metabolic, endocrine and vascular adrenergic receptors. In man, under most circumstance, noradrenaline levels in plasma are several fold higher than adrenaline unlike some animal species. In several studies, using different approaches, there is very little evidence, except during heavy physical exercise, that concentrations of noradrenaline achieved in plasma would significantly and directly influence arterial pressure or heart rate. When noradrenaline was infused intravenously to normal volunteers plasma concentrations had to increase by several fold to cause any change in systolic blood pressure (Fitz-Gerald et al., 1979). During Long-term intravenous infusions of noradrenaline to conscious dogs, an increase in circulating noradrenaline from 3.0 to 10.0 nmol/l was not associated with significant changes in blood pressure (Casals-Stenzel et al., 1979).

Plasma noradrenaline closely reflects short-term changes in sympathetic activity and is directly related to short-term changes in systolic blood pressure and heart rate within individuals (Watson et al., 1979a) (Fig. 1). However, as can be seen in figure 1 there were wide inter-individual differences in the position of this relationship which will make it difficult to compare groups of subjects.

The relationship between blood pressure and plasma noradrenaline either resting supine or standing in patients with essential hypertension remains controversial (Louis et al.. 1973; die Champlain et al., 1977; Lake et al., 1977). Great caution must be exercised over conditions of sampling, age, sex and race of patients and choice of patients and control groups in addition to analytical factors before interpretation of the results (Jones et al., 1979a). In a large scale population study no relationship was noted between blood pressure and plasma noradrenaline (Jones et al., 1978). The importance of the choice of control group is illustrated in figure 2. Mean supine plasma noradrenaline in a group of young healthy laboratory controls consisting of medical and paramedical personnel was 1.42 ± 0.12 nmol/l and significantly lower than either normotensive patients or essential hypertensives studied under identical conditions (2.60 ±

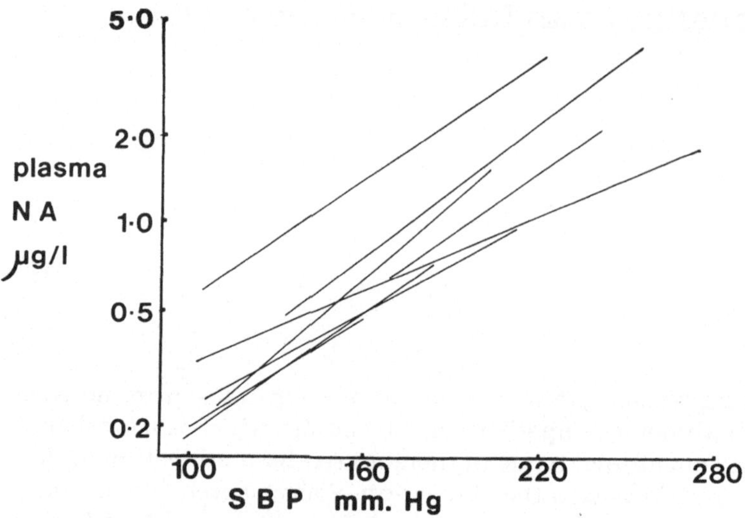

Fig. 1. Relationships between systolic blood pressure and simultaneous venous plasma noradrenaline in eight essential hypertensives. Each line is derived from a single subject with five to twelve measurements made under conditions of physical activity. The correlation coefficient (r) ranged from 0.52 to 0.91 and was significant (p < 0.05) in all cases

0.41 and 2.42 ± 0.24 nmol/l respectively). The striking difference in variance in the laboratory controls is lost on assuming the erect posture (Fig. 3) when the differences are lost (Jones et al., 1979a). In the population study referred to above (Jones et al., 1978) blood pressure was normally distributed and plasma noradrenaline revealed a log normal distribution with a wide range. The differences between trained laboratory staff and untrained patients whether normotensive or hypertensive may reflect underlying anxiety in the latter groups.

In the population study referred to above (Jones et al., 1978) blood pressure was normally distributed and plasma noradrenaline revealed a log normal distribution with a wide range. The differences between trained laboratory staff and untrained patients whether normotensive or hypertensive may reflect underlying anxiety in the latter groups.

Several other factors may serve to confound assessments of peripheral sympathetic activity based on plasma levels of noradrenaline. The transmitter is usually measured for reasons of convenience in peripheral venous plasma and this may not reflect transmitter overflow from haemodynamically important tissues such as the heart and resistance vessels.

Studies were performed of plasma noradrenaline simultaneously sampled from multiple arterial and venous sites during isometric and dynamic exercise and at rest (Table 1). Although there are differences, particularly between pulmonary

66

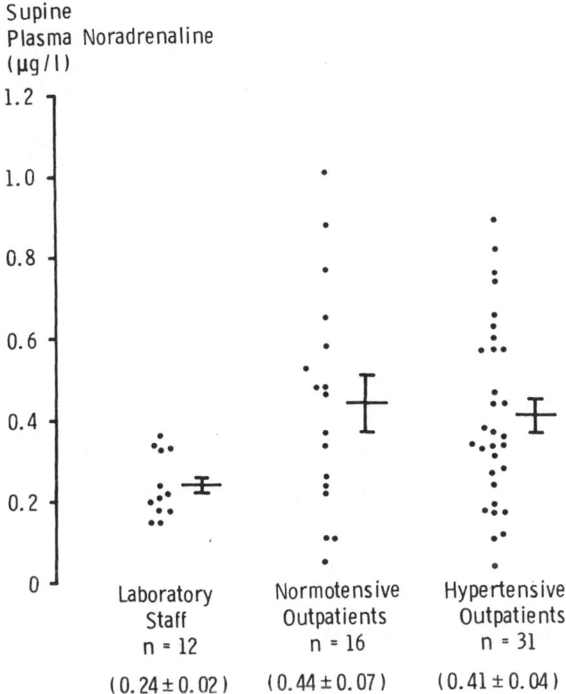

Fig. 2. Supine plasma noradrenaline after ten minutes rest in laboratory staff, normotensive outpatients and essential hypertensive patients. The mean (± SEM) is shown. Mean age of the laboratory controls was 31 + 2 years and 41 ± 3 and 47 ± 2 years respectively for normotensive and essential hypertensive patients (Jones et al., 1979a)

artery levels and other sites, during dynamic exercise, analysis of variance confirmed that although there were significant differences between subjects and between activities (rest, handgrip and bicycling), there was no consistent difference between the sites sampled (Watson et al., 1979b). Similar conclusions were drawn from studies in which noradrenaline was measured at several different venous levels in patients with essential hypertension. At rest the only significant difference was that noradrenaline levels in the hepatic vein were significantly lower than other sites, presumably a consequence of catecholamine uptake and metabolism by the liver (Jones et al., 1979b).

Several mechanisms contribute to the clearance of noradrenaline from plasma in addition to hepatic uptake. Peripheral tissue both neuronal and non neuronal can clear noradrenaline by specific uptake mechanisms with subsequent metabolism. Previous studies have utilised radio labelled precursors or noradrenaline to devise dynamic measures of synthesis, release or clearance of transmitter. Recently we have examined the kinetics of continuously infused noradrenaline to assess inter-individual variation in noradrenaline kinetics in volunteers (Fitzgerald et al., 1979). Plasma noradrenaline was measured during short term

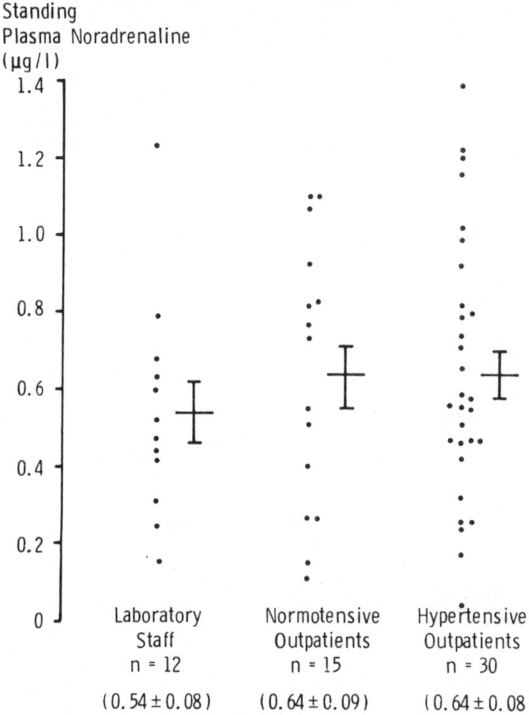

Fig. 3. Plasma noradrenaline (mean ± SEM) after three minutes standing in laboratory staff, normotensive outpatients and patients with essential hypertension (Jones et al., 1979a)

step up infusion of noradrenaline and prolonged (10 hour) infusions. In the latter study noradrenaline infusion at 0.06 μg/kg/min for 10 hours to 5 normotensive volunteers raised plasma noradrenaline from 1.2 nmol/l to over 7 nmol/l at steady state. The mean increase in blood pressure was 21.8 mm Hg systolic and 14.1 mm Hg diastolic. The clearance of noradrenaline ranged from 27.9 to 100 ml/kg/min and was little influenced by acute haemodnamic changes. There was also a wide range in volume of distribution (0.09-0.40 litres/kg) (Mean 13.5 litres) but less variation in half-life in plasma (1.45-2.9 minutes) (Table 2).

There was no difference between plasma half life after short term (5 x 10 min) infusions and a long term (10 hour) study. The endogenous circulatory input of noradrenaline was calculated in both studies from the steady state plasma level and the clearance. This index of catecholamine production ranged from 0.33 to 1.96 μg/min but the mean value was similar in short term (0.83 ± 0.33 μg/min) and long term (0.85 ± 0.32 μg/min) studies (Table 2). This would correspond to an endogenous input into the circulation of 1.2 mg/day which represents around 15-20% of the total urinary output of catecholamines and

68

Table 1. Plasma noradrenaline (nmol/l ± SEM) at different vascular sites at rest and during exercise

	System artery	Femoral vein	Pulmonary artery	Antecubital vein
Resting	1.60 ± 0.77	1.60 ± 0.59	2.43 ± 0.53	2.30 ± 0.95
Handgrip (isometric exercise)	1.65 ± 0.47	2.36 ± 0.83	2.66 ± 0.95	2.89 ± 0.89
Bicycling (dynamic exercise)	4.67 ± 1.24	4.37 ± 1.18	6.67 ± 2.60	4.43 ± 1.06

Mean plasma noradrenaline at four sites at rest and during isometric and dynamic exercise in six patients undergoing cardiac investigation (Watson, Page, Littler, Jones and Reid, 1979)

Table 2. Kinetic parameters and endogenous noradrenaline production in five normotensive subjects during intravenous noradrenaline infusion (mean ± SEM with range in brackets) supine

	Volume of distribution (litres)	Half-life (mins)	Clearance (litres/min)	Endogenous noradrenaline production (μg/min)*
Short term infusion (50 mins)	—	1.67 ± 0.40 (0.57 - 2.40)	4.32 ± 0.91 (1.80 - 6.58)	0.83 ± 0.33 (0.33 - 1.95)
Long term infusion (10 hours)	13.51	2.09 ± 0.34 1.45 - 2.90)	4.46 ± 1.02 (2.08 - 7.25)	0.85 ± 0.32 (0.36 - 1.96)
P		NS	NS	NS

* Endogenous noradrenaline production calculated as clearance x supine basal plasma noradrenaline

thus suggests that some 15-20% of noradrenaline released from sympathetic nerve endings may reach the systemic circulation.

A striking observation in these studies is the wide interindividual differences in clearance of noradrenaline which would be likely to confound direct interpretation of resting plasma concentration as an index of sympathetic activity. Preliminary studies in hypertensive subjects (FitzGerald, personal communication) indicate that although resting plasma levels were higher than controls, plasma half-life was longer, clearance reduced and the calculated endogenous input of noradrenaline into the circulation was not significantly different in the two groups.

In conclusion plasma noradrenaline measurements can provide useful information on sympathetic activity in the short term, particularly within individuals. Several factors however limit the usefulness of plasma noradrenaline in studies between groups. Small effects of age and substantial effects of physical activity and anxiety are added to considerable interindividual differences in clearance of noradrenaline. Further studies are warranted to investigate the contribution of changes in clearance of noradrenaline to observed differences in plasma levels.

Acknowledgement. While these studies were being undertaken the author was supported as a Senior Fellow in Clinical Science by The Wellcome Trust. The contributions of Drs. H. Jones and G. FitzGerald and other colleagues at Hammersmith Hospital are gratefully acknowledged. Figures 2 und 3 are reproduced by kind permission of Clinical Science. Mrs. Mary Wood kindly typed the manuscript.

References

Casals-Stenzel J, Tree M, Reid JL, Hamilton C, Brown JJ, Fraser R, Lever AF, Millar JA, Morton JJ, Robertson JIS (1979) Prolonged noradrenaline infusion in the conscious dog: Relation of plasma noradrenaline to arterial pressure. Circ Res (in press)

Champlain J de, Cousineau D, Ameringen MR van, Marc-Aurele J, Yamaguchi N (1977) The role of the sympathetic nervous system in experimental and human hypertension. Postgrad Med Suppl 3 53 : 15

FitzGerald GA Hossman V, Hamilton CA, Reid JL, Davies DS, Dollery CT (1979) Interindividual variation in the kinetics of infused noradrenaline in man. Clin Pharmacol Ther (in press)

Jones DH, Hamilton CA, Reid JL (1978) Plasma noradrenaline, age and blood pressure: a population study. Clin Sci Mol Med Suppl 4 55 : 735

Jones DH, Hamilton CA, Reid JL (1979a) The choice of control groups in the appraisal of sympathetic activity in essential hypertension. Clin Sci (in press)

Jones DH, Allison DJ, Hamilton CA, Reid JL (1979 b) Selective venous sampling in the diagnosis and localization of phaeochromocytoma. Clin Endocrinol 10 : 179

Lake CR, Zeyler MG, Coleman MD, Kopin IJ (1977) Age adjusted plasma norepinephrine levels are similar in normotensive and hypertensive subjects. N Engl
  J Med 296 : 208
Louis WJ, Doyle AE, Anavekar S (1973) Plasma norepinephrine levels in essential hypertension. N Engl J Med 288 : 599
Watson RDS, Hamilton CA, Reid JL, Littler WA (1979a) Plasma noradrenaline
  and systolic blood pressure during physical activity in hypertension. Hypertension (in press)
Watson RDS, Page AJF, Littler WA, Jones DH, Reid JL (1979 b) Plasma noradrenaline at different vascular sites during rest and isometric and dynamic
  exercise. Clin Sci (in press)

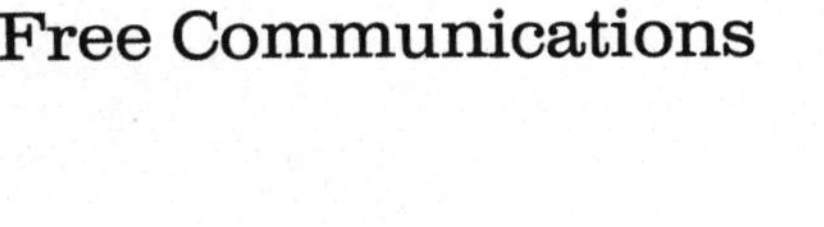

Free Communications

The Central Peptidergic Stimulation Syndrome:
A Role for Brain Peptides in Central Mechanisms of Blood Pressure Regulation

D. GANTEN, R. W. ROCKHOLD, T. UNGER, G. SPECK, B. SCHÖLKENS

Summary

Angiotensin II (ANG II) and enkephalins (ENK) occur in brain tissue and they increase blood pressure when injected into the brain ventricles. Stimulation of ANG II receptors by exogenous administration of the peptide or endogenous stimulation of its biosynthesis leads to the release of antidiuretic hormone (ADH) and adrenocorticotrophic hormone (ACTH) and to an increase of sympathetic tone ("central peptidergic stimulation syndrome"). ENK produce similar humoral effects and the humoral pattern of increased ADH, ACTH and sympathetic tone has also been found in spontaneously hypertensive rats (SHR). It is concluded that central peptidergic stimulation can contribute to be maintenance of high blood pressure in SHR. Such a conclusion is supported by the fact that 1) SHR are supersensitive to intraventricular ANG II and ENK, 2) in SHR the brain renin-angiotensin system (RAS) is stimulated while plasma renin is decreased, and 3) intraventricular ANG II receptor blockade results in the lowering of blood pressure in SHR.

Current Concepts of Hypertension

The current concepts trying to explain the pathogenesis of hypertension focus on peripheral organs such as the kidney, blood vessels and the heart. Thus, it has been proposed that high blood pressure results from the reduced capacity of the kidneys to excrete salt and water in amounts that are proportional to the intake [1, 2]. An enhanced vasoconstrictor response of blood vessels to pressor hormones has been suggested as being not only a consequence of, but also a cause for, hypertension [3]. Moreover, an overactivity of the sympatho-adrenal and sympatho-neuronal system with its consequences on blood vessels, heart and kidney function is considered of importance for the development and maintenance of hypertension [2].

These and other hypotheses do not exclude one another and may in fact be complementary. Computer models are believed by some authors to provide an analysis of cause-effect-relationships if proper input of peripheral pathophysiological data is assured [1]. No provision for an important role of the brain has been allowed in these cybernetic models of hypertension. Indeed, if this were to be done, the computer program would be dominated by a black box, i.e. the brain, since no quantitative data on disturbances in brain function and their consequences on blood pressure are known.

None of the present concepts gives a satisfactory explanation as to why peripheral organs dysfunction and why normally efficient counter-regulatory mechanisms are unable to bring blood pressure back to control levels by re-adjustment of peripheral organ function.

The brain plays a major role in the control, integration and coordination of heart function, vascular resistance and excretory activity of the kidney. This is achieved by direct synaptic contact of the central nervous system with peripheral organs via sympathetic and parasympathetic innervation. It is also achieved by the release of hormones from the brain which may have blood pressure effects by themselves, e.g. ADH [4], opioid peptides [5, 6] or which are releasing factors for other blood pressure regulating hormones (e.g. ACTH, gonadotropins). Epinephrine and norepinephrine have been shown to be involved in central mechanisms of blood pressure regulation, and significant changes of both transmitters have been described in different forms of experimental hypertension [7, 8].

In addition to these neurotransmitters, the neuropeptides have also demonstrated pressor effects [9]. We suggest that several peptides such as angiotensin, opioid peptides, substance P and others found in the brain may be of importance for the control of the activity of the autonomic nervous system, the release of hypothalamic and pituitary hormones and, thereby, central mechanisms of blood pressure regulation.

Spontaneously Hypertensive Rats

The pathophysiological mechanisms underlying the development and maintenance of high arterial blood pressure are different in the various strains of rats with genetic and spontaneous hypertension. In spontaneously hypertensive rats of the strokeprone strain (sp-SHR), plasma volume and blood volume were found to be diminished from the early onset of hypertension [2]. This makes it unlikely that retention of salt and expansion of intravascular volume represent the trigger mechanism for hypertension in these animals [2]. On the other hand, it has been shown that sympathetic nervous activity and plasma catecholamines are increased in these rats. This explains the increased sympathetic vascular tone and total peripheral resistance and an initial acceleration of heart rate in SHR [10]. The influence of stimulated sympathetic activity on kidney function has been shown by the delay of high blood pressure development following denervation of the kidneys in young SHR [10, 11]. The rise of blood pressure which occurs as the consequence of an increased sympathetic vascular tone, cannot be prevented by pressure diuresis and natriuresis, since the same increased sympathetic activity reduces the sodium and water excreting capacity of the kidney. Thus, salt and fluid homeostasis is maintained at the cost of blood pressure regulation [2].

In the sp-SHR, increased levels of ACTH, i.e. corticosterone, have also been measured [2]. This further increases the sensitivity of vascular smooth muscle to vasopressor agents such as catecholamines and ADH. Elevated levels of ADH in the plasma of SHR have also been reported [4]. Apart from its volume-retaining effect, ADH has been proposed to be also a pressor hormone [12]. The concomitant increase of corticosterone, catecholamines and ADH in SHR therefore represents a self-potentiating mechanism to increase blood pressure (Fig. 1). Furthermore, corticosterone has recently been reported to increase brain angiotensinogen concentrations which, in turn, could increase central ANG II synthesis [13].

Brain Peptides

Several peptides which were previously believed to occur in peripheral tissue exclusively, e.g. vasoactive intestinal peptide, gastrin and angiotensin, have now been discovered in the brain [14]. Peptides such as endorphins, enkephalins, substance P, kinins, neurotensin, have a wide distribution in the peripheral tissue and also occur in brain tissue [14].

It has been suggested that the peptides act as neurohormones in the brain, being secreted into the extracellular space or into the cerebrospinal fluid, thereby stimulating distant receptors or modifying synaptic events at low peptide concentrations [15]. This would result in a sustained regulation of activity of multiple nerve cell aggregates and in a complex concerted output [9, 15].

The information available to date would also be compatible with a classical neurotransmitter role of brain peptides. Neurotransmitters induce an activation of single neurone activity and simple, limited output. It is also conceivable that, in the same neurone and by the same peptide, a transmitter and neurohormonal mode of action could be in effect simultaneously, depending on whether a postsynaptic membrane with receptors adjacent to the peptide-releasing varicosity or synapse is present (transmitter) or not (neurohormone). As neuromodulators, peptides can exert long-term effects on neurotransmitter action and an overlap of peptide distribution and catecholamines has been reported for several brain peptides [14].

We suggest that the neurohormone concept is particularly suited to explain some of the brain peptide effects on blood pressure. This is supported by the finding of high peptide concentrations in the median eminence which is an important area for the control of neuroendocrine secretory processes [14].

Cardiovascular and Humoral Effects of Brain Peptides

Of all the peptides recently discovered in the brain, very little work has been done on their cardiovascular effects.

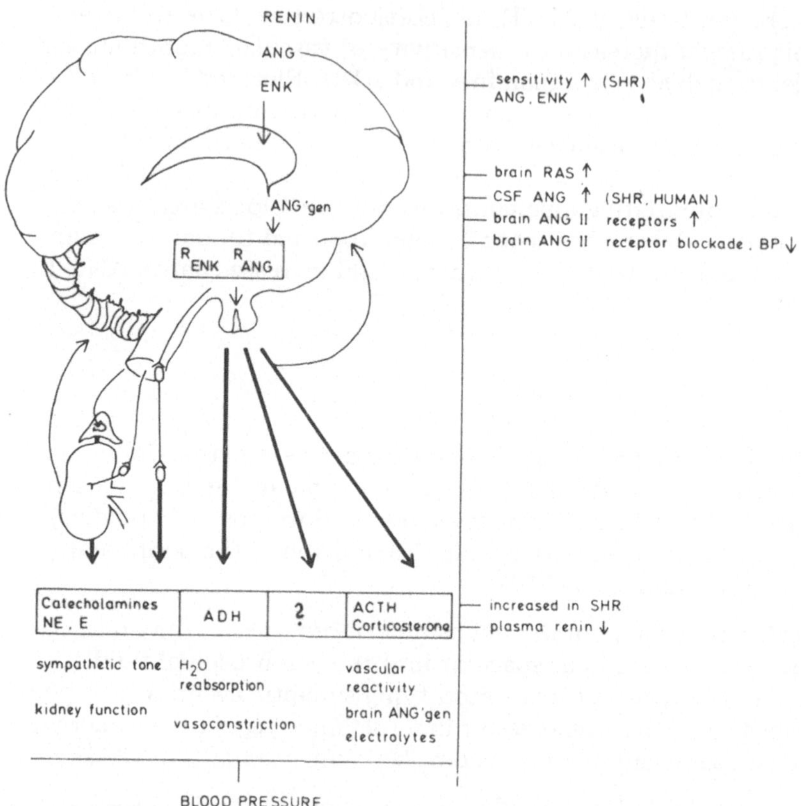

Fig. 1. General outline of possible mechanisms, leading to an elevation of blood pressure following stimulation of central peptide receptors: R_{ENK} = enkephalin receptors, R_{ANG} = angiotensin receptors. The effects on the release of hormones from the pituitary and adrenal gland following central peptidergic stimulation is indicated by the arrows. The evidences for a pathophysiological significance of these mechanisms is indicated on the right

Angiotensin

ANG II has a dual function as a true hormone circulating in the plasma and as a local tissue peptide [9]; it produces blood pressure increases when injected intravenously or into the brain ventricles. In the brain, it acts mainly on circumventricular organs such as the organum vasculosum lamina terminalis, the area postrema, the subnucleus medialis and others [16].

Most of the angiotensin effects have been studied by injection of synthetic peptide into the brain ventricles or into specific brain regions. In addition, angiotensin is generated within the brain itself. Due to the extremely high concentrations of angiotensinogen in cerebrospinal fluid, renin purified from kidney, brain or other extrarenal sources and injected into the brain will lead to angiotensin I (ANG I) formation, and brain converting enzyme will then convert ANG I to ANG II which stimulated specific brain ANG II receptors [17-19]. ANG II is thus the first peptide for which endogenous biosynthesis in the brain has been shown in vivo.

In such experiments with stimulated ANG II biosynthesis, it has been confirmed that intraventricular ANG II generation leads to an increase in the secretion of ACTH [20], an elevation of plasma corticosterone [20] and also increased plasma norepinephrine and epinephrine levels in plasma [19, 20], dopamine remains unchanged [20]. The parallel increases of epinephrine and norepinephrine indicate that both the sympatho-neuronal and sympatho-adrenal axis may be stimulated by brain ANG II. This latter conclusion is supported by the recent finding that the enzyme tyrosine hydroxylase in the adrenal gland is stimulated subsequent to centrally induced ANG II biosynthesis [21].

The partial dependence of pressor responses elicited by intraventricular ANG II on the release of ADH has been demonstrated by the dose-dependent increase of plasma ADH in control rats and by the reduced pressor responses to intraventricular ANG II in rats with hereditary hypothalamic diabetes insipidus which have a decreased capacity of ADH synthesis [9].

In summary it follows that endogenous brain ANG II increases arterial blood pressure by the stimulation of the release of ADH, ACTH, epinephrine and norepinephrine. In addition, other mechanisms may be involved.

Opioid Peptides

It is known that pain- and stressful situations are strong stimuli for the release of opioid peptides and entail acute and long-term effects on blood pressure, but little work has been done on the hemodynamic effects of these peptides. Like angiotensin, opioid peptides occur in plasma as circulating hormones and they also occur in high concentrations in the median eminence. Opioid peptides and ACTH have a common high molecular weight precursor, and beta-endorphin is secreted in equimolar quantities with ACTH into the blood [22, 23]. We have reported that enkephalins produce blood pressure increases following administration into both the lateral brain ventricles and the systemic circulation. These effects can be separated from blood pressure lowering effects which appear to be mediated by morphine receptors in the medulla oblongata [5, 6, 9, 19].

The central pressor responses of enkephalins as those of ANG II are ADH-dependent. Pressor responses to enkephalins were diminished or absent in rats with hereditary inability to produce ADH [19]. A role of enkephalins in the regulation of vasopressin secretion is supported by a report on the presence of enkephalin-positive cell bodies in the paraventricular and supraoptic nuclei of the hypothalamus projecting to the posterior pituitary [22]. This also suggests

that enkephalins may be released into the blood stream together with vasopressin and oxytocin. The pressor effects of intraventricular ENK were accompanied by increases in heart rate which may have been caused by a stimulation
of sympathetic tone. In addition, it was found that the baroreceptor reflex is
blunted following intraventricular ENK [21].

Thus stimulation of opioid peptide receptors appears to produce increases in
sympathetic tone and ACTH as are observed following the stimulation of brain
ANG II receptors. The blood pressure effects of ENK are clearly dependent on
the capacity of ADH synthesis [19].

Central Peptidergic Stimulation in SHR

The hemodynamic actions of intraventricular ANG II and ENK have been tested in sp-SHR. These rats exhibited a supersensitivity to both peptides and responded with greater blood pressure increases than normotensive control rats
[20]. The humoral pattern of increased ACTH (i.e. corticosterone), ADH and
sympathetic tone in SHR, as discussed above, is similar to the one observed
following stimulation of brain ANG II and ENK receptors. Thus, the increased
ACTH, ADH and sympathetic tone in sp-SHR ("central peptidergic stimulation
syndrome") (Fig. 1) is in agreement with the concept of central ANG II and
ENK contributing to the development and maintenance of high arterial blood
pressure in these rats.

This concept is supported by data indicating increased levels of immunoreac-
tive angiotensin in cerebrospinal fluid of SH rats and patients with essential
hypertension [9, 24]. We have also found that brain renin was elevated in the
A1, A2, A5, and A6 region of young sp-SHR. These noradrenergic brain areas
are important for blood pressure regulation [7, 8, 14]. The speculation that
brain angiotensin influences catecholamine turnover in these areas is substan-
tiated by the known effects of ANG II on catecholamine synthesis and release
[9], and by unpublished observations that induction of brain ANG II biosynthesis has marked effects on epinephrine, norepinephrine and dopamine beta
hydroxylase in specific brain regions [21]. Furthermore, the decreased plasma
renin in sp-SHR is compatible with an increased activity of brain renin, since a
negative feedback has been demonstrated between plasma renin and brain renin
[9].

Pharmacological interferences with the peptide systems further support the
conclusion of central peptidergic stimulation participating in the maintenance
of high blood pressure in sp-SHR: Blockade of ADH by ADH antibodies led
to a reduction of arterial blood pressure in these rats [12] and blockade of central ANG II receptors by saralasin produced significant blood pressure decreases
in sp-SHR even after nephrectomy [9, 25]. These effects were especially marked
following long-term intraventricular administration of saralasin [20].

Thus, the concept of central peptidergic stimulation may not only contribute
to our understanding of the pathophysiology of the hypertensive disease, but

it may also lead to novel antihypertensive drugs which could be designed to block the synthesis of pressor peptides and/or enhance the action of depressor peptides.

References

1. Coleman Jr TG, Guyton AC, Young DB, Clue JW de, Norman Jr RA, Manning Jr RD (1975) The role of the kidney in essential hypertension. Clin Exp Pharmacol Physiol Suppl 2 2 : 571-581
2. Dietz R, Schömig A, Haebara H, Mann JFE, Rascher W, Lüth JB, Grünherz N, Gross F (1978) Studies on the pathogenesis of spontaneous hypertension of rats. Circ Res Suppl 1 43 : 98-106
3. Folkow B (1975) Relationship between physical vascular properties and smooth muscle function; its importance for vascular control and reactivity. Clin Exp Pharmacol Physiol Suppl 2 2 : 55-61
4. Crofton JT, Share L, Shade RE, Allen C, Tarnowski D (1978) Vasopressin in the rat with spontaneous hypertension. Am J Physiol 235 : H361-H366
5. Simon W, Schaz K, Ganten U, Stock G, Schlör KH, Ganten D (1978) Effects of enkephalins on arterial blood pressure are reduced by propranolol. Clin Sci Mol Med Suppl 4 55 : 237s-241s
6. Bolme P, Fuxe K, Agnati LF, Bradley R, Smythies J (1978) Cardiovascular effects of morphine and opioid peptides following intracisternal administration in chloralose-anesthetized rats. Eur J Pharmacol 48 : 319-324
7. Chalmers JP (1975) Brain amines and models of experimental hypertension. Circ Res 36 : 469-483
8. Grobecker H (1976) Die Rolle peripherer und zentraler adrenerger Neurone bei der Entstehung der experimentellen Hypertonie. In: Ganten D, Dietz R, Lüth B, Gross F (eds) Beta-Adrenerge Blocker und Hochdruck. Stuttgart, Thieme, pp 4-14
9. Ganten D, Stock G (1978) Humoral and neurohumoral aspects of blood pressure regulation: Focus on angiotensin. Klin Wochenschr Suppl 1 56 : 31-41
10. Schömig A, Dietz R, Rascher W, Lüth JB, Mann JFE, Schmidt M, Weber J (1978) Sympathetic vascular tone in spontaneous hypertension of rats. Klin Wochenschr Suppl 1 56 : 131-138
11. Liard J-F (1977) Renal denervation delays blood pressure increase in the spontaneously hypertensive rat. Experientia 33 : 339-340
12. Möhring J (1978) Neurohypophyseal vasopressor principle: Vasopressor hormone as well as antidiuretic hormone? Klin Wochenschr Suppl 1 56 : 71-79
13. Printz MP, Lewicki JA, Wallis CJ (in press) Brain angiotensinogen: Origin and evidence for an influence by adrenal corticosteroids. Symposium on Enzymatic Release of Vasoactive Peptides, Heinsheim, 1979. New York, Raven
14. Hökfelt T, Elde R, Fuxe K, Johansson O, Ljungdahl A, Goldstein M, Luft R, Efendic S, Nilsson G, Terenius L, Ganten D, Jeffcoate SL,

Rehfeld J, Said S, Perez de la Mora M, Possani L, Tapia R, Teran L, Palacios R (1978) Aminergic and peptidergic pathways in the nervous system with special reference to the hypothalamus. In:Reichlin S, Baldessarini RJ, Martin JB (eds) The hypothalamus. New York, Raven, pp 69-135

15. Barker JL, Smith TG (1977) Peptides as neurohormones. In: Cowan WM, Ferrendelli JA (eds) Approaches to the cell biology of neurones. Society for Neuroscience Symposia, Vol II. Bethesda, Society for Neuroscience, pp 340-373

16. Phillips MI, Felix D, Hoffman WE, Ganten D (1977) Angiotensin-sensitive sites in the brain ventricular system. In: Cowan WM, Ferrendelli JA (eds) Approaches to the cell biology of neurons. Society for Neuroscience Symposia, Vol II Bethesda, Society for Neuroscience, pp 308-339

17. Sirett NE, McLean AS, Bray JJ, Hubbard JI (1977) Distribution of angiotension II receptors in rat brain. Brain res 122 : 299-312

18. Snyder SH (1978) Peptide neurotransmitter candidates in the brain: Focus on enkephalin, angiotensin II and neurotensin. In: Reichlin S, Baldessarini RJ, Martin JB (eds) The hypothalamus. New York, Raven, pp 233-244

19. Ganten D, Speck G (1978) The brain renin-angiotensin system: A model for the synthesis of peptides in the brain. Biochem Pharmacol 27 : 2379-2389

20. Ganten D, Unger T, Rockhold R, Schaz K, Speck G (in press) Central peptidergic stimulation: Its possible contribution to blood pressure regulation. Symposium on Radioimmunoassay, Applications in Cardiovascular Medicine. Amsterdam, Elsevier

21. Parvez H, Guerce A de, Stock G, Ganten D (to be published)

22. Rossier J, Battenberg E, Pittman Q, Bayon A, Koda L, Miller R, Guillemin R, Bloom F (1979) Hypothalamic enkephalin neurones may regulate the neurohypophysis. Nature 277 : 653-655

23. Nakanishi S, Inoue A, Kita T, Nakamura M, Chang ACY, Cohen SN, Numa S (1979) Nucleotide sequence of cloned cDNA for bovine corticotropin-β-lipotropin precursor. Nature 278 : 423-427

24. Kaneko Y, Ohnishi T, Fujishima S, Tanaka K, Umemura S (1979) Relation of angiotensin II concentrations in cerebrospinal fluid to systemic blood pressure levels in essential hypertension. 6th Scientific Meeting of the International Society of Hypertension, Göteborg, June 11-13, 1979

25. Mann JFE, Phillips MI, Dietz R, Haebara H, Ganten D (1978) Effects of central and peripheral angiotensin blockade in hypertensive rats. Am J Physiol 234 : H629-H637

Glandular Adenylate Cyclase System in Genetic Hypertension – Age-Dependent Response to Catecholamines[1]

G. SCHMID, A. HEIDLAND

Introduction

Various approaches have been made to evaluate the role of central and peripheral catecholaminergic mechanisms as to their effect on the pathogenesis of high arterial blood pressure in spontaneously hypertensive rats (SHR). Both sympatho-neural and sympatho-adrenal malfunctions are involved in causing and possibly maintaining arterial hypertension in SHR and yet, the experimental evidence that has been published to date is often divergent and the underlying mechanisms are still not completely defined.

Moreover, the age of the animals seems to be a particular determinant in the abnormal sympathetic nervous function of SHR. In young SHR for example, increases in cardiac norepinephrine turnover and splanchnic sympathetic discharge have been noticed (Okamoto et al., 1967; Yamori, 1974 and 1976). The discrepancy in cardiac norepinephrine turnover disappears when the animals reach the age of 15 weeks (Yamori, 1976; Howe et al., 1978). Higher plasma norepinephrine concentrations and stepped-up dopamine-β-hydroxylase activities can also be observed in young SHR. However, the importance of plasma norepinephrine levels as an index of sympathetic nervous activity is confined since they do not offer any information concerning the sensitivity of the specific adrenoreceptor system.

Recently, a method was described which enables the assessment of β-adrenoreceptor function (Schmid and Heidland, 1979) demonstrating target cell signal transformation with in vivo experiments on rats. This method is based on the measurement of cAMP excretion in parotid glands which are known to be chiefly regulated by their heavy supply on catecholamines.

To obtain more insight into β-adrenoreceptor function in arterial hypertension, in the present study salivary cAMP output was investigated in young (6-8 weeks) and older (16-18 weeks) SHR, before and during isoproterenol stimulation. The results were compared with those of normotensive control animals of the same age. In addition, adenylate cyclase activity measurements in parotid gland tissue were carried out during *in vitro* studies employing young and older SHR and controls. In

---

[1] Supported by the Deutsche Forschungsgemeinschaft, SFB 92 (Biomund)

these experiments, basal as well as isoproterenol and fluoride stimulated adenylate cyclase activities were evaluated.

Methods

Animals

Wistar Kyoto (WKy) rats were used which are genetically related to SHR and acknowledged as the best control strain available up to now, as well as spontaneously hypertensive rats (SHR). WKy and SHR were divided into two groups according to age: group I = 6-8 weeks, group II = 16-18 weeks old.

In Vivo Studies of cAMP Excretion in Parotid Saliva

Parotid saliva was collected as described in detail by Schmid et al. (1979). Salivary flow was stimulated by pilocarpine application at an initial dose of 7 mg x kg^{-1} followed by a continuous infusion at the rate of 0.045 μg x kg x min^{-1}. Fractionated collection of saliva began 20 minutes after pilocarpine application. Each sample corresponded to a 10 minute collecting period. After determining the extracted volume, the samples were immediately frozen. After cAMP extraction from the saliva specimens, the nucleotide was measured radio-immunologically.

In Vitro Studies on Adenylate Cyclase Activity of Parotid Gland Homogenates

Determination of adenylate cyclase activity was carried out as described by Schramm and Naim (1970).

Results

Effect of Age on cAMP Content (Without and During Isoproterenol Application) in Parotid Saliva of Normotensive Rats

When salivary flow was continuously stimulated with pilocarpine (0.045 μg x min^{-1} x kg^{-1}), the excretion rate of salivary cAMP from both parotid glands ranged between 20-30 fmoles x min^{-1} both in young and old rats. No significant difference in salivary cAMP output was found in these two groups of rats (Fig. 1).

Figure 2 additionally shows the effect of isoproterenol on the salivary cAMP excretion rate of these animals. Isoproterenol was infused intravenously at a rate of 4 μg x kg^{-1} x min^{-1}. The cAMP excretion rate immediately increased at the beginning of isoproterenol infusion in both groups of animals and reached a maximum output within 10 min. In young normotensive Wistar rats,

84

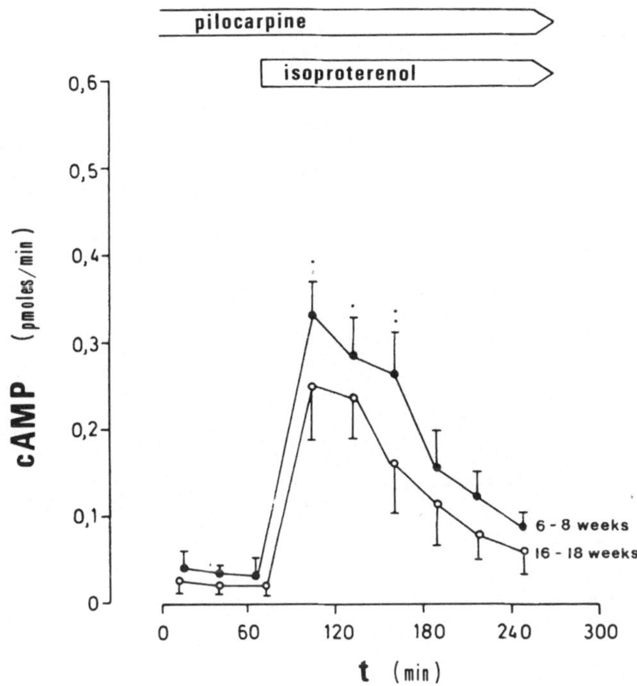

Fig. 1. Effect of age on cAMP excretion in parotid saliva of both glands in normotensive rats.
●——● = 6-8 weeks and ○——○ = 16-18 weeks old WKy rats.
Mean ± SD, n = 8 animals per group.
x = p < 0.05, xx = p < 0.01
Pilocarpine was infused subcutaneously at a dose of 0.045 μg x min^{-1} x kg^{-1} ,
isoproterenol was applied intravenously at a dose of 4 μg x kg^{-1} x min^{-1}

cAMP excretion increased from 20-30 fmoles/min to about 340 fmoles/min,
i.e. by a factor of 14. The maximal increase of cAMP output in older rats was
only 11 fold with about 270 fmoles/min. In both normotensive control groups,
cAMP excretion rates decreased from the normal level although isoproterenol
infusion was continuously administered at the same rate. The isoproterenol
stimulated cAMP excretion rate was still higher in young animals than in old
ones. There was no significant difference in salivary cAMP excretion rate
between standard Wistar and Wistar Kyoto controls.

*Age-Dependent Effects of Isoproterenol on cAMP Excretion in Parotid Saliva
of SHR*

Salivary flow was stimulated with pilocarpine at the same dose as used on normotensive controls. Isoproterenol was intravenously infused at a rate of 4 μg x
kg^{-1} x min^{-1} as mentioned above. The basal cAMP output (during pilocarpine

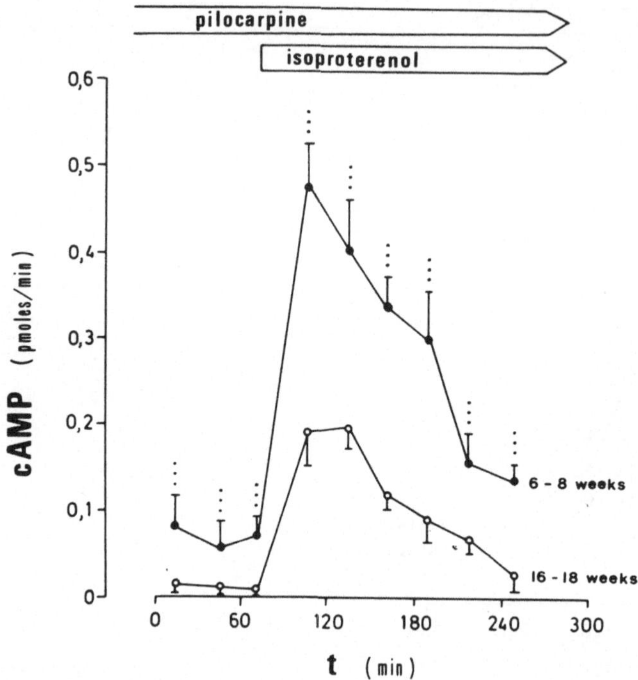

Fig. 2. Effect of age on cAMP excretion in parotid saliva of both glands in spontaneously hypertensive rats.
●——● = 6-8 weeks and ○——○ = 16-18 weeks old SHR.
Mean ± SD, n = 8 animals per group.
x = p < 0.05, xx = p < 0.01 and xxx = p < 0.001
Pilocarpine and isoproterenol were infused as described in Figure 1

application) as well as the isoproterenol induced cAMP excretion into the saliva was greater in young SHR than in controls of the same age. Basal salivary cAMP output was 150% higher in SH rats than in controls. Isoproterenol application induced a rise in the cAMP excretion rate to about 480 fmoles/min, a maximum output which was 150% higher than in young controls.

Opposite effects were seen in older SHR (16-18 weeks). Although the basal cAMP output in parotid saliva did not significantly differ in old SH rats compared to normotensive controls of the same age, isoproterenol induced cAMP excretion decreased to about 78% of the control amount, i.e., to about 200 fmoles/min. Isoproterenol induced cAMP of the old controls was only 90% of the amount produced by the young of the same strain. In contrast to this slight difference in the normotensive control groups, the old SHR strain excreted only about 50% of the young control output.

In Vitro Determination of Adenylate Cyclase Activity Without and During Fluoride or Isoproterenol Stimulation of Parotid Gland Homogenates from Young and Old WKy and SH Rats

The results are shown in Figure 3. Parotid gland adenylate cyclase activity of young WKy rats was taken as 100%. The 16-18 week old WKy rats did not demonstrate a significant alteration in parotid gland adenylate cyclase activity without or during fluoride, or isoproterenol stimulation.

Young SHR (6-8 weeks) exhibited a significantly higher activity of adenyl cyclase both with and without isoproterenol stimulation. Old SHR (16-18 weeks) demonstrated opposite effects with decreased adenylate cyclase activites after fluoride or isoproterenol stimulation.

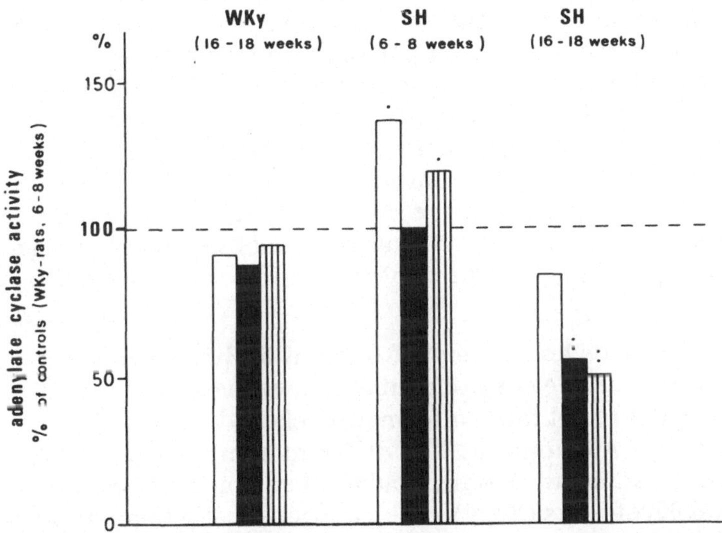

Fig. 3. Adenylate cyclase activities (basal as well as during fluoride and isoproterenol stimulation) in parotid gland homogenates of both young (6-8 weeks) and older (16-18 weeks) WKy- and SH-rats. The adenylate cyclase activities in parotid glands of the young WKy-rats were signified as 100%.
n = 6 animals per group.
x = p < 0.05, xx = p < 0.01 and xxx = p < 0.001

Discussion

Cyclic AMP was found to be contained in rat parotid saliva. Stimulating salivary flow with pilocarpine caused an excretion rate of salivary cAMP ranging between 20-30 fmoles/min as total output from both parotid glands. The glands themselves are considered to be the main source of salivary cAMP.

87

In particular, there is no evidence for an origin of salivary cAMP from plasma (Schmid, 1979). Former results from in vitro (Malamud, 1969; Schramm and Naim, 1970) and in vivo studies (Schmid and Heidland, 1979) strongly emphasize the fact that cAMP formation in parotid glands as well as cAMP excretion in parotid saliva reflect β-adrenoreceptor activation.

Isoproterenol application at a rate of 4 μg x kg^{-1} x min^{-1} enhanced cAMP output in parotid saliva of young (6-8 weeks) standard Wistar rats demonstrating a rise from a basal rate of 20-30 fmoles/min to about 340 fmoles/min, i.e., a 14-fold increase. Pilocarpine-stimulated cAMP excretion rates of 16-18 week old rats of the same strain were similar to those of the younger rats. When administering isoproterenol to this older group, the induced salivary cAMP excretion increased to only about 270 fmoles/min which signifies a 11-fold rise. This diminished cAMP response to isoproterenol application with respect to the age of the animals might suggest an age-dependent function impairment of the β-adrenoreceptor adenylate cyclase complex. This possibility bears more weight for consideration in view of the fact that a parallel study demonstrated no significant differences between parotid gland weights or their respective catecholamine contents when comparing young and old rat groups. It must be taken into consideration, however, that there might be some differences in body composition and hormonal environment between young and old animals which would pose a problem in selecting the suitable active dose of isoproterenol for the two groups. If the same dose is given to young and old alike, the slight difference of cAMP output might not necessarily hinge on an age-dependent activity of the gland β-receptors and their response to isoproterenol.

A major problem in studying catecholaminergic functions of SH rats concerns the lack of appropriate normotensive control animals (Lovenberg et al., 1973; Yamabe et al., 1973). In order to get more information clarifying the influence of rat strains on salivary cAMP output, two different control strains were used in our experiments, the standard Wistar population commonly used in our laboratory and Wistar Kyoto rats (WKy) which are genetically related to SHR and believed to be the best control strain available at present. When drawing a comparison between these two strains, no significant differences in cAMP output before or during isoproterenol application was noticed.

Collating normotensive controls with SH rats, two contrary deviations in salivary cAMP output depending on animal age were found. The basal and isoproterenol induced salivary cAMP output was increased in young 6-8 week old rats which could be caused by the higher plasma catecholamine levels in these animals or the accelerated firing rate of their sympathetic nervous system. The resulting stepped-up cAMP saliva excretion correlates well with formerly published data on young SH rats. Plasma noradrenaline concentrations and dopamine-β-hydroxylase activities are found to be increased in young SH rats (Grobecker et al., 1976; Nagaoka and Lovenberg, 1976) which might be the cause of the increased basal cAMP excretion rate. Since tyrosine hydroxylase, dopamine-β-hydroxylase and phenylethanolamine N-methyltransferase activities in the adrenal glands of these young animals are decreased, this status might

suggest that the domain of activity is situated in peripheral sympathetic noradrenergic nerves.

Enhanced cAMP response to isoproterenol by young SH rats requires the presence of an additional disorder in the signal transformation system of the sympatho-adrenal system in these animals. Exposure of β-adrenergic target cells to
increased catecholamine stimulation usually causes a subsiding sensitivity of the
appropriate β-adrenoreceptor function (Remold-O'Donnell, 1974). In young
SH rats however, both sympathetic activity and response to sympathetic stimuli (as judged by isoproterenol stimulation) are augmented. The reason for this
hypersensitivity in the β-adrenergic signal transformation system of the target
cells of the young animals is unclear. Formerly published data on enhanced
catecholaminergic functioning target tissue reactivity might support our findings. Our in vitro studies measuring adenylate cyclase activities subsequent to
isoproterenol or fluoride stimulation as well as basal activity evaluation (i.e.,
without neurotransmitter stimulation), indicate — in agreement with the in
vitro studies — an increment in the adenylate cyclase complex sensitivity
towards catecholamines without showing changes in the adenylate cyclase
capacity after fluoride stimulation of the catalytic subunits in the cAMP
complex. This result offers additional support to the possibility that along
with an enhanced sympathetic activity in young SH rats, their receptor system
reacts hypersensitively to catecholaminergic agonists. Therefore, in addition
to higher basal level activity, the degree of sympatho-adrenal system responsiveness of the target cells probably contribute to the development of hypertension in SH rats.

Whereas normotensive controls only display a slight decrease in cAMP response
to isoproterenol stimulation, the difference in output is highly significant com
pared to older SH rats. 16-18 week old SH rats show a decreased response with
lowered cAMP output subsequent to isoproterenol application when compared
to younger animals of the same strain or to normotensive controls of the same
age. Decreased basal cAMP output of older SH rats correlates well with the data
of Amer et al. (1974) and Ramanathan and Shibata (1974) which indicate a
decreased cAMP level in heart tissue and vascular walls. The decrease might be
caused by a lowered sympathetic discharge and/or a smaller rise of plasma
catecholamine levels found in the animals. However, in our investigations the
response to isoproterenol stimulation was reduced as well. This phenomenon seems
to be related to a subsensitivity in the presence of an augmented catecholamine
stimulation which also exists in other catecholaminergic systems. Our in vitro
studies indicate that this reduction is not exclusively evoked by an impaired
function in the signal transformation complex. Since the fluoride stimulated
adenylate cyclase activity is reduced as well which suggests a diminished responsiveness of the catalytic subunit in the adenylate cyclase complex, it should
be taken into consideration that the actual amount to transformation units
migth also have decreased. A similar reduction of the number of β-adrenorecep-
tors has been reported in the heart (Woodcock et al., 1978).

Acknowledgement. I thank Mrs. A. Wolpert, Miss Ch. Ullrich, Miss M. Stehr and Miss I. Müller for their skillful technical assistance.

References

Amer M, Gomoll AW, Perhach Jr JL, Ferguson HC, McKinney GR (1974) Aberrations of cyclic nucleotide metabolism in the hearts and vessels of hypertensive rats. Proc Nat Acad Sci USA 71 : 4930

Grobecker H, Saavedra JM, Roizen MF, Weise V, Kopin IJ, Axelrod J (1976) Peripheral and central catecholaminergic neurons in genetic and experimental hypertension in rats. Clin Sci Mol Med 51 : 377s

Howe PRC, Provis JC, West MJ, Chalmers JP (1978) Changes in cardiac norepinephrine in spontaneously hypertensive and stroke-prone rats. J. Cardiovasc Pharmacol 5 : 16

Lovenberg W, Yamabe H, Jong W de, Hansen CT (1973) Genetic variation of the catecholamine biosynthetic enzyme activities in various strains of rats including the spontaneously hypertensive rat. In: Usdin E, Snyder S (eds) Frontiers in catecholamine research, Pergamon, Oxford

Malamud D (1969) Adenyl cyclase activity in isoproterenol stimulated mouse salivary glands. J Cell Biol 43 : 84

Nagaoka A, Lovenberg W (1976) Plasma norepinephrine and dopamine-β-hydroxylase in genetic hypertensive rats. Life Sci 19 : 29

Okamoto K, Nosaka S, Yamori Y, Matsumoto M (1967) Participation of neural factors in the pathogenesis of hypertension in the spontaneously hypertensive rat. Jap Heart J 8 : 168

Ramanathan S, Shibata S (1974) Cyclic AMP blood vessels of spontaneously hypertensive rat. Blood Vessels II : 312

Remold-O'Donnell E (1974) Stimulation and desensitization of macroplaye adenyl cyclase by prostaglandins and catecholamines. J Biol Chem 249 : 3615

Schmid G, Heidland A (to be published) Evaluation of β-adrenergic activity by determination of cAMP-excretion rate in parotid saliva. — In vivo experiments in rats.

Schmid G (1979) Cyclisches 3', 5'-Adenosinmonophosphat in Gehirn und Speicheldrüse bei arterieller Hypertonie. Habilitationsschrift, Würzburg

Schramm M, Naim E (1970) Adenyl cyclase of rat parotid gland. Activation by fluoride and norepinephrine. J Biol Chem 245 : 3225

Woodcock EA, Funder JW, Johnston CI (1978) Decreased cardiac β-adrenoreceptors in hypertensive rats. Clin Exp Pharmacol Physiol 5 : 545

Yamori Y (1974) Contribution of cardiovascular factors to the development of hypertension in spontaneously hypertensive rats. Jap Heart J 15 : 194

Yamori Y (1976) Neurogenic mechanisms of spontaneous hypertension. In: Onesti G, Fernandes M, Kim KE (eds) Regulation of blood pressure by the central nervous system. Grune and Stratton, New York, pp 65-76

Effects of Somatostatin on Pressor Responsiveness to Angiotensin and Catecholamines in Essential Hypertension

J. ROSENTHAL, I. ARLART, H. JÄGER

Summary

The pressor response to angiotensin has been linked to the sympathetic nervous system which is said to have a pivotal function in essential hypertension.

In order to assess the contributing roles of these two systems studies were carried out before and during administration of Somatostatin (S) which has been shown to suppress stimulated renin concentrations and to lower blood pressure in essential hypertensives with high renin.

Five normal volunteers and 18 patients with essential hypertension were subjected on different days in a randomized fashion to the following protocols:
a) Basal conditions: i.v. infusion of S (250 μg priming dose, then continous infusion of 250 μg/h over 60 min);
b) Stimulation studies: i.v. infusion of either Orciprenaline (O) (0,03 mg/min) or Angiotensin II (A) (5 ng/min);
c) Administration of S as in (a) followed 10 min later by infusion of one of the substances ad described under (b).
Before and during the studies blood pressure and heart rates were monitored and venous blood collected for determination of plasma renin activity (PRA).

Following administration of S under basal conditions, mean arterial blood pressure (MAP) and heart rate (HR) remained essentially unchanged in all normal volunteers and hypertensives; renin was unaffected in the normals but tended to be lower in the hypertensive group. O produced in all volunteers and patients increments of MAP, HR and PRA of varying degree, whereas A raised blood pressure and HR but lowered PRA. Combination of S and O reduced the rise in PRA by 43%, MAP by 23% and HR by 16% compared with O alone in the normals and similar blunted responses were observed in the hypertensive group; combination of S with A was different in that blood pressure and heart rate changes in normals and essential hypertensives resembled Orciprenaline responsiveness with renin decreasing to undetectable levels under the double infusion.

The results indicate that the inhibitory action of S on the cardiovascular and humoral responses to O and A involve the sympathetic nervous system conceivable by receptor interactions via decreased Ca^{2+}-diffusion.

Regulation of blood pressure and responsiveness of the cardiovascular system
to various stimuli are governed and modulated by ultrastructural and biochemical aspects of cardiac and smooth muscles, by catecholamine metabolism —
neuronal and extraneuronal storage —, electrolytes and drug receptors.

The interrelationship of these different regulatory mechanisms are poorly understood and investigations along these lines are difficult to perform. One or
more important aspects involve specific cellular sites for Na-Ca-interactions
which are considered to be ultimately decisive for performance of contractile
proteins: The possible sites at which Na could influence force development by
smooth muscles are summarized in Table 1 and they are believed to include
extracellular — membrane bound — and intracellular mechanisms with or without involvement of autonomic nerve terminals.

Table 1. Specific Cellular sites for Na^+-Ca^{++} Interactions

---

Possible sites at which Na^+ could influence force development by smooth muscle:

1. the cell membrane active Ca^{++} extrusion pump
2. passive "channels" in the cell membrane permeable to Ca^{++}
   a) receptor regulated
   b) membrane potential regulated
   c) resting membrane leak
3. Ca^{++} binding sites at the inner surface of the plasmalemna
   a) receptor regulated
   b) membrane potential regulated
   c) dependent on stability of the phospholipid bilayer
4. Ca^{++} binding sites on the outer surface of the sarcoplasmatic reticulum
5. the sarcoplasmatic reticulum Ca^{++}-ATPase
6. the sarcoplasmatic reticulum Ca^{++} release gates
7. Ca^{++} binding sites on mitochondria
8. the mitochondrial Ca^{++} pump
9. the mitochondrial Ca^{++} leak
10. Ca^{++} binding sites on soluble Ca^{++} buffer molecules
11. Ca^{++} sensitive sites on the regulatory proteins of the contractile apparatus
12. autonomic nerve terminals

Against the background of these considerations and repeatedly demonstrated
evidence that Ca sequestration influences cardiovascular responsiveness [1]
pertinent studies were carried out by our group.

Previously we had been able to show that somatostatin (S), a cyclic tetrade-
capeptide which inhibits the spontaneous release of pituitary growth hormone
and some other hormones and which is found in the gastrointestinal tract, the

central nervous system and some peripheral sympathetic noradrenergic and primary sensory neurones, diminishes together with Furosemide in high renin essential hypertensives (HREH) plasma renin activity (PRA), blood pressure (BP), cardiac index (CI) and stroke index (SI), thus revealing a negative inotropic effect [2].

More recent findings in isolated organs have confirmed these results in spontaneously beating auricles of guinea pigs and demonstrated dose-response curves for S with different concentrations of calcium: lower calcium concentrations resulted in significantly stronger decreases in the amplitude of spontaneous contractions [3].

Table 2 summarizes the most important results of these in vitro experiments; other findings, not mentioned here, have indicated a species specifity for the action of S which is not surprising in view of the many synthetized analogues with selective metabolic and cardiovascular effects that are becoming increasingly available [3].

In further pursuit of our experiments we aimed at investigating the pressor responses to A and O during administration of S. We performed studies in humans who were treated in a randomized fashion on different days with either angiotension or the β-agonist orciprenaline alone, with S alone or with the combination of S and A or O. Table 3 summarizes the details of the protocols.

Table 2. Negative inotropic action of Somatostatin (S)

---

1. S exerts dose-dependent negative effect in guineapig auricles
2. negative inotropic effect not inhibited by practolol, phentolamine, methysergide, diphenydramine, cimetidine, atropine and indomethacine
3. negative inotropic effect potentiated by reduction in Ca^{2+} concentration
4. on a molar basis S equipotent with acetylcholine as a negative inotropic agent
5. S inhibits selectively the positive inotropic action of neurotensin
6. S interacts with specific receptors located in cardiac cell membranes. S/receptor interaction may cause decreased Ca^{2+} diffusion and/or transport

---

Source: Quirion, Regoli, Rioux & St-Pierre (1979) [3]

Figure 1 shows the results with orciprenaline in essential hypertensives and in normotensive controls: in both groups S depressed BP and PRA slightly, orciprenaline stimulated renin and raised BP and HR, and the double infusion diminished the orciprenaline response to renin by 43%, to HR by 16% and to mean arterial pressure (MAP) by 23%.

Upon studying these results after the essential hypertensives had been renin-profiled [5] the data revealed suppressibility of renin under S only in the high renin essential hypertensives (HREH) together with decreased responsiveness of BP under double infusion; the changes in the low renin essential hyperten-

Table 3. Protocols

1. Basal conditions: i.v. infusion of somatostatin (250 µg priming dose, followed by continous i.v. infusion of 250 µg over 60 min)
2. Stimulation studies: i.v. infusion of either orciprenaline (0.03 mg/min) or angiotensin II (5 ng/min) over 60 min
3. Administration of somatostatin as in 1. followed 10 min later by infusion of one of the substances described under 2.

Monitoring of blood pressure and heart rate, determination of plasma renin activity (4) before and during infusion

5 normotensive volunteers, 18 patients with essential hypertension (with determination of renin status)

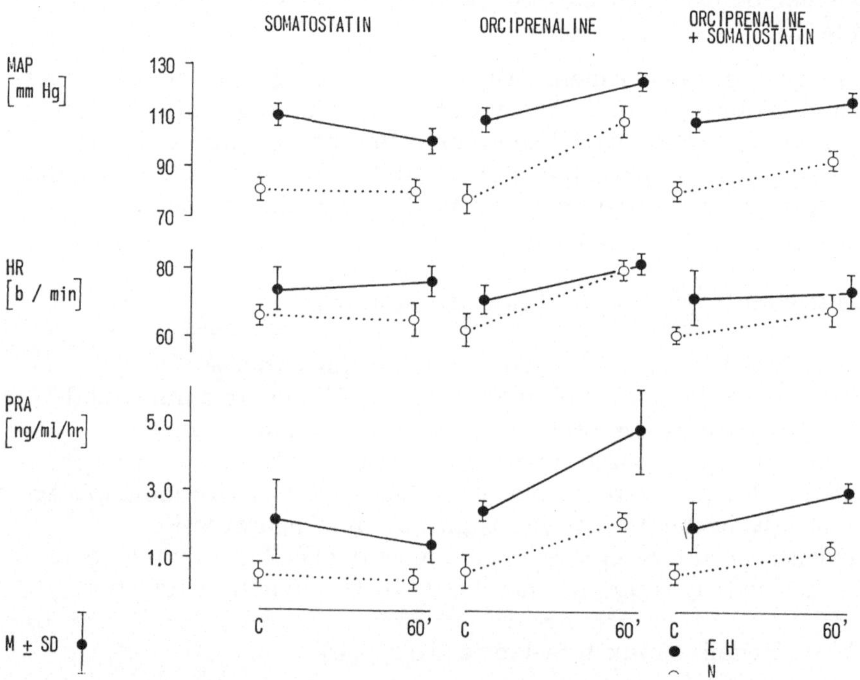

Fig. 1. Short-term effects of somatostatin, of orciprenaline, and of orciprenaline under somatostatin infusion on mean arterial pressure (MAP), heart rate (HR), and plasma renin activity (PRA) in normotensive volunteers (N) and patients with essential hypertension (EH) during 60 min observation periods (C = control values)

sives (HREH) together with decreased responsiveness of BP under double infusion; the changes in the low renin essential hypertensives (LREH) were negligible and indeterminate in the normal renin essential hypertensives (NREH) (Fig. 2).

94

The angiotensin studies in both groups demonstrated increases of BP and decreases of BP and decreases of renin and virtually no changes under double infusion for MAP but more pronounced decreases of renin in the essential hypertensives (Fig. 3).

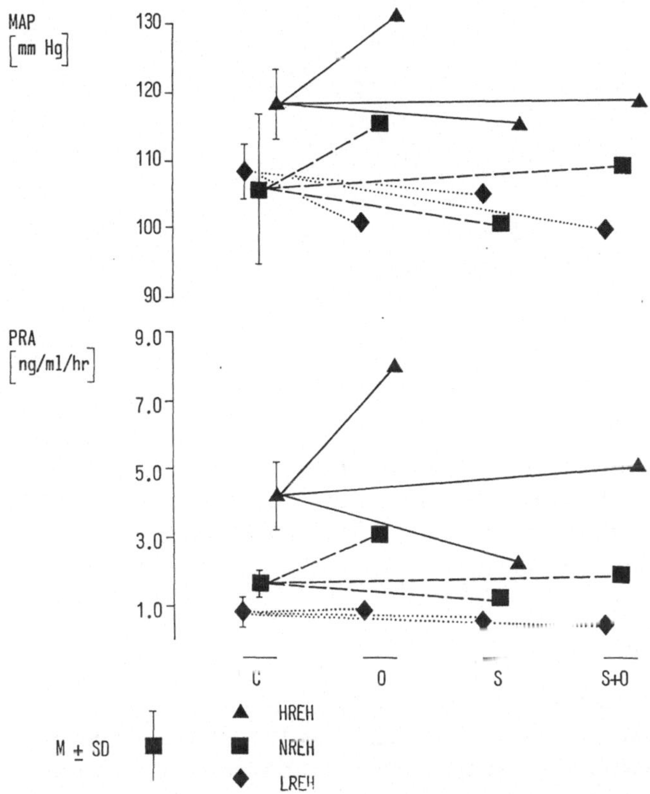

Fig. 2. Changes of mean arterial pressure (MAP) and of plasma renin activity (PRA) in high renin essential hypertension (HREH), normal renin essential hypertension (NREH), and low renin essential hypertension (LREH) before (C = control values) and under administration of orciprenaline (O), of somatostatin (S), and the double administration of somatostatin and orciprenaline (S+O) (computed values over a 60 min observation period)

Again, the evaluation of these results according to renin status revealed the responsiveness of the HREH with respect to renin but the lack of influence on the blood pressure raising effect of angiotensin under the double infusion (Fig. 4).

The physiological significance of all these findings remains to be determined. The concentrations of S required to elicit the described effects are unlikely to be found in the circulating blood, at least under physiological conditions.

95

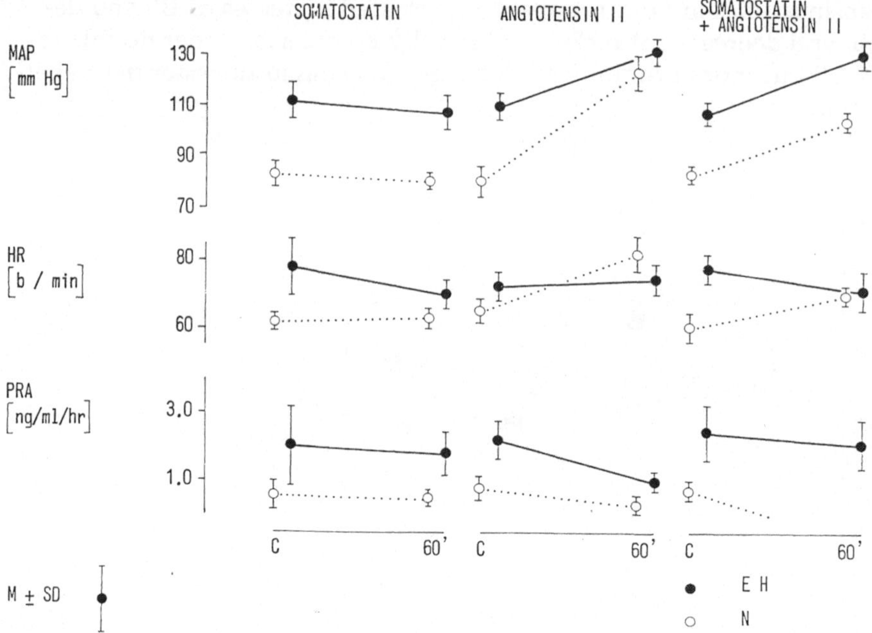

Fig. 3. Short-term effects of somatostatin, of angiotensin II, and of angiotensin II under somatostatin infusion on mean arterial pressure (MAP), heart rate (HR), and plasma renin activity (PRA) in normotensive volunteers (N) and patients with essential hypertension (EH) during 60 min observation periods (C = control values)

However, large amounts of S may be released from the pancreas and gastro-intestinal tissues into the portal and caval veins and reach the heart; moreover, S was found to depress the spontaneous firing of neurones in various brain areas.

These results raised the possibility that S acts as a naturally occurring neuro-transmitter or neuromodulator in the central and autonomic nervous system.

The mechanism by which S exerts its action could be seen in relation to de-creased calcium diffusion and/or transport into cardiac and smooth muscle cells indicating that S interferes with the excitation-secretion mechanisms.

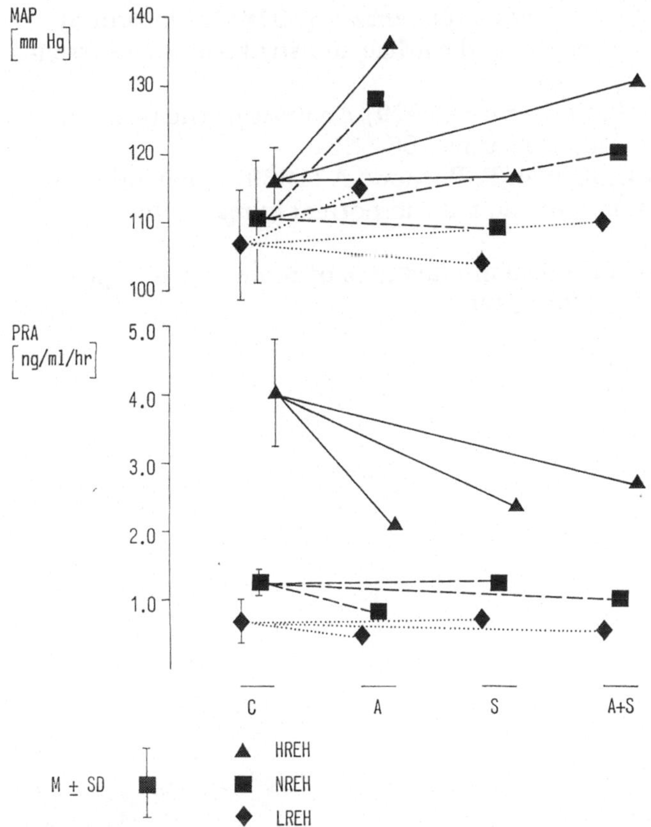

Fig. 4. Changes of mean arterial pressure (MAP) and of plasma renin activity (PRA) in high renin essential hypertension (HREH), normal renin essential hypertension (NREH), and low renin essential hypertension (LREH) before (C = control values) and under administration of angiotensin II (A), of somatostatin (S), and the double administration of somatostatin and angiotensin II (S+A) (computed values over a 60 min observation period)

References

1. Reuter H, Blaustein MP, Haeusler G (1973) Na-Ca exchange and tension development in arterial smooth muscle. Philos Trans R Soc Lond [Biol] 265 : 87

2. Rosenthal J, Raptis S, Zoupas C, Escobar-Jimenez F (1978) Inhibition by somatostatin of renin, blood pressure and cardiac and stroke index in essential hypertension. Circ Res 43 : I-69
3. Quirion R, Regoli D, Rioux F, St-Pierre S (1979) Analysis of the negative inotropic action of somatostatin, J Pharmac 66 : 251
4. Haber E, Koerner T, Page LB, Kliman B, Purnode A (1969) Application of a radioimmunoassay of plasma renin activity in normal human subjects. J Clin Endocrinol 29 : 1349
5. Brunner HR, Gavras H (1975) Clinical implications of renin in the hypertensive patient. J Am Med Ass 223 : 1091

Acute Effects of Labetalol on Haemodynamics and Response to Emotional Stress in Hypertensive Patients

J. Bahlmann, J. Brod, P. Pretschner, W. Hubrich

The effects of the treatment of hypertensive patients with beta-blocking agents which proved very effective can be counteracted and even neutralized by the prevalence of a reflex alpha-stimulation. Eight years ago, an agent was introduced under the name of labetalol of which it is claimed that it blocks both the alpha- and beta-receptors [3, 22]. Its beta-blocking properties are thought to be more effective than the alpha-blocking ones [23]. Peroral and intravenous administration of labetalol lowers the blood pressure of normotensive and hypertensive subjects [16, 23], this being due in the first place to a lowering of the total peripheral vascular resistance whilst the heart rate remained unaffected or slightly fell and the cardiac output decreased. At the same time the orthostatic reflex was slightly blocked [9] but the drug was tolerated in most probands without undue difficulties. While several studies were devoted to the effect on the arterial side of the circulation, few studies deal with the effects on the venous side.

In our previous studies we have found that the venous compliance in essential and renal hypertension is reduced [6]. It was also established that the reduction of the venous compliance contributes to the circulating homeostasis during the emotional stress reaction [7]. We have, therefore, investigated the haemodynamic response to intravenous labetalol in subjects with essential and renal hypertension studying, in addition to central haemodynamics, the behaviour of the vessels of the forearm. Also the effect of labetalol on the haemodynamic response to emotional stress was investigated.

Methods

The studies were carried out in 20 patients with hypertension (blood pressure exceeding in rest on several occasions 145/95 mm Hg) of which in nine it was essential and in eleven it was due to a chronic renal disease (three glomerulonephritis, seven chronic pyelonephritis and one hypoplastic kidney). Eleven men and nine females (average age 40 years) were involved in the study. Their hypertension was in stage I or II (WHO). None of these patients had anaemia (mean haemoglobin 15 g/100 ml), chronic renal failure, heart failure or malignant hypertension and their glomerular filtration rate averaged 114 ml/min. The

differential diagnosis of hypertension was based on the past history and the
criteria described previously [5].

All the subjects were investigated after a night's fast in a quiet laboratory in the
morning. All medication was stopped at least three weeks prior to the investigation. The details of the applied techniques were described on previous occasions [6, 7]. Briefly summarized, these consisted in the simultaneous measurements of the cardiac output by the dyedilution technique, the intravascular
measurements of the arterial and central as well as peripheral venous blood
pressure, forearm blood flow by occlusion plethysmography and forearm vascular volume by a combination of plethysmography with an isotope technique.
From these values the vascular resistances were calculated in the conventional
way. Venous distensibility was measured at an occluding cuff pressure of
30 mm Hg and was defined as forearm vascular volume per 1 mm Hg forearm
venous pressure.

Plasma renin activity was estimated by a radioimmunological method (normal
range in our labortory 0.6 to 4.0 ng angiotensin/ml/1 hour). Blood samples for
renin were drawn from the central venous catheter twice during the control
period and during the first and third experimental period following labetalol.

The Valsalva manoeuvre lasted for 15 s and we aimed at an elevation of central
venous pressure by 30 mm Hg. We assessed the changes of heart rate during
and after the Valsalva manoeuvre, the increase in blood pressure in the post-
Valsalva period (overshoot) and the duration of the overshoot.

Three resting control periods of 10 min duration were followed by a Valsalva
manoeuvre which was repeated twice. Labetalol was injected as soon as the
baseline was regained through the central venous catheter in 1 min in a dose
ranging from 0.6 to 1.6 mg/kg body weight. We aimed at lowering of the blood
pressure by at least 10% of the control value. If this was not achieved within
10 min, a small supplementary dose of labetalol was added (5 cases with 0.1-0.5
mg labetalol/kg body weight). The labetalol effect was followed for 30 to 45
min. After this two Valsalva manoeuvres were carried out at a 3 min interval.

We waited again until the base line was restored and then a standardized emotional stimulus of 5 min duration in the form of strenuous mental arithmetic
was applied [4, 7]. Venous occlusion started at the beginning of the second
minute of the mental arithmetic and was continued for the following 4 min.
As a basis for comparison we used our recent data on the effect of the emotional stress on central and peripheral haemodynamics in hypertensive subjects
[7].

For the statistical analysis of the labetalol effect on haemodynamics the paired
t-test was used. The comparison of the emotional response in untreated and
treated subjects was based on the unpaired t-test.

Consent was obtained from each informed subject and the study was approved
by the committee for Drug Research in Man of our Medical School.

Results

Basic Haemodynamics Before and After Labetalol

The results of a typical experiment in a hypertensive (WHO II) patient suffering from chronic pyelonephritis and nephrolithiasis is shown in Figure 1. The blood pressure which averaged initially 196/110 mm Hg started to fall already in the course of the 2nd following the injection of 100 mg labetalol (1.6 mg/kg body weight). During the subsequent 38 min the blood pressure was maintained at 150/90 mm Hg (a decrease of 46/20 mm Hg), whilst the mean blood pressure decreased from 139 to 115 mm Hg. This decrease was due entirely to a drop of the total peripheral vascular resistance from 2850 to 2130 dynes $\cdot$ sec $\cdot$ cm $^{-5}$. The cardiac output changed very little from 3.9 to 4.3 l/min and the heart rate remained unchanged. There was no change of the central venous pressure and the peripheral venous pressure slightly decreased. The venous distensibility and vascular volume of the forearm were very low from the start, which is in keeping with our data on these parameters in patients with renal hypertension, and were only slightly further reduced by labetalol. Forearm blood flow slightly rose which was due to a marked drop of the forearm vascular resistance from 70.5 to 39 dynes $\cdot$ sec $\cdot$ cm $^{-5}$. The plasma renin activity decreased from 2.2 to 1.55 ng angiotensin/ml/hour.

The statistical analysis of the data of both groups of patients has shown that there is no basic difference in the response to the acute administration of labetalol in either type of the hypertensive subjects. Their data represented in Figure 2 and are discussed as one collective. The significant drop of the blood pressure in all its three components (systolic, diastolic, mean) was due to a significant reduction of the total peripheral vascular resistance. The cardiac index, stroke index and heart rate did not change significantly. Also the central and peripheral venous pressures remained unaltered in most subjects with the exception of a slight fall in renal hypertensives. The forearm vascular volume increased in one half of the subjects whilst in the remainder it either fell or remained unaltered, so that the overall change was not significant. The changes of the venous distensibility were inhomogenous and statistically insignificant. There was an uniform and significant drop of the forearm vascular resistance. However, in view of the drop of the perfusion pressure the changes of the forearm blood flow were small and the upward trend was statistically insignificant. The plasma renin activity fell significantly in all subjects.

Valsalva Manoeuvre Before and After Labetalol

There was no difference (Fig. 3) in both groups in the rise of the central venous pressure during the Valsalva manoeuvre before and after labetalol, so that the stimulus was the same. It is obvious that both the acceleration of the heart rate during the test and the overshoot of the systolic blood pressure after cessation of the stimulus were markedly diminished. Also the duration of the systolic overshoot was greatly reduced.

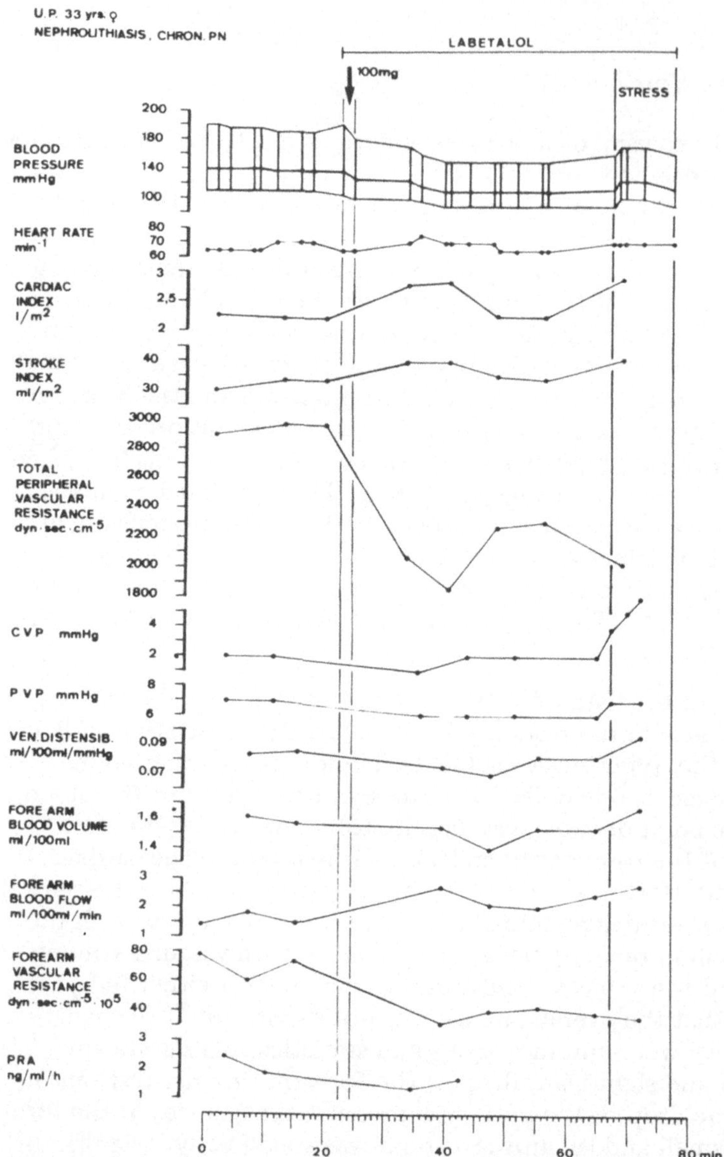

Fig. 1. Effect of intravenous labetalol on blood pressure and haemodynamics in a patient with renoparenchymatous hypertension (CVP = central venous pressure; PVP = peripheral venous pressure; ven. distensib. = venous distensibility of the forearm; PRA = plasma renin activity

Emotional Stress Under Labetalol

In untreated subjects (Fig. 4) both with essential and renoparenchymatous hypertension an acute emotional stimulus produced a significant rise of the

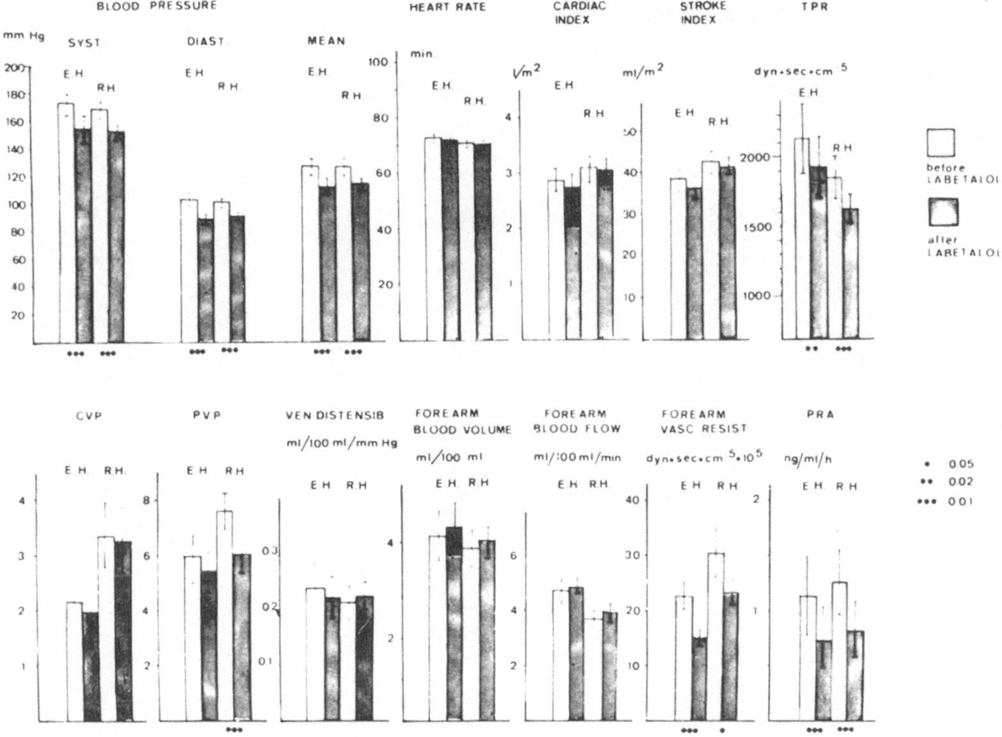

Fig. 2. Effect of labetalol on central and peripheral haemodynamics in essential (E.H., n = 9) and renal (R.H., n = 11) hypertension. (Abbrevations as in Figure 1. Data is given as mean ± standard error and statistical significance by asterisk.)

blood pressure (systolic, diastolic, mean), heart rate and cardiac output [7]. The change of the total peripheral vascular resistance was insignificant. Central and peripheral venous pressures rose. The volume of blood in the vessels of the forearm changed only slightly and venous distensibility decreased. Forearm vascular resistance dropped and along with the rise of the perfusion pressure this produced a marked rise of the forearm blood flow.

In hypertensive *subjects treated* with labetalol the emotional rise of the blood pressure also occurred, but was slightly blunted for the diastolic pressure in essential and renal hypertensives and for the systolic and mean pressure in essential hypertensives. This rise started from a lower level, so that it usually only reached the control blood pressure before labetalol was given. However, the heart rate and cardiac output rose to a significant lesser extent in both types of hypertension. The total peripheral vascular resistance reduced by the previous administration of labetalol did not change significantly during the stress period. The rise of both the central and peripheral venous pressure was reduced in the treated essential hypertensives whilst in the renal hypertensives the rise of central venous pressure was larger after labetalol and the increase in the peripheral venous pressure was almost the same.

103

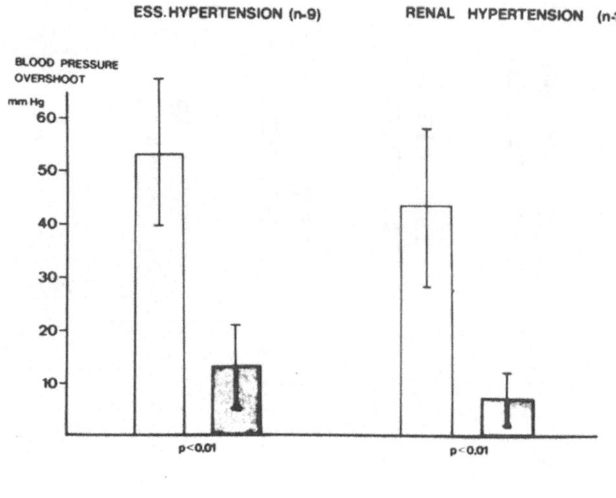

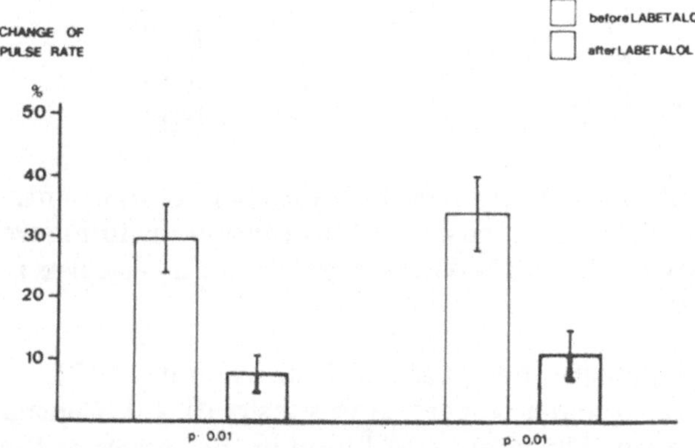

Fig. 3. Effect of labetalol on the reflex tachycardia during and blood pressure overshoot after the Valsalva manoeuvre in hypertensive patients

The forearm vascular volume and the venous distensibility which hardly changed during emotional stress in both groups of untreated hypertensives increased markedly in 4 out of the 6 essential hypertensives and in 6 out of the 8 renal hypertensives in whom the parameter was studied after labetalol. Unlike in untreated subjects there was no significant change in the forearm vascular resistance in both groups. The consequence of this was that the rise of the forearm blood flow was very small, even if regular and, therefore, significant.

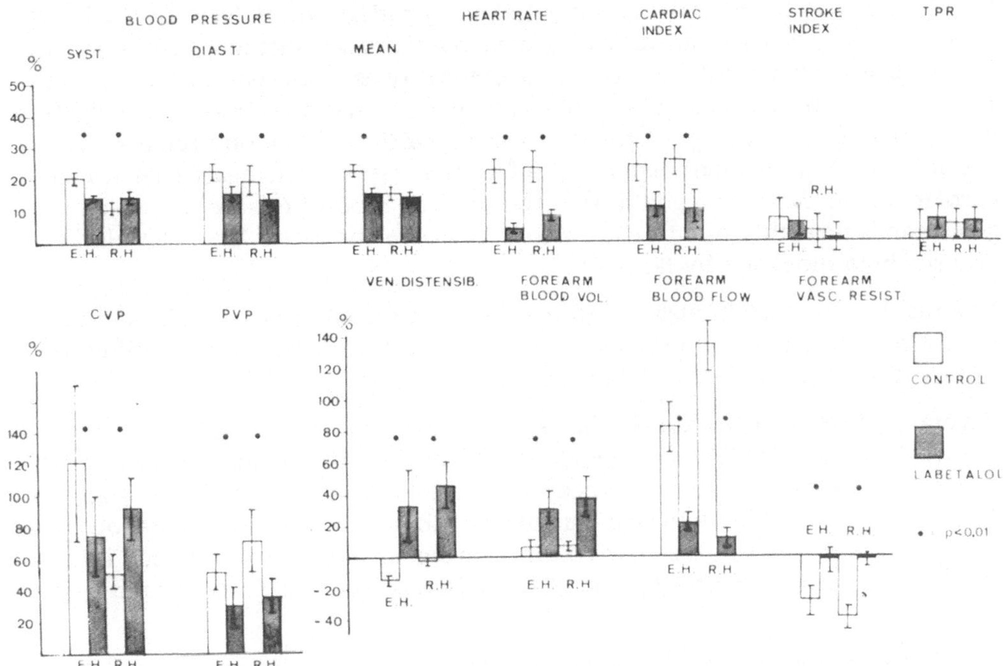

Fig. 4. Effect of labetalol on the blood pressure change and haemodynamic response to acute emotional stress in essential (E.H.) and renal (R.H.) hypertension. Control data of E.H. and R.H. taken from 7. (TPR = total peripheral vascular resistance; CVP = central venous pressure; PVP = peripheral venous pressure; ven. distensib. = venous distensibility of the forearm; forearm blood vol. = forearm blood volume; forearm vasc. resist. = forearm vascular resistance. Data is given as mean ± standard error and statistical significance by asterisk.)

Discussion

In our investigation, we found that the vasodilation in the muscles, which is a prominent feature of the haemodynamic response to an acute emotional stress [4, 7], is almost completely suppressed by labetalol. This vasodilation is under normal circumstances brought about by the beta-adrenergic activity [10, 17] and by sympathetic cholinergic fibres [2, 11]. These are the only vasodilator effects mediated by the sympathetic system. The active parasympathetic vasodilating activity is limited only to the nose, face, tongue and male genitals [14] and these areas are too small to be of a major haemodynamic importance. We must, therefore, conclude that the drop of total peripheral vascular resistance which was responsible in our study, in accordance with others [16], for the decrease of blood pressure after labetalol could have been produced only by a reduction of the alpha-sympathetic vasoconstrictor tone. This included, as we have shown, also the vasoconstrictor tone in the skeletal muscles.

105

Reducing the blood pressure by pure vasodilation, the beta-sympathetic fibres to the heart should be reflexly activated and produce an increase of the heart rate and of the cardiac output as happens regularly for instance after diazoxide [1]. This, after labetalol, did not occur obviously as a consequence of its beta-blocking action, whose high degree has been demonstrated in our investigation by the strong suppression of the reflex tachycardia and blood pressure overshoot in the Valsalva manoeuvre. The fact that neither the heart rate nor the cardiac output have changed during the drop of blood pressure under such a blockade is probably due to the balance between the reflex beta-stimulation and the beta-blockade by labetalol.

The regular decrease in plasma renin activity in the treated subjects corresponds to the known data on the effect of beta-blockade and also to the findings of others [26] on the effect of labetalol in this respect.

Several features of the data on the venous side of the circulation after labetalol are worth recording: The very small and irregular drop of the central and peripheral venous pressure; the absence of changes of venous distensibility and forearm vascular volume in one half of the subjects; an increase in venous distensibility and forearm vascular volume during emotional stress which is in striking contrast to the behaviour of these two parameters in untreated hypertensives.

This unquestionable rise of the venous distensibility and forearm vascular volume recorded during emotional stress in two thirds of all observations is not easily explainable. This rise is the opposite to what we have found about the compliance of the capacitance system of the forearm in untreated hypertensives both unstressed and under an acute emotional stress [7]. One may question whether results gained on the capacitance vessels of the forearm can be generalized to the whole body, the more so as great differences in the innervation of veins between various species and also between various regions of the body are well known [20, 21, 24]. These differences, and also the fact that natural and synthetic catecholamines [15] contain different proportions of alpha- and beta-activity possibly explain the divergent results of some of the investigators. Whereas it is claimed [18] that both the alpha- and beta-adrenergic stimulation is venoconstrictor, there is more evidence in the opposite direction [13, 19, 25]. It was demonstrated for labetalol that it antagonizes the local venoconstrictor action of noradrenaline and vasodilator response to isoprenaline in normal subjects [9]. Therefore, an alpha- and beta-blockade of the action of the catecholamines on the veins during emotional stress would be expected to leave the venous distensibility unaffected but not to increase it. There is, however, a difference in the vasoactive effects of the circulating catecholamines and catecholamines liberated at the sympathetic nerve terminals [12]. In addition it has been demonstrated, that isolated veins pretreated with an alpha-blocking agent react to adrenaline and isoprenaline in high dosage with a venodilation [8, 13]. On the other hand, beta-blockade either prevents the venodilation or enhances the venoconstriction by the catecholamines [13, 25]. In case of the alpha- and beta-blocker labetalol the alpha-blockade on the veins would, therefore, appear to be dominating during an emotional stress.

106

Summary

The effect of an intravenous bolus of labetalol (0.6-1.6 mg/kg body weight) on central and peripheral haemodynamics was studied in 20 hypertensive subjects.

The blood pressure reduction was entirely accounted for by the fall of the total peripheral vascular resistance including the vascular resistance in the muscles.

The peripheral vasodilation was not counteracted by a reflex rise of the cardiac output and also the reflex tachycardia and overshoot of blood pressure in the Valsalva manoeuvre were greatly diminished.

Central and peripheral venous pressure, vascular volume of the forearm and venous distensibility were affected only insignificantly by labetalol. The vascular resistance of the forearm fell markedly but due to the parallel drop of the perfusion pressure the blood flow was not significantly affected.

The emotional rise of the blood pressure was not prevented but it was slightly smaller and started from the lowered level. The usual rise of the cardiac output was blunted and was balanced by a slight increase in the total peripheral vascular resistance.

Labetalol completely abolished the emotional vasodilation of the muscle.

Contrary to the usual slight drop of the venous distensibility and a minute change of a forearm vascular volume in untreated subjects, an acute emotional stress in treated subjects produced a rise in both these parameters.

References

1. Bahlmann J, Brod J, Cachovan M (1978) Effect of diaxozide on capacitance vessels. Eur J Clin Pharmacol 13 : 321-323
2. Barcroft H, Brod J, Hejl Z, Hirsjärvi EA, Kitchin AH (1960) The mechanism of the vasodilatation in the forearm muscle during stress (mental arithmetic). Clin Sci 19 : 577-586
3. Boakes AJ, Knight EJ, Prichard BNC (1971) Preliminary studies of the pharmacological effects of 5-(1-hydroxy-2-((1-methyl-3-phenyl propyl) amino)-ethyl)-salicylamide (AH 5158) in man. Clin Sci 40 : 18-19
4. Brod J, Fencl V, Hejl Z, Jirka J (1959) Circulatory changes underlying blood pressure elevation during acute emotional stress (mental arithmetic) in normotensive and hypertensive subjects. Clin Sci 18 : 268-279
5. Brod J (1971) Study of renal function in the differential diagnosis of kidney disease. Br Med J 3 : 135-143
6. Brod J, Bahlmann J, Cachovan M, Dahlgrün HG, Hundeshagen H, Feldmann U (1977) Haemodynamics of hypertension in chronic renal disease. Contrib Nephrol 8 : 100-108
7. Brod J, Cachovan M, Bahlmann J, Bauer GE, Celsen B, Sippel R, Hundeshagen H, Feldmann U, Rienhoff O (1979) Haemodynamic changes during acute emotional stress in man with special reference to the capacitance vessels. Klin Wochenschr 57 : 555-565

8. Bucher TJ, Müller-Schweinitzer E, Stürmer E (1973) In vitro demonstration of the existence of β-adrenoceptors in human saphenous and canine femoral veins. Naunyn Schmiedebergs Arch Path Pharmacol 280 : 153-160

9. Collier JG, Dawnay NAH, Nachev CH, Robinson BF (1972) Clinical investigation of an antagonist at α- and β-adrenoceptors — AH 5158 A. Br J Pharmacol 44 : 286-293

10. Eliasch H, Rosen A, Scott HM (1967) Systemic circulatory response to stress of simulated flight and to physical exercise before and after propranolol blockade. Br Heart J 29 : 671-683

11. Eliasson S, Folkow B, Lindgren P, Uvnäs B (1951) Activation of sympathetic vasodilator nerves to the skeletal muscles in the cat by hypothalamic stimulation. Acta Physiol Scand 23 : 333-351

12. Glick G, Epstein SE, Wechsler AS, Braunwald E (1967) Physiological differences between the effects of neuronally released and bloodborne norepiphrine on beta-adrenergic receptors in the arterial bed of the dog. Circ Res 21 : 217-227

13. Guimaraes S, Osswald W (1969) Adrenergic receptors in the veins of the dog. Eur J Pharmacol 5 : 133-140

14. Knoche H, Addicks K (1977) Vegatatives Nervengewebe und Gefäßsystem. In: Sturm A, Birkmayer W (eds) Klinische Pathologie des vegetativen Nervensystem. Vol II. Fischer, Stuttgart, p 765

15. Kobinger W (1965) Über die unterschiedliche Beeinflussung von Widerstands- und Kapazitätsgefäßen durch verschiedene Sympathicomimetica. Naunyn Schmiedebergs Arch Path Pharmacol 252 : 103-121

16. Koch G (1976) Haemodynamic effects of combined α- and β-adrenoreceptor blockade after intravenous labetalol in hypertensive patients at rest and during excercise. Br J Clin Pharmacol Suppl 3, 3 : 725-728

17. Konzett H, Strieder N, Ziegler E (1968) Die Wirkung eines β-Receptorenblockers auf emotionell bedingte Kreislaufreaktionen, insbesondere auf die Durchblutung des Unterarmes. Wien Klin Wochenschr 80 : 953-959

18. Lochner W, Müller-Ruchholtz ER, Lösch HM, Grund E (1978) Kreislaufwirkungen einer Beta-Blockade bzw. Beta-adrenergen Stimulation unter besonderer Berücksichtigung des kapazitiv-venösen Systems des großen Kreislaufs. In: Mäurer W, Schömig A, Dietz R, Lichtlen PR (eds) Beta-Blockade 177. Thieme Stuttgart, p 148-156

19. Mellander S, Johansson B (1968) Control of resistance, exchange, and capacitance functions in the peripheral circulation. Pharmacol Rev 20 : 117-196

20. Meyer HE, Abboud FM, Ballard DR, Eckstein JW (1968) Catecholamines in arteries and veins of the foreleg of the dog. Circ Res 23 : 653-661

21. Rice AJS, Leeson CR, Long JP (1966) Localization of venoconstrictor responses. J Pharmacol Exp Ther 154 : 539-545

22. Richards DA, Woodings EP, Stephens MDB, Maconochie JG (1974) The effects of oral AH 5158, a combinded α- and β-adrenoceptor antagonist, in healthy volunteers. Br J Clin Pharmacol 1 : 505-510

23. Richards DA, Prichard BNC, Boakes AJ, Tuckmann J, Knight EJ (1977)

Pharmacological basis for antihypertensive effects of intravenous labetalol. Br Heart J 39 : 99-106
24. Sutter MC (1965) The pharmacology of isolated veins. Br J Pharmacol 24 : 742-751
25. Webb-Peploe MM, Shepherd JT (1969) Beta-receptor mechanisms in the superficial limb veins of the dog. J Clin Invest 48 : 1328-1335
26. Weidmann P, Chatel R de, Ziegler WH, Flammer J, Reubi F (1978) Alpha and beta adrenergic blockade with orally administered labetalol in hypertension. Am J Cardiol 41 : 570-576

Round Table Discussion:
Does the Renin-Angiotensin System Play a Signigicant
Role in Human Hypertension?

Chairman: F. Gross, Heidelberg
Panelists. H.R. Brunner, Lausanne; A.F. Doyle, Heidelberg, Australia;
J.H. Laragh, New York; A.F. Lever, Glasgow

Gross: Ladies and gentlemen: I'm glad that we have an opportunity to start this
round table discussion the title of which is put into a question: Does the renin-
angiotensin system play a significant role in human hypertension? Now we may
remember the Bible where it is written that our talk should be "yes, yes" or
"no, no", and what is more is of evil. So I think we could be very short, but
I'm afraid we won't be able at the end of this two hours' discussion to give a
clear answer to the question put before us. You all know our four panelists.
For those who are new in this "Club" here, I should like to introduce Dr.
Brunner from Lausanne, Dr. Laragh from New York Cornell University, Dr.
Doyle from Melbourne and Dr. Lever from Glasgow. You see already, when
you compare these five — including myself — contributors to the discussion,
that the mean age of this group is a little higher than the mean age of those
who spoke this morning on catecholamines and the sympathetic nervous system. This demonstrates that most of us here who present data this afternoon
have been in the field already for a long time. So we are an "old generation"
of hypertensiologists whereas this morning a "younger generation" had the
floor. Of course, I take out Dr. Brunner who is, let us say, a "grand child" of
the old hypertensiologists.

When the renin-angiotensin system became related to the regulation of salt or,
more precisely, sodium balance, the possible role of angiotensin as a vasopressor agent was neglected or even suppressed, at least by some of us. Of course,
nobody tried to deny that there are renin-dependent forms of hypertension,
the renin-secreting tumor, some forms of renovascular hypertension and malignant hypertension, although in the latter case, when a secondary hyperaldosteronism develops — and we well remember John Laragh's contribution in
1960 to this topic — increased renin secretion may be the consequence rather
than the cause of high blood pressure inducing a vicious circle. When the vicious circle is turned on the enhanced production of angiotensin pushes blood
pressure higher up, which has the consequence that more sodium is lost which
results in a further stimulation of the renin system and so the vicious circle is
maintained.

The unsettled problem is still the significance of the renin-angiotensin system
in primary or essential hypertension. Does the renin-angiotensin system play
any role in inducing blood pressure increase in essential hypertension? I should

like to say if the renin-angiotensin system would be responsible for the increase in blood pressure, we could finish our discussion, and then, of course, primary hypertension would not be primary any longer, but be a form of secondary hypertension. But if the renin system is stimulated by sodium depletion or diuretics it may, under these conditions, contribute to the maintenance of high blood pressure or may also contribute to the further increase of high blood pressure. A methodological question arises here. How well do the plasma concentrations of either renin or angiotension inform us on the activity of the renin-angiotensin system, especially on the intrarenal action of angiotensin? We have discussed a similar problem this morning when we talked all the time on catecholamine plasma levels and when we heard how little they have to do with what may be going on in the synaptic cleft. What conclusions can be drawn from the so-called low, normal or high plasma renin activity and what is the possible role of extrarenal renin, especially with respect to the regulation of blood pressure?

The study of the renin-angiotensin system revealed the interrelationship between the regulation of blood pressure and sodium balance. But one wonders if that interrelation is so tricky that in a larger number of human beings chronic elevation of blood pressure occurs as a consequence of the stimulation of the system by salt depletion or negative sodium balance. The fact that in populations who are on a low salt diet and therefore should have a stimulated renin-angiotensin system, hypertension is rare or absent indicates the usefulness of the control of sodium balance by that system. The therapeutic effectiveness of the converting enzyme inhibitor captopril in the treatment of high blood pressure is a strong argument in favour of the pathogenic significance of the renin-angiotensin system. But things are certainly not as easy as they appear to be and we will hear quite a bit of this complex interrelation during our discussion. However, before we come to that, it may be useful to define the position of the renin-angiotensin system and to review the opinions of the panel members. It may be advisable to start with simple things, facts which are relatively clear. Here we can refer to various types of secondary hypertension, especially to the renovascular hypertension and subsequently we may go on to the more tricky field of essential hypertension. I think the order of the introductory presentations would be that first Dr. Lever would speak, then Dr. Doyle, then Dr. Laragh, and then Dr. Brunner. And I would now like to ask Dr. Lever to introduce the topic of secondary hypertension.

Lever: Peter Wolff, Mr. Chairman, ladies and gentleman. What role does renin or angiotensin play in the pathogenesis of hypertension? To outline some of the ways in which it might play a role, I've sketched at the end of that board three different mechanisms. The first is the well-known, direct vasoconstrictor action which was first to be shown and is best known. It comes on within a minute or so of injection of angiotensin II. It could be exerted in vivo by blood borne angiotensin II, producing vasoconstriction. Equally it could be exerted by locally generated angiotensin II, within the kidney blood vessels or within blood vessels elsewhere. Second, there is the very marked, slowly progressive pressor effect which comes on when initially subpressor doses of angiotensin are given over a long time. The mechanism of the slow effect is quite unknown, it probably involves the central or peripheral nervous system.

112

I'm going to talk about essential hypertension and then about renal hypertension, asking whether or not renin-angiotensin is involved in pathogenesis? I shall consider three questions: Is the plasma level of the angiotensin II increased in essential hypertension? If it isn't, is the pressor response to increment of endogenous or exogenous angiotensin increased? And then finally, does blood pressure fall when inhibitors of the renin-angiotensin mechanism are given?

First of all the plasma levels. I've plotted here plasma angiotensin II-values in normal subjects on a fixed dietary intake of sodium in a metabolic ward with samples taken at 9 o'clock in the recumbent position. In Conn's syndrome angiotensin II is suppressed and nobody is surprised about that. In essential hypertension with so-called normal renin (and most of the 63 patients on that graph with essential hypertension have normal renin) the mean value is between 20 and 21 picograms/ml. It's also between 20 and 21 picograms/ml in the control group. So there is no excess of angiotensin II in the peripheral plasma of patients with essential hypertension compared with normal. In low-renin hypertension, there is, as you would expect, a low level of angiotensin II. In renal artery stenosis there is higher than normal concentration but many of the patients with undoubted surgically-curable renal artery stenosis have levels of angiotensin II well within the normal range.

That's the first bit of evidence. There is not an excess of angiotensin II in blood in most forms of hypertension in our experience, and I think many others would agree with that. Now, is there an increased sensitivity or responsiveness? We heard a bit about the matter this morning.

The way in which we test responsiveness is shown in the next slide. We infuse angiotensin in a step-wise increasing dose, 2 ng/kg/min for an hour,   , stepping up to 4, then to 8 ng/kg/min. Blood samples are taken in the control period and at the end of each of these increments of angiotensin infusion. We are then in a position to correlate plasma angiotensin II concentration before and during the infusion with concurrent blood pressure. A dose-response curve can be made. Is this dose-response curve in normal subjects different from the dose-response curve in essential hypertension?

This shows the increment of blood pressure before and during the angiotensin infusion plotted against concurrent plasma angiotensin II concentration. You see the two curves, essential hypertension and normals are very close together. I accept that essential hypertensive patients do lie slightly above the normals at some points, but all that this elevation could explain is a 4 or 5 mm Hg difference of mean arterial pressure for a given plasma concentration of angiotensin II. I suggest that is not enough to explain the larger difference of blood pressure by enhanced sensitivity. So there is not a major increase of sensitivity or responsiveness to angiotensin II in essential hypertension. A third line of evidence comes from inhibitor infusion studies. We have some experience with saralasin and the next slide shows the results in eleven essential hypertensive subjects infused with saralasin at 10 μg/kg/min. No change in arterial pressure occurred after one hour of infusion. Now one could say that the agonist res-

ponse from the saralasin exactly balanced the depressor effect that would have
occurred in the absence of an agonist effect, but we do get a very good correlation between plasma angiotensin II before the infusion and the drop of blood
pressure during infusion and we do reduce blood pressure in this way quite
markedly in patients with renal artery stenosis, when angiotensin II concentrations is raised. The test is effective in one form of hypertension but not in another. So I suggest that the failure of one specific inhibitor to reduce blood
pressure, the absolute normality of the plasma concentration of angiotensin
II, and the lack of an altered response to angiotensin II in essential hypertension make it very unlikely indeed that an altered direct vasoconstrictor effect
(this first effect I spoke of earlier), is responsible for essential hypertension. I
am not suggesting that angiotensin is not acting in some other way that we are
not testing. What I am suggesting is that it is not acting as a direct vasoconstrictor agent in this first way to produce essential hypertension or to maintain it.

So much for essential hypertension, what about renal hypertension? Here I
have to say something about the slow developing pressor effect of angiotensin.
You remember that if an infusion of angiotensin in larger dose is given over a
week or so, in the rabbit blood pressure rises within minutes, the elevation can
be maintained thereafter for a week and, when the infusion is stopped, the
blood pressure falls promptly. If, on the other hand — and Dickinson was the
first to do this — the infusion is given at a rate which is initially subpressor
and then continued for the same period blood pressure climbs gradually, and
in the rabbit it reaches approximately the same level that can be achieved with a
moderately high dose of angiotensin given by acute direct infusion. This has
been confirmed in the dog and in man (by Laragh and by Oelkers). It has been
shown recently in the rat by Miss Alison Brown and here the slow effect is so
marked that at the end of an infusion lasting seven days she can obtain higher
level of blood pressure than can be achieved by a high angiotensin infusion given
acutely. Now, the implication of that is very interesting. If you can achieve two
pharmacological effects with angiotensin II, one with low dose, the other with
higher dose, the first is more likely to be important physiologically. Thus, a
small increase of plasma angiotensin II maintained for a long time may have a
larger effect on blood pressure than a larger increase for a short time. Now, to
what extent are these two phenomena responsible for maintenance of renal
hypertension? We have arbitrarily divided renal hypertension into a number of
phases, and the first two are shown here schematically. If a clip is placed on a
renal artery of an animal — and that animal is conscious at the time (the clip
can be applied from the outside) — blood pressure rises acutely within minutes.
That increase can be maintained for weeks. Plasma levels of renin and, more
important, angiotensin II rise acutely after the clip over the first few hours, but
after a day or two begin to decrease towards the normal range, in most cases
they don't actually reach in the normal range, they remain above it. Now, if we
test the response to so-called specific inhibitors of the renin-angiotensin mechanism at these two different times, we get a rather different picture. If the inhibitors saralasin, teprotide, captopril are given at this early stage we get complete reversal of the hypertension which, because of the diversity of the inhi-

bitors, rather suggests that angiotensin is wholly responsible for the elevation of
blood pressure at this stage. If the inhibitors are given later, different things
may happen. If plasma angiotensin concentration is raised the fall of blood
pressure with inhibitor is large. If angiotensin is lower the fall is less.

If you make dose-response curves in a conscious dog after putting a clip on one
renal artery measuring angiotensin II and blood pressure, you get a clear regression. That is shown here. — If you take the same dog on another occasion and
infuse angiotensin II into a peripheral vein and measure the increment of arterial angiotensin II with blood pressure and angiotensin II rising together, you
get another regression line. The two regressions superimpose exactly. I suggest
that this means that the rise of angiotensin II after renal artery stenosis is suf-
ficient to cause the rise of blood pressure by the direct pressor effect. This,
with the inhibitor evidence, gives a fairly convincing answer to the question:
does the direct vasoconstrictor effect of angiotensin II ever cause hypertension?
I think the answer is "yes". It causes hypertension for few hours or days after
renal artery constriction in animals at least, and possibly in man, also. Thereafter, a rather interesting change occurs. Hypertension, as I have said, persists, but
the renin decreases, the response to inhibitor is now more variable. If you do serial
dose-response studies during the development of renal hypertension, the curve moves progressively upwards. The implication here is that, if angiotensin is producing hypertension in the chronic phase, it could only be doing so by sustaining
a higher level of blood pressure for a given plasma level of angiotensin II.

Angiotensin must be able to alter its own dose-response curve. Dr. Bean has
tested this by infusing dogs for two weeks with 2 ng/kg/min of angiotensin II
— a low dose in dogs. There was a progressive rise of blood pressure. Dose-response studies were done before, during and after the slow pressor effect. Dur
ing the effect there was an upward shift in the dose-response curve. Thus, angiotensin is able to alter its own dose-response curve in the manner found in
chronic renal hypertension. This means that angiotensin II is a potential candidate as a cause for renal hypertension. Interestingly, Dr. Casals has done the
same experiment with noradrenaline which did not raise blood pressure progressively when given by constant infusion in low dose and it does not shift
its own dose-response curve. So the effect with angiotensin is not a general
property of all vasoconstrictor substances. Now, the human equivalent of long-
term infusion of angiotensin in the dog obviously is renin secreting tumor.
The patient with renin-secreting tumor does not have a value of blood pressure
similar to that of a normal subject infused with angiotension — he has a level
of blood pressure much higher than can be accounted for by the direct vasoconstrictor action of angiotensin. Now, as renin-secreting tumor raises blood
pressure by secreting excess renin which forms excess angiotensin II, it would
appear that angiotensin II raises blood pressure in man by more than its direct
vasoconstrictor effect. We suggest that the second mechanism is the slow developing response.

Now, finally, the inhibitors. We noticed when we stopped the prolonged infusion of angiotensin II in dogs that blood pressure decreased slowly, much more

slowly than when we stop an acute infusion. This raised the possibility that we
were missing an effect of inhibitors on renal hypertension because we were not
giving them over a long enough period to reverse the second slow-acting pressor
effect. Dr. Riegger, who is in the audience, did an experiment in rats where saralasin was infused for eleven hours and I think many of you may have seen the
results.

This compares dextrose-infused renal hypertensive rats with dextrose-infused
normotensive rats all having measurements of blood pressure for eleven hours.
These were the controls. Next saralasin is given as a bolus and then continued
as infusion for eleven hours. Blood pressure decreased slowly with complete
reversal of the hypertension. We have done similar experiments with teprotide in
the rats and got similar results. The interesting thing with man and the rat is
that the higher the plasma angiotensin II level before the inhibitor is given, the
bigger the acute fall of pressure. However, if the renin and angiotensin levels are
normal as they were in almost all those rats, then the slow blood pressure fall
is greater.

The next slide shows two patients with renal artery stenosis. In the top panel
we have a lady with severe renal artery stenosis, marked narrowing of the vessel, with plasma angiotensin II of 800 pg/ml. In the bottom panel, an almost
equally hypertensive lady with a plasma angiotensin II of 20. So there is a
very big difference between their endogenous angiotensin levels before the inhibitor was given in both cases in exactly the same way as single tablets of 25
mg. In this woman it produced a very marked fall in pressure which was maintained for the rest of that day. She was given some salt, because she was sodium-
depleted as well at that time and the improvement was maintained thereafter
with captopril up to 450 mg/day. The point I'd like to make is that after operation her blood pressure was about the same as it had been at the end of the
long-term captopril treatment. The second lady was quite interesting because
she had a normal plasma angiotensin II and her renal vein renin ratio — for those
who are foolish enough to believe these measurements produce anything in
terms of prognosis — was 1.05, in other words: she had a negative renal vein
renin ratio. We gave her captopril and nothing very much happened to her blood
pressure on the first day, but when we persisted with 450 mg for 60 days her
blood pressure decreased gradually. She then had an operation — reconstruc-
tion of renal artery — and as in the other woman, she has a similar blood pressure after operation as at the end of her captopril. Now, I think the lesson in
these two women is that if there are two components of the pressor action, a
direct one and a slow one, and if plasma angiotensin II is very high the main
effect will be the direct one. Blood pressure will fall rapidly when inhibitors
are given. If you have a normal level of angiotensin II the slow-acting effect
will predominate and blood pressure will fall slowly when inhibitors are given.

The question we are asked was "Is there a significant role for angiotensin II in
hypertension generally?" In essential hypertension I don't think there is a significant role as an acute vasoconstrictor but this does not exclude other roles
for angiotensin II. In renal artery stenosis I think most people here would agree

116

that in the early stages there is good evidence for a role as an acute vasoconstrictor. After the chronic stage develops, we have to propose that something
else in addition is at work. We believe that much of the evidence suggested it
could be a slow-developing pressor effect of angiotensin II. Thank you very
much.

Questions

Weidmann: The relationship between angiotensin II infusion and blood pressure response from our data some of which I have just shown this morning
appears to be different in borderline hypertension and established essential hypertension and the hyperreactivity which we found is in borderline and I think
we have the same tendency in established hypertension that the difference becomes really extremely small. So, this is just a suggestion. Perhaps we should
look at the two things differently.

Lever: I am not suggesting that you haven't shown a difference. We did not
find one, but I would suggest if there is a difference, it is not a big one. I think
we agree on that.

Seldin: I'd like to ask Dr. Lever if in the rats or in the patients there was any
evidence of a weight gain during the period following the acute hypertensive
episode, a weight gain that might bei construed as evidence of prior salt depletion? And second, if during the period where the chronic effect you alluded
to prevailed, where the diuretics were tried and whether, if so, they gave a
dramatic lowering of the blood pressure?

Lever: The lady who didn't receive salt and did have her blood pressure lowered gradually by captopril had exchangeable sodium measured before and at the
end of treatment. It didn't change at all. Dr. Riegger's rats were infused with
saralasin for 11 hours and they did not show an increase in urinary sodium as
compared with controls receiving dextrose. Yes, when we failed with captopril
(which was not in renal artery stenosis but in chronic renal failure), and we
added a diuretic we did get a large fall of blood pressure.

Seldin: I simply would like to point out that if volume expands owing to whatever reason, say the administration of angiotensin II via aldosterone, the rat or
the patient would ultimately come into balance, so that intake would reflect
output and weight gain would be a much more reliable evidence for the steady-
state extracullular volume than would urinary sodium under such circumstances. I recall that Grollman at one time clipped the renal artery — I think it was
of a rat — and put a figure-of-8 ligature around the contralateral renal artery
and again developed an angiotensin-type hypertension for one week or two
which then persisted following the fall of angiotensin to normal and which was
rapidly corrected by diuretic measures. I merely raise the question of the role
of sodium so that a volume hypertension in a certain sense plays a role in re-
placing and masking what orginally started out as angiotensin-hypertension.
And we have seen several patients with bilateral renal artery stenosis, severe
hypertension, low renin, by any criteria very low, whose renins rose to the normal range as their blood pressure fell to normal following surgery.

Bühler: Did you do any aldosterone measurements in your essential hypertensives during chronic angiotensin II infusion? What does aldosterone do?

Lever. Yes. The aldosterone response to acute angiotensin II infusion in essential hypertension is greater than in normal, quite a lot greater.

Bühler: So this could be an additional factor for your slow-onset effect?

Lever: No, I don't think so because, in the dog, as blood pressure rose slowly the aldosterone decreased. That was the experience I think of the Mississippi group as well. In other words: I don't think aldosterone would explain the slow pressor response.

Doyle. I think the question of the renin-angiotensin system and its role in essential hypertension has undergone a transformation since the introduction of captopril. I believe that up to recently it's been fairly clear that the role of the renin-angiotensin system by which I refer to the direct vasoconstrictor effect in man has been very limited indeed. But I think the introduction of a substance which at least, among other actions, inhibits the formation of angiotensin II from angiotensin I, has given new results which make it necessary to re-evaluate the whole situation. The data which I have to show today is from animal experiments. It has no direct relevance to man, but it may throw some light on the actions of captopril and perhaps on some of the aspects of the renin-angiotensin system in patients.

In the two-kidney Goldblatt-hypertensive rat, which is a model in which one kidney is clipped and the other left intact, it's generally agreed that the plasma renin activity rises quite sharply in the majority of animals and these data confirm that in our experiments that is the case. On the other hand, almost everybody who studied this model has found a number of animals in whom the plasma renin activity appears to be within the normal range.

McDonald, Boyd and Peart in this particular model found that the fall of blood pressure that they could induce with injections of saralasin correlated very closely with the plasma renin activity at the time. And they were able to divide their animals into two groups: Those who had a fall of blood pressure of less than 20 mm Hg and those who had a fall of blood pressure of greater than that.

When they looked at these animals, namely those with a fall of less than 20 mm Hg, they found that the fall of blood pressure induced by saralasin was small as by definition, and that subsequent nephrectomy reduced the blood pressure very considerably. In the animals who had a big fall of blood pressure with saralasin again subsequent nephrectomy reduced the blood pressure to lower levels so that it would appear from those kinds of experiments using saralasin that the plasma renin activity is a good guide to the extent to which the renin-angiotensin system is affected in this model. However, as Dr. Lever has already told you, Dr. Riegger at that time in Glasgow, showed that long-term infusions of saralasin could reduce the blood pressure in most two-kidney animals.

The data I'd like to present today are related now to the effects of captopril rather than to saralasin.

In the two-kidney Goldblatt-hypertensive model, the renins of which you saw
in the first slide, the administration of 10 mg/kg of captopril by mouth — that's
a big dose — induces an immediate fall in blood pressure which is sustained for
between 24 and 72 hours, whereas in the sham-operated animals it induces no
fall in blood pressure.

If we look at the relationship between plasma renin activity and the blood pressure change induced by captopril, it is clear that there is no relationship at all,
it doesn't resemble that slide from McDonald, Boyd and Peart at all. So, animals who have low plasma renin and animals who have high plasma renin had
equally large falls in blood pressure.

If in the two-kidney Goldblatt-animal the opposite kidney is removed, there is
an immediate fall of plasma renin to normal levels or even slightly below and
this shows the change in plasma renin which occurred in a group of two-kidney
hypertensive animals after 3 days.

When in these animals who had subsequently had contralateral nephrectomy,
saralasin was again given there was no significant fall in blood pressure, but the
response to captopril was abolished. So, these data would seem to indicate that
captopril appears to be working by a mechanism related to the renin-angiotensin system, even though it often works or appears to work in animals who have
normal plasma renin activity.

In the spontaneously hypertensive rat which also has low levels of plasma renin
captopril also, in this instance at a dose of 20 mg/kg, induces an immediate and
quite prolonged fall of blood pressure which is not seen in the corresponding
normotensive Wistar-Kyoto rat. We were interested in the possible mechanism
of this and following the work of Thurston and Swales in which they demonstrated some response to saralasin after nephrectomy we decided to look at the
effects of nephrectomy in these animals in terms of the response to captopril.

As you can see from this slide, there was a persisting fall of blood pressure in
the one hour-nephrectomized SHR, but not in the Wistar-Kyoto rat, and this
occurred in spite of the fact that the plasma renin levels had fallen to virtually
zero over the period of the observations. I may say that this fall in blood
pressure is identical to that occurring in intact animals. This shows that in the
intact animal there is after the administration of a small intravenous dose of
captopril a progressive fall of blood pressure over 3 hours and this occurs in
the 1-hour-nephrectomized rats and it also occurs in the 24-hour-nephrecto-
mized rats and I think this is of importance because — as Thurston and Swales
have suggested — the vascular renin appears to disappear within 3 or 4 hours
and is certainly mostly gone by 24 hours. It is clear that these results might
imply that captopril is working by some non-renin mechanism but it might also
imply that captopril is working by a renin-mechanism independent of the
kidneys.

In order to test this we looked at the effect of infusions of captopril in the intact and in the anephric SHR. As you can see in the intact animal, saralasin
induces a fall in blood pressure and so it does in the anephric animal although

less than in the intact. This is probably not surprising since this particular animal receives an infusion of almost 2 ml of saline over that period of times. So, these data appear to suggest to us that captopril, and indeed saralasin, might be working in the SHR through a mechanism related to the renin-angiotensin system, but not, of course related to the kidneys since it persisted in the nephrectomized animal. And the obvious candidate, as we heard from Dr. Ganten this morning, is the central nervous system.

Dr. Hutchinson who worked with Dr. Ganten is familiar with his technique and set up this model of the intact SHR with arterial and venous cannulas and with a cannula leading to the intracerebral ventricles.

This slide shows that the intracerebral injection of 2 mg/kg of captopril produces a sustained fall in blood pressure of the SHR; this is not reproduced by the vehicle, it does not occur in the Wistar-Kyoto rat and is much larger than that seen on intravenous infusion. I think there are two possibilities: firstly that captopril is operating by a mechanism independent of the renin-angiotensin system or secondly that the renin-angiotensin system, as suggested by Dr. Ganten this morning, may be in part responsible via actions which are not related to the kidney, and in this incidence of course, intracerebrally. I think that these data, of course, can't be taken directly over to man, but I am sure that the data that we are going to hear from Dr. Brunner and Dr. Laragh and the data we have already heard from Dr. Lever has already suggested that captopril may work in patients without obvious evidence of renin-dependent hypertension. I think, it is early to say, but I believe that the introduction of captopril has put a new dimension into our interpretation of the actions of the renin-angiotensin system.

Questions

Ganten: I have a comment. There has been a recent paper by Philips from Iowa who confirmed what you showed that captopril lowers blood pressure in nephrectomized spontaneously hypertensive rats after i.v.t. administration, not after i.v. administration, and I might add that we have measured arterial wall renin in spontaneously hypertensive rats which is increased. You mentioned that it has disappeared after 24 hours. There appear to be two renin activities in the vascular wall, one is taken up from the plasma and then adsorbed to the vascular wall, and the other probably synthezised in the vascular wall.

Brod: Can't you explain these effects just by any more bradykinin in blood?

Doyle: Yes, I think you might. I don't think you could explain the saralasin effect as possible, but I really think, it is too early to say how this antihypertensive drug works. If you look back at methyldopa, if you look at prazosine, if you look at hydralazine, the ultimate effects of all these drugs appear to be rather different of that which their inventors dreamed.

Gross: Well, former errors should not be repeated. — I was surprised that in the nephrectomized rat saralasin produced a fall in blood pressure, because in the normotensive rat or in positive sodium balance it increases blood pressure.

Brunner: With saralasin and with teprotide we don't get a blood pressure fall in nephrectomized rats.

Gross: A rise, I would expect.

Brunner: A rise.

Gross: You see, the discrepancies start already.

Laragh: Ladies and gentlemen, in particular Dr. Peter Wolff: I am extremely pleased to be here and I guess I ought to be pleased for the opportunity to present for you a different perception of a situation than you have just heard with the preceeding two speakers. I hope that this will make for some useful intellectual constructivity. I think that the renin-angiotensin-aldosterone system should be viewed as a true biological control system. It regulates sodium balance and blood pressure as I will show you, and if it is a true control system all of the measurements of renin or angiotension or aldosterone must be closely related to the setting in which they are taken. In other words, there is no question about the fact that most essential hypertensive patients have normal angiotensin levels and we have known for 20 years that most of them have normal renin levels. The point of view is only what has changed. The knowledge base, not the fact. Those "normal" angiotensin II levels, I will try to point out to you, are not normal for the high blood pressure or the state of sodium balance. If I can demonstrate that, then I would like in turn to make an analogy. We all have known that values are normal according to the absolute measurement. In diabetes mellitus all the insulin levels are normal at rest. Everybody knows that, too. But there is an inappropriate relationship between the insulin and the glucose and I think that in considering hypertension and if you will accept the concept that the renin-angiotensin-aldosterone system is a true control system — again I repeated that — then you can perhaps re-think what these measurements really mean in different patients. Now, I am going to start by showing you an experiment in humans and these studies were done in humans before the animal studies that you have heard about today.

This is a 35 year old normal woman. And before we did this study we got into the renin-angiotensin field by showing — as Dr. Gross indicated — that there were massive amounts of aldosterone in human malignant hypertension and that this was due to renin we hypothesized. I would differ here again with Dr. Gross when he states that renin is a consequence because I think I can show you that if you erase the renin you will erase the malignant syndrome. It is the ultimate vector, it maybe a consequence of something else, and we have to figure out why it gets high. In malignant hypertension, if you erase the renin by total nephrectomy, by saralasin, by captopril or propranolol, the syndrome goes away and it is therefore renin-dependent. The same is true for most human Goldblatt hypertension which is surgically curable, — of the one-kidney form. Having been convinced of that, the real question is, could angiotensin II bet the vector? I am talking about the ultimate agent for some or all of the hypertension in human essential hypertension. Is there any vasoconstrictor substance that we know of that could be the vector? The only two that are possible are angiotensin and noradrenaline. That's all we have. So we ask this question. — This is a 35 year old woman on the balance ward given angiotensin by constant infusion. This was published in the JCI in 1965. As you see here, the idea was to take this woman and raise her pressure from 100/60 to 130/80 and hold it there. That's what we wanted to do: Mild chronic hypertension. In those days we didn't know too much about the diurnal rhythm in pressure and so we kept it up during sleep and everything. The woman wore a tubing in her arm and walked around and had a constant sodium diet. Now note what happened, — and we did this in many people — she went into positive sodium balance and gained about 2 kg over the first 5 days and then went into escape, a term first introduced by Don Seldin, where the sodium balance becomes neutral again and at the end of the infusion she natriuresed. Now, as we would expect we can relate the sodium retention to the marked stimulation of aldosterone. The secretion rate is very high as she is retaining sodium. Contrary to what had often been thought that angiotensin produces tachyphylaxis and wasn't a good candidate to cause hypertension because in time it would fade out — what this study shows is exactly the opposite happens in the human. As the infusion proceeds and as the sodium balance becomes positive you have to give less and less and less angiotensin, so that at the end of 5 days we were using a fifth of the original dose to keep the pressure up. This is volume-related, sodium balance becomes positive, and the amount of angiotensin needed drops. You can visualize from this experiment that if we were able to keep it on you might end up with hypertension consequent to very small amounts of A II. We estimated that the infusion rate at the end of this time was close to producing what the normal values for plasma angiotensin are estimated to be. So, angiotensin fits the model for causing hypertension chronically in relatively small amounts. Now, does noradrenaline fit this model?

No. In the same study we gave noradrenaline to normal subjects and on the last day we had to give twice as much noradrenaline to keep the pressure up, whereas with angiotensin you get an increasing sensitivity associated with positive sodium balance. Noradrenaline doesn't stimulate aldosterone and it produces paroxysms of natriuresis as the pressure rises and you end up using much more drug to keep up the blood pressure — something which some of you who are old enough to remember who are working on coronary care units know already namely that when you give levophed you have to give more and more to keep up the blood pressure after several days and finally you get no response. Angiotensin does not have that characteristic.

Then to investigate the differences between angiotensin and noradrenaline we used cirrhosis with ascites as a model for extreme sodium depletion and there you see 16.4 μg/ml of A II had to be given to get the pressure up, 20 times as much as the normals, they are very anergic, and then when you do get the pressure up in man with this huge dose it produces a natriuresis, a very big one, and so as you keep on giving the infusion you have to give more and more drug. You start out at 9 times as much and you go up to 16 showing the relation again to salt balance and showing here an effect of very high doses on distal tubular sodium excretion, an effect that Ochwadt in his country has

shown with micropuncture with very large doses of angiotensin. But, once
again, noradrenaline doesn't do it, noradrenaline has the same feature here, so
it never causes sodium retention. So, of the two known substances angiotensin
fits and is plausible as a factor to sustain chronic hypertension in human
subjects. It's plausible in amounts close to the normal range. Noradrenaline does
not seem to fit the requirement.

That study in that woman and some other volunteers gave us the first links
which suggested to us how the renin system works in all of us and suggested to
us what we call our vasoconstriction-volume analytical model which we use to
study our patients. This analytical concept ist useful. Because it turns out that
while there may be thousands of inputs on your blood pressure and mine, and
these include prostaglandin, emotions, cyclic AMP etc., there are finally only
two things that can change your blood pressure: The size of the container
between the aortic valves and the capillaries and we call this the *vasoconstriction*
factor, and the amount of liquid filling that container, and that's the *volume*
factor. And the renin system exerts major control over both of these. As the
figure indicates, at the same time over the next 24 hours this reaction occurs
and with hydraemia, salt and water retention volume rises until it feeds back
and turns itself out. But if you look at this system in this way it's rather neat
because the volume factor is flow and flow is what life is all about. The first
defense of any threat is to vasoconstrict. But then the chronic defense is to
bring back flow and open up the microcirculation. Now, if these two factors
are the key elements in pressure and if we can measure renin activity and aldosterone, if we are going to find out what's going on in patients we have to
relate them to the concurrent state of volume as best as we can. We use the
urinary sodium measurement routinely and constant salt diets whenever possible.

We measure renin in this setting because it's obvious that renin activity is mov-
ing all the time in all of us according to this relationship and it depends on
analyzing the renin in relation to the sodium to decide what is abnormal. If
that is the case, then we would expect that the renin-sodium profile would
reveal a spectrum of patients, some with a lot of vasoconstriction due to renin,
and we think that's what malignant hypertension is, and some with a lot of
volume, and we think that's what low renin patients are who are diuretic-sensitive.
In between there may be mixtures of these two pathophysiological components. There is a great deal of evidence to indicate that in different people the
vasoconstriction and volume components are quite different. Now, can the
renin measurement show us that and can we prove that the renin measurement
is dynamically interacting with the state of blood pressure?

The first thing we had to get was an agent that would block renin. And the first
agent that came along, was the beta-blocker propranolol. This is a key study in
exposing the role of renin done by Dr. Fritz Bühler when he was with us. It
shows a malignant hypertensive woman with a very high renin level of 40 in
whom propranolol treatment alone was given to this critically ill woman with
papilledema and paralysis of one arm and one leg. There was a total correction,

130/65 in a few days, but the key thing is the associated pharmacological surgery. Renin which was 40 came down to sub-normal levels preceeding the blood pressure drop. Aldosterone which as high because renin was high also came down. Potassium, which was low, as it usually is in untreated malignant hypertension, was low because aldosterone was high. It came up without any repletion being necessary and sodium balance exhibited no change because even though the blood pressure dropped 100 points really dropping renal perfusion in this situation the aldosterone was choped off at the same time and so sodium balance as is the case in more than half of people receiving propanolol is not affected by the blood pressure drop.

The next slide shows the subsequent study of Bühler, which he couldn't wait to complete, of 94 patients with profiled essential hypertension. No other drug but propranolol was given to them. The essence of it is that the high renins had a tremendous benefit, as a group, the normal renins an intermediate benefit. And what fits the theory is that propranolol does not work very well in low-renin patients, in fact sometimes it's pressor as we have shown subsequently. So, it selectively works according to the height of the renin level and this effect is also related to the degree to which renin is reduced. Now the propranolol issue has been a testy one because everyone has said that this is a beta-blocker which interacts with lots of other things in the circulation and how can we attribute so much of its action to renin? That's a very reasonable and fair criticism. However, the facts are that many workers in the early research could not show lowering of renin levels with beta-blockers. We now know these data were incorrect due to the presence of large amounts of inactive renin which the method used did not take account of. And I think now the data indicate from all over the world, — one thing that beta-blockers really do as a species is maredly reduce plasma renin levels. Besides that, the CNS theory of antihypertensive action has more or less ben exploded even by those people who work on it, as evidenced by a recent review by Frank Ganong. And the cardiac output concept of propranolol's hypotensive action is also untenable since beta-blockers lower cardiac output whether or not they lower pressure and since this action wouldn't lower pressure anyway, theoretically. Now, whatever the case, — and there may be other factors in beta-blocker's action — most of its action, until proven otherwise, can be reasonably assigned to its antirenin effect which is a very impressive one and easy to demonstrate. The most recent evidence on this point comes from Arthur Guyton's laboratory where David Young has been showing that captopril and propranolol are identical in their action on the high-renin malignant hypertensive dog, moreover both drug fail completely to lower the pressure in the angiotensin infusion dogs, testifying not only to the similarity of captopril and propranolol, but to the very strong likelihood that the major action of both is against renin.

Let's take a quick squint at this propranolol problem and then finish up with the angiotensin blocking drugs. How does the renin system participate in normal blood pressure control? Well, we are convinced it does and I am going to the whole story here. I want to show you how important we think sodium balance is for revealing any of these phenomena. Shown on the slide are normal

124

people, people like you and I in the laboratory. In fact, I failed to volunteer, but the rest of people in our lab did so. What they did was to go on a tilt table. When you and I go on a tilt table on a normal or high salt intake your renin shoots up to 1.5 fold or so. Nothing happens to your blood pressure. If you then give intravenous propranolol and go on the tilt table again renin goes down by 50 percent but still nothing happens to the blood pressure on the tilt table. Then we put these normal people on a low sodium diet and the renin goes from 1 to 5 — a classic sodium depletion response. And then they go on a tilt table again and defend their pressure, but now the renin goes up rather sharply. Then we asked the question how much of that renin response is beta-adrenergic-mediated? So we gave intravenous propranolol to all four sodium depleted subjects and all four fainted on the tilt table and the blood pressure collapsed, falling towards zero. Thus, propranolol erased renin secretion and it erased the defense of posture. This is a very fine example I think of how propranolol acts and how the beta-adrenergic system defends blood pressure with the final mediator being renin. Now, propranolol we don't think blocks all of renin secretion. It blocks the baro-receptor mediated component, it doesn't block the macula densa-activated renin secretion.

Propranolol may act as suggested from a study done by Steve Atlas and Jean Sealey to block the conversion of inactive renin to active renin. Their study simply shows that the change in inactive renin is directly related to the degree to which propranolol lowers the pressure with inactive renin rising commensurably. Other investigators, including Dr. Schalekamp, who is here, have shown that propranolol does affect the ratio between active and inactive renin, but this study has the added dimension of showing that this is related to the degree of pressure drop induced by the drug. More recently, Dr. Sealey has shown that renal kallikrein which lines the distal tubules and is absent in the proximal tubule is a potent activator of renin. Now, whatever the mechanisms, propranolol is an antirenin drug. You can argue about whether it's 90% or 92%, but most of the evidence today allows to construct the working hypothesis that this is the main way in which it lowers blood pressure.

I left the blocking drug story to Hans Brunner. But what we had to find out and what we have learnt from the blocking drug story is that a plasma renin measurement really does mean something. In fact it is a direct measure of how much vasoconstriction renin is inducing in you and me and in patients with high blood pressure. And this is a slide of 89 patients published in the New England Medical Journal by Dave Case of our group in 1976. What it shows is when you give the intravenous nonapeptide converting enzyme inhibitor the degree to which the blood pressure is dropped by this nonapeptide is predictable from the control renin level. The higher the renin level the greater the drop. This means that the renin is doing something in these people. It's not just floating around, it is actually a direct index of how much squeeze it's putting on the arterial system. When you relate this to the sodium excretion you have an index which tells you how appropriate or inappropriate the renin activity is for this state of sodium balance and then you have a way of analyzing patients for abnormal behavior. Now, the teprotide or nonapeptide story has been completely retraced in chronic studies that Dr. Brunner will tell you about. Before summing up on my own little talk here I would like to make some comments about some other things that Dr. Doyle said. First of all, I would like to quote other people's work because we haven't done some of this, but Dr. Antonaccio at Squibb tells me that they cannot show any effect of captopril on blood pressure in nephrectomized animals. They have given 100 mg/kg to rats of captopril and they have given it to SHR where it gives a tiny effect, perhaps due to vascular renin. So there is one reason to look for alternative explanations to those presented by Dr. Doyle. We cannot show any effect of captopril in nephrectomized humans nor can we show any action of propranolol. And propranolol and captopril do not act in primary aldosteronism either, another low-renin state. We have eight patients so that I can be pretty sure in telling you whatever the actions of captopril or propranolol are on blood pressure that they don't work in the low renin model nor do they work in the DOCA rat. So these findings are at striking variance with Dr. Doyle's report. Similarly, in Goldblatt hypertension in humans we are nearly always able to identify the renin factor by measuring it. It is in them that saralasin and captopril reveal it, if you take into account the agonistic action of saralasin. In terms of the correlations between captopril and the control renin level — we have over 100 patients now — there isn't any doubt about the fact that the activity of captopril in human subjects is closely connected to the height of the control renin level. Low renin patients show some response, but don't forget they have some renin.

Questions

Oelkers: Probably renin is important for the maintenance of blood pressure, but I think a patient treated with propranolol is not a very good example because you take him one of his most important counterregulation mechanisms, namely the increase in heart rate.

Laragh: Oh sure, you take that away, too. But it's probably the renin that accounts for the blood pressure collapse. Maybe the heart rate, too. I think that's a fair question. Yet slowing or speeding the pulse per se will not necessarily influence blood pressure.

Brunner: We have done the same study before, not with a tilt-table, but putting people upright. They were also normal subjects, normal sodium intake, and then salt depletion, but we didn't use propranolol, we used saralasin. When you put normal salt-depleted subjects upright and give saralasin they faint. So that, I think, could be an answer to your question.

Thurau: John, could you comment on your concept of the determinants of blood pressure? I unterstand vasoconstriction as peripheral resistance. I don't understand what you mean by volume as a determinant of blood pressure.

Laragh: By volume, and this is a hard problem for any of us to define, because it's a non-measurable volume, what I am referring to is the volume of fluid between the aortic valves and the capillaries, the volume that fills the vascular tree. We have called that the arterial volume. It's a function of cardiac output, but it's more than that. It's the volume that distends the arterial bed.

126

Thurau: But it's not measurable?

Laragh: No. — But that does not make it invalid.

Thurau: The other questions is: You presented this case where you showed the sodium retention during angiotensin II infusion and related it to the increase in aldosterone. Do you have any data that, if you block aldosterone or you take the adrenals out, angiotensin still is leading to sodium retention? In other words: Is it necessary that aldosterone is involved in this retention?

Laragh: Well, — most people agree — the sequence is angiotensin stimulates aldolsterone secretion and I think that accounts for part of the sodium retention. I think another part, as Mc Caa and Guyton and others have shown, is due to renal vasoconstriction of the A II. Both are causing sodium retention.

Seldin: I'd like to say a word about this enigmatic volume. It's quite clear that patients with AV shunts do not have hypertension in a sense. I mean a patient with Beri-Beri, with thyrotoxicosis in a high output state, with anaemia in a high output state. They have plenty of salt retention, their cardiac output is high and arterial filling is excessive. It's quite clear that there must be a critical part of the circulation, presumably beyond the resistance vessels, where a receptor-sensing system is available and which expresses itself in a hypertensive way. It's true that in classical heart failure you do get salt retention. In the low output states arterial filling is reduced, but, on the other hand, in cirrhosis of the liver 60% of the patients have a high cardiac output, nobody has hypertension and there is massive salt retention. In some sense, therefore, there are a whole group of clinical circumstances where arterial filling is excessive, salt retention is massive and there is no hypertension. We are clearly specifying a receptor system. — I think this is the key point in the whole problem of the control of sodium excretion. The second point I'd like to make is that the titration of the renin-angiotensin system with some concept of volume can be exposed with diuretics in a certain sense. In other words, one can have trivial levels of angiotensin which may be excessively high given a certain expanded volume. And under circumstances where the volume is shrunken angiotensin may disproportionately rise and then expose as you point out a saralasin or any other inhibitor effect. I do think, therefore, that the finding of a low renin or a low angiotensin is no evidence whatsoever, that the driving force behind the hypertensive process may not still be the renin-angiotensin system masked by salt retention in a setting where a steady-state doesn't allow for unrelenting salt retention and escape allows for sodium balance, but at a set where volume is overexpanded and renin suppressed.

Laragh: I think that's a key point, Don. If the renin-angiotensin system is at fault in such a hypertension where the renin ends up being very low, when you suck off the fluid you should re-expose the defect and it should be above normal and you should be able to see that, much like in chronic renovascular hypertension of the one-kidney form. The renin is low or normal, but if you volume-deplete them it shoots up above. And I think actually that could be a productive way for us to look at it.

Gross: I think we have to face here again the problem that what we measure in plasma is not really representin in every respect the activity of the renin system.

Laragh: It correlates pretty well with what happens with the blockade.

Gross: Not always. — Dr. Doyle, is there any explanation for the difference in rats between Melbourne and Princeton? I mean with respect to taking out the kidneys and responding to captopril or saralasin?

Doyle: I think more perhaps relevant than the differences between what happens to rats, is the astonishing difference it appears to happen to patients. I think the unsupported assertion, that propranolol operates exclusiverly on the renin-angiotensin system is to me astonishing.

Laragh: I am sorry Dr. Doyle is astonished. He misquoted me because I think it's largely due to renin, not exclusively as he said. I'd like to say it's probably most of its action and if you could tell us how else it might do, I'd love to hear about it.

Brunner: I am slightly in a difficult position because I think a lot has been said already, but I will still try in my role as grandchild of this group to retrace a little bit some evidence we have gathered with experimental and clinical studies using antagonists of the renin-angiotensin system there is nothing new about. Our results suggest to us that the renin-angiotensin system participates actively in maintaining the elevated blood pressure of many hypertensive patients. The approach using inhibitors to study the role of a pressor system is rather straight-forward, I think. If the pressor system participates in maintaining a certain blood pressure level its blockade should lead to a drop in pressure. To extra-polate that the measured blood pressure reduction reflects precisely the pres-sor effect of the system one has to imply of course that the inhibitor is 100% specific and has no pressor or depressor action of its own. I would like to start like some speakers before me with some studies with saralasin that we have started in 1971 when I was still in Dr. Laragh's lab together with Dr. Gavras.

These are rats of the two-kidney one-clip Goldblatt type, that means that they have a clip on one renal artery and the contralateral renal artery is left intact and you see when we infused saralasin into these two-kidney animals there was a clear and significant drop in blood pressure. And when we stopped saralasin blood pressure went up again. Thus, in this model with high renins (because it had been shown before that this model has high renin levels at 6 weeks, when this experiment was carried out) we concluded that the renin system partici-pates actively in maintaining the elevated blood pressure, since to my know-ledge nobody has seriously challenged the specificity of saralasin as an angio-tensin II-antagonist.

Now we want to look at patients, and here you have a high renin patient, ac-tually the first high renin patient to whom we gave saralasin back in 1970. It's a young lady with malignant hypertension, very high renins, blood pressure 140 diastolic. When we infused saralasin blood pressure dropped, when we stopped saralasin it went right up, and repeating saralasin infusion we dropped blood pressure again. We thought that this was really the first direct — or indirect if you want — evidence that the renin-angiotensin system can participate actively in maintaining an elevated blood pressure in a human being. Now, of course, high renin hypertension is not so frequent as you know as well as I.

When we infused saralasin to high renin patients we got a clear drop in blood pressure. However, when we infused it to normal and low renin patients there was hardly any change in blood pressure and this has been confirmed in hundreds of patients. So, on the basis of this, of course, one could conclude that the renin plays only a role in a very slight minority of hypertensive patients with high renins, but in the majority of the hypertensive patients it has nothing to do with the hypertension. An alternate explanation which we tend to favour is that the renin participation is actually masked in these normal and low renin patients by the inherent agonistic or pressor effect of saralasin. So, we then wanted, of course, to use other compounds and we chose to continue or studies with teprotide and captopril, two inhibitors of the converting enzyme which inhibit the generation of angiotensin II.

This is just to show some studies with captopril and you see you can lower blood pressure with captopril alone in patients with essential, renovascular, and renal hypertension. Of course, the highest drop we observed was in renovascular hypertension, but we saw also some drop in blood pressure in essential hypertension and even in patients with renal disease, although the drop was small.

Even if captopril, as has been mentioned before, lowers blood pressure in low renin patients, there is a clear correlation between the renin and the blood pressure drop induced by captopril. And, of course, the higher the renin the bigger the drop in blood pressure. I would like to point out that in two patients with primary hyperaldosteronism for instance there was no blood pressure drop whatsoever with captopril. Now, why is the effect of the converting enzyme inhibitor greater or more important than that of saralasin? Of course, one might argue that the blood pressure-lowering effect of converting enzyme inhibition is not specific, that is, it is not related to blockade of the renin system. As you know, converting enzyme is identical with kininase II and some have claimed that accumulating bradykinin could be responsible for the blood pressure reduction by captopril or teprotide. Now, some people have found increases in bradykinin levels, but several groups have not found an increase. I would just like to mention the NIH-group, Dr. Hökfelt in Scandinavia and Dr. Johnston from Australia who didn't find any increase in bradykinin levels. On the other hand, some have found increases in bradykinin levels, but the increase was not sustained and I guess, we are more interested in sustained rather than in just acute or transient changes. Now, of course, that doesn't completely rule out a role for bradykinin because even if bradykinin levels are not increased in the plasma that doesn't mean that the bradykinin could not play a role at some other particular place in the body. Now, you have just heard these beautiful experiments by Dr. Doyle showing a decrease in blood pressure of nephrectomized animals. We did similar experiments.

Dr. Jaeger of our group has given teprotide to nephrectomized rats maintained on a normal sodium diet or salt-depleted. And you see he had a transient blood pressure decrease in normal animals on a normal sodium diet, but a sustained decrease in normal animals on a low sodium diet. In the nephrectomized animals neither on normal sodium nor after salt depletion did he get any decrease in blood pressure with teprotide. As you have heard Dr. Laragh has not found a decrease in nephrectomized man with captopril. I just come back quickly to this patient with primary hyperaldosteronism. When we gave captopril (this is one of the two patients we have studied so far) you see there is no decrease in blood pressure. However, when we put this patient for 4 weeks on 600 mg of spironolactone he got some decrease in blood pressure, but he was not normalized. When we then gave captopril, we got some further decrease in blood pressure, but meanwhile renin had gone up, although the renin was not high afterwards — it was double or more than double as high as before.

We have tried different ways to know whether teprotide has a non-specific blood pressure-lowering effect, that means angiotensin II-independent. Dr. Jaeger gave angiotensin II infusions in rats, salt-depleted and on normal sodium, and with this, of course, he increased the blood pressure. I would call this a pure angiotension II-dependent hypertension. Then he gave teprotide in the salt-depleted rats and in those on normal sodium diet and he got no blood pressure reduction. Of course, when you infuse angiotensin II, teprotide cannot interfere with that angiotensin effect, because we can only stop the generation of endogenous angiotensin II. Meanwhile we have done some similar experiments which are slightly more sophisticated with chronic infusions of angiotensin II. Dr. Textor who is right now working with us infuses rats for 10 days with angiotensin II and then treats them with captopril and he sees no blood pressure-lowering effect of captopril, whatsoever. So, in other words, as hard as we try, we have not been able to find so far a nonspecific effect of these drugs teprotide and captopril — and when I say non-specific I mean an effect which is not dependent on the renin-angiotensin system. Accordingly, we conclude that until we have some good evidence for an angiotensin-independent blood pressure-lowering effect of converting enzyme inhibition, we feel that blood pressure reduction obtained with captopril reflects to a major degree active participation of the renin system in blood pressure regulation.

I just want to show you quickly here our first follow-up of 16 patients treated for up to 1 year with captopril. All had captopril, 8 needed in addition a diuretic. But all these get less diuretic than they had before when they had other drugs which did not lower the blood pressure completely. You can keep the blood pressure under control for 1 year and longer. And when one then remembers that most hypertension can be normalized by either captopril alone or combined with diuretics I believe that the renin-angiotensin system plays an important role in clinical hypertension. Thank you.

Questions

Distler: You showed one patient with primary aldosteronism receiving 100 mg captopril for 100 minutes and he had no hypotensive effect. I wonder whether this patient wouldn't have had any effect if you had given it for a prolonged period of time, say for days or weeks, and in higher doses?

Brunner: Higher doses? I don't think there is any evidence that you need more than 25 mg to get a bigger effect. I think there is no evidence, whatsoever, so far. I don't know if anybody challenged that. Now, for a longer period? With 50 or 100 mg you would not get a 12 hour duration of blockade. I take that criticism, but actually in the other patient who got it for 2 weeks there was no blood pressure reduction.

Oelkers: Dr. Brunner, you have shown that after acute administration of captopril you get in normal-renin patients no significant drop in blood pressure. But with chronic treatment you get a fall in blood pressure. But I doubt whether this means that renin or angiotensin does play a role in the generation of hypertension in these patients. Isn't the treatment with captopril in some way, besides lowering angiotensin levels, also a very mild reversible form of chemical adrenalectomy? These patients have probably decreased aldosterone levels and they shouldn't be able as normal subjects to conserve sodium.

Brunner: Yes, this is an important effect. Indeed you get a decrease in aldosterone and indeed I think the fact that you don't get salt retention when you lower blood pressure which you see usually with most other antihypertensive drugs, that's a significant contribution. Now, on the other hand, I would still say angiotensin II has been responsible for the stimulation of aldosterone, so there you have another angiotensin effect. I would still maintain that this is due to angiotensin because it's the angiotensin II-dependent part of aldosterone that I also influence.

Oelkers: But that's normal, we all have it.

Laragh: I think if I understand your question, than it is a key one. No one has found that normal-renin patients have a delayed response, their response is as good on day 1 as it is on anyone else. But everybody has an improvement in response and that probably didn't come out. I think you found that too, Hans. Because the aldosterone benefit takes weeks and the aldosterone begins to fall to almost Addisonian levels which is I think another terrific biological evidence of blockade of the renin system, urinary aldosterone excretion may be 1 or 2 or 3 μg/day in chronic therapy. And it's not until 10 days or 2 weeks that we believe we see the full expression of captopril. But there is no difference to normal renin or even some low renins.

Brunner: I would also point out that I believe that this reduction in aldosterone is very important for the diuretic effect if you have to add a diuretic. Diuretics are particularly effective, it seems to us, in association with captopril. Most patients need much less diuretics afterwards, I would maintain that this also is an angiotensin effect, an indirect one by aldosterone.

Gross: But what I don't understand is that you may have patients who don't respond to captopril or respond very poorly, and then you give a diuretic and they respond. So you have to turn on the renin system in order to obtain a clear-cut effect of captopril. I think there are figures from Cleveland group,

Bob Tarazi presented them, according to which lowering of blood pressure with captopril alone occurred in 20% to 30% of patients, whereas after adding a diuretic the response was about 70%. So, we have to turn on the renin system, to obtain a distinct effect of captopril.

Brunner: Well, I think Dr. Seldin has already discussed this and he said this probably much better than I have been trying to say this for a long time. Now, I think that first of all these figures vary. Some say you need a diuretic in about 30%. I guess, it depends on what kind of population you are dealing with. I can tell you we need a diuretic probably in about 50% of our patients, but we have a lot of patients with renal failure. You say, you have to turn on the renin, I say it differently. I say that these patients that need diuretics, are patients who have too much sodium to start with. When I block the renin system I identify those who have too much sodium and then I can titrate how much sodium to have to get off to get them normotensive. I think, using these inhibitors is the best way to identify how much sodium a patient has in excess to start with. But, of course, this remains a matter of debate whether it was too much to start with or whether there is depletion, at the end. I would claim that at the end they are not depleted, they are just where they should be.

Gross: But after some time of administering a diuretic one should be able to take off the diuretic and the patients should be maintained with captopril alone.

Brunner: No, because I think they have some renal excretory defect of sodium and when I stop the diuretic they will tend at a normal blood pressure to retain sodium until they become hypertensive again.

Gross: But then you need for the explanation an additional defect; that is then not only a renin story, but that's rather a kidney story.

Brunner: I was not saying that all hypertension is only a renin defect, certainly not.

Gross: No, you said only 90%.

Möhring: When you would do the same thing in a normotensive subject, why dont't you see as much fall in blood pressure? Your answer is because in hypertension this system is reset, it's imbalanced between renin, but nobody has measured that. You argue now with your effect that it must be like that. That's an argumentation which is already implied in what you studied. I think that's not allowed. There would be an alternative that — I am now just phantasizing maybe — the cardiovascular reflex systems in hypertension are less active if you go up or down. You do the same thing with captopril for instance as in a normotensive organism. But your cardiovascular reflex systems opposing now this fall in blood pressure work with a lesser gain. So you get a greater fall in blood pressure. That would be an alternative suggestion and there is also lot of litera ture consistent with this notion. I just question now if we really know that in hypertension the system is reset what you imply in your argumentation for interpreting your data.

Brunner: I am not sure I talked about resetting. I talked about sodium retention. All comes down to the point, what is a normal amount of sodium in the body and how do you measure it?

Möhring: My argument is just you say that in hypertension the relation between what John Laragh called the vasoconstrictor side and the volume side is not appropriate, right? and you interprete in that way your findings. I think that's an argumentation which is circular.

DeQuattro: I have a question regarding again the interrelationships of the renin-angiotensin system and the sympathetic nervous system. You have studied a lot of high renin patients with either saralasin or captopril. Have you studied some high renin hypertensives who don't have renal sequelae? Have you looked at any of those and seen not a good response to saralasin or to captopril? Or have you looked at their plasma catecholamines? I am interested because we had 8 patients that we divided, 4 with high renin and high catecholamines and 4 with high renin and normal catecholamines. The high renin-high catecholamines did not respond well to saralasin. So, the point was that perhaps their high renin was related to a sympathetic drive and just blocking the renin system would not lower the blood pressure.

Brunner: I didn't analyze the data in this way. We just looked at catecholamines in the whole bunch, and we didn't see a change. To answer the question about saralasin: We had some patients with high renins who did not respond to saralasin, certainly. But those in our hands were mostly again patients who had some decrease in glomerular filtration rate.

Seldin: I think it's possible to imagine two models which would accomodate both points of view. One model accounts for the kind of thrust that characterizes Dr. Brunner and Dr. Laragh and also some of the other points of view that have been mentioned. I think one can also imagine a group of hypertensive patients, as Dr. Gross suggested, who may have essentially a renal disease. In this model one would imagine that they tend to stabilize their sodium balance at a high extracellular volume. They have an increased avidity for sodium as the basic disorder. Under such circumstances when they come into a steady-state they might have an expanded extracellular and blood volume, an increased effective arterial blood volume, and their blood pressures might be high and their renins suppressed. By the way, this needn't be only a primary tubular disorder; conceivably it might be linked with catecholes. For example without going into detailed renal physiology, Brenner in a beautiful series of studies has shown that norepinephrine will cause sodium retention if it does not raise the blood pressure. In other words, if you manipulate the model in such a manner that you get mild levels of norepinephrine you get post-glomerular vasoconstriction and sodium retention without necessarily raising blood pressure. Well, one model then might be a primary defect with salt retention, either secondary or tubular, in which the steady-state is characterized by low renin. A second model might involve a primary defect in the renin-angiotensin system, but secondary salt retention masks that in the way that several people have alluded to. So, what you look at the steady-state is hypertension with low renin, but they might have different origins. I would be interesting if someone would do a careful sodium balance with diuretics because if the primary defect were in the renin-angiotensin system you should get an amplified rise in renin-angiotensin as you shrink volume toward normal. Whereas, if the primary defect was sodium retention, as volume comes toward normal it should normalize and it might be possible to sort out these different effects if one did the proper studies.

Gross: Thank you very much, Dr. Seldin, for this attempt to unify the various opinions.

Lever: The measurements of plasma volume, of ECF volume, of exchangeable sodium, and of total body sodium in hypertensive patients with low renin are not increased, nor is there an overbrisk response of renin to the sodium-depleting effects of diuretics. I would like it to be true, but it isn't.

Seldin: I think one can get very significant volume changes which can't be measured. Let me give you an example. Supposing you have a patient with nephregenic diabetes insipidus. You give a diuretic, the diuretic is chlorothiazide. The patients or the rat comes into a steady-state. Urine volume is markedly reduced, no antidiuretic hormone is involved, but you can't measure any change in volume. What I am trying to argue is that there is a volume contraction, the volume contraction is seen by the kidneys, but it can't be measured. In chronic administration of thiazide to lower blood pressure in a steady-state once again where sodium intake equals sodium output, you can't measure reliably any change in either extracellular or plasma volume, but there are inferential reasons for believing that the plasma volume is shrunken (as judged by the response of systems like the renin-angiotensin system and the antidiuretic hormone system). So, I am not as disconcerted as you are by the measurements which failed to show that there is any measurable shrinkage in extracellular volume and in plasma volume. I think if you look at the whole functioning system there is plenty of indirect evidence to suggest it. We measured extracellular volume by radiosulphate, which is sort of a better measure — at least theoretically, don't misunderstand — than total body sodium which measures various intracellular and transcellular compartments. We could never show any change in the steady-state where intake equals output, but there is plenty of indirect evidence.

Reubi: Perhaps I may offer my own contribution to medical philosophy. First, when we talk about blood pressure we measure the blood pressure within large arteries and the only way the blood pressure can be increased in the large arteries is either by a vasoconstriction in the arterioles or by an increased flow of blood within the artery. Because the concept that you are filling a plastic tube in pressing fluid inside — I think that's a purely static concept which is not valid at all. So, I don't like the expression volume hypertension. In other words, if you have a volume hypertension you have either an increased cardiac index or an increased arteriolar resistance. Admittedly this can be due to an increased volume as far as an increased cardiac index is concerned, but you should be able to measure this increase in volume. Or this can be due to an increase in the sodium content of the arterioles. That would be another possibility. But perhaps you should be able to measure it, too. When you are operating

with volume hypertension you cannot measure anything and I think that's the
weak point. If you compare this to the situation in renal disease: In renal disease usually the exchangable sodium is increased if the patient is hypertensive
or the blood volume is increased. So I think Guyton's concept may be valid in
renal disease, but not in essential hypertension because we can imagine that if
primary sodium retention would be responsbile for the hypertension in essential hypertension we can imagine that the kidney has other ways of getting rid
of excess sodium than just by increasing the systemic blood pressure. Now, just
a general comment. We are discussing regulatory mechanisms, catecholamines,
renin, sodium and so forth. I think this is not the problem, probably. The problem is why is in essential hypertension the regulation defective? If you have an
increase in renin why don't you have a decrease in volume? If you have an increase in catecholamines, why don't you have simultaneously an increase in
prostaglandin or something like that? I think there is no doubt about the
reality of all the described mechanisms, but they don't bear much relationship
to the etiology and pathogenesis of essential hypertension.

Laragh: I wish I could say things as incisively as Don Seldin can. — I am an
old space measurer, too, and there is no volume measurement that's good enough
to pick up what we are looking for. But not withstanding that, I went to the
trouble with Tom Pickering of reviewing every volume study in every hypertensive ever made in the world where renins were measured. And it comes
out that the volumes are high in low renin hypertension in more than half
of the studies and in the other they are normal, but they are never low and
everybody who ever studied high renin hypertension finds the volumes quite
low, including Dr. Weidmann. There is no volume study which is against it.
All we are dealing with is a failure to demonstrate which doesn't mean much
in science. Now, let me tell you something else about the volume. There are
some important things we do know about low renin hypertension. One is,
the body perceives volume depletion by the high renin, aldo, and ADH. When
you give a diuretic so you can see it. Secondly, everybody that has ever
studied low renin patients finds they have lower haematocrits, lower ureas
and lower uric acids, and high renins have the opposite and high total proteins,
so that I don't think we are operating in a vacuum. There is nothing against
the idea. It may be circuitous reasoning, but if we don't have a functional basis
to differentiate patients we can't have a hypothesis to work with.

Gross: But, John, don't you simplify too much when you ascribe so much to
volume alone? Isn't there also something like sodium distribution, for example
an increase in intracellular sodium which has nothing to do with volume?

Laragh: There can be a lot, but my definition is based on the fact that a diuretic corrects the hypertension and don't forget when you stop the diuretic I never saw a patient in the world who didn't gain 2 kg. They are chronically depleted. It's an operational definition. I can go to sodium in the artery wall, I like
Louis Tobian's theory, but that's another layer of conception. The first layer
is to find out which patients have which properties and then study them.

Vetter: I think when we are discussing renin we often implicate that the group
of high renin patients and those of low renin patients represent homogenous
groups. I follow Dr. Seldin, this is not true. We have collected some 100 patients
over the years and the number is so great as to separate them in age-different
groups. We found out that in younger patients or in early stage of hypertension there is always a strong inverse correlation between blood pressure and
renin secretion. When the patients are becoming older, there is a conversion of
this correlation so that the older patients always show, as a group, a positive
correlation between renin and blood pressure. There is also a marked and for us
astonishing sex difference in the middle age groups. Men show the conversion
from this inverse correlation to a positive correlation at early years. We have
interpreted this that this is probably a change in renal vascular system. That
means that when we are comparing the blood pressure, younger people with
low renin state have always high blood pressure and high-renin younger people
have a moderate blood pressure. There is quite a difference in the older people:
Low renins have a moderate blood pressure and high renins a severe blood pressure. Also aldosterone secretion dissociated early from renin. So it is typical for
the younger low-renin patients that there is an appropriate high aldosterone
secretion perhaps indicating that volume factor.

Drayer: When I joined Dr. Laragh's group a couple of years ago, we studied 83
patients with low-renin hypertension and 42 with high-renin hypertension and
within each sub-group there was no correlation at all between renin and age.
Moreover, the age of the low-renin patients obviously as many others have published was higher than that of the high-renin patients. But the age at which the
hypertension started in the patients was different. There was a similar duration
of hypertension in both groups. So it is not unlikely that low-renin patients
will get their hypertension at on older age.

Gross: Let's not complicate the story by age too much now. I think we should
come to an end and I wonder if members of the panel would like to have a last
word.

Lever: My last point would be this: If blood pressure is controlled by say 3 or
4 systems, by catecholamine shall we say, by sodium, or by angiotensin, and if
one of them is removed by a specific agent and blood pressure falls, it does not
follow logically that the blood pressure was elevated by overactivity in that
system in the first place. Much of the assumptions that have been sweeping
through this room this afternoon and earlier are based on the fact that a response to a specific agent which is positive necessarily implicates the mechanism
concerned. I suggest that it doesn't necessarily though I believe that in the case
of the SQUIBB-inhibitors a lot of useful information has been obtained. My
second point — last one — is that we have, much to our disappointment, recently found that captopril lowers blood pressure by a mechanism which is not related to the decrease of angiotensin II. In other words there is some other mechanism at work. We did this by infusing dogs with angiotensin II producing our
dose-response curves, giving captopril and then making another dose-response
curve during captopril. If the only way in which captopril lowered blood pres-

sure was by lowering angiotensin II the two dose-response curves should coincide. They didn't. There was a big difference between the two. We are not the first people to observe this. I think the Bostonians have noted it as well. So there is another mechanism involved. A fascinating new observation made independently by Moncada and by Dollery is that if you give indomethacin to animals receiving captopril its blood pressure lowering effect is eliminated. And the implication obviously is that prostaglandin of one sort or another is involved in the blood pressure-lowering effect. Many of you may know more of this. It was reported quite recently.

Gross: Would you answer the question: Does the renin-angiotensin system play a significant role in human hypertension?

Lever: Yes, I think it does in the early stages of renal hypertension and probably in the chronic stages. I don't know whether it causes essential hypertension, but I think the evidence is strongly against it acting as a direct pressor agent.

Doyle: I think it's really very difficult to answer the question as to whether the renin-angiotensin system does play a more significant role in essential hypertension than most people thought. I think it is obviously very difficult to evaluate exactly how this system might operate. Clearly, the renin-angiotensin system has profound effects. It has effects on glomerulo-tubular balance so that the renin-angiotensin system can itself alter sodium. It has effects on thirst, so the renin-angiotensin system clearly must have its own effects on volume. I think it's really unbelievably naive to suppose that measuring the circulating levels of this material which is in many instances a local hormone is going to tell you precisely whether it's acting in the system or not. Now, I think the real difficulty now arises from the fact that the captopril appears to provide entirely new aspects. If one could be certain that captopril is operating exclusively through the renin-angiotensin system I think the answer would have to be "Yes, the renin-angiotensin system is much more important in human essential hypertension than most people supposed 2 or 3 years ago". One is always left with the doubt that it may not be operating entirely through the renin-angiotensin system. I think, until the pharmacology of the material has better worked out I believe that we have to keep an open mind.

Laragh: I think the experience today indicates that essential hypertension has entirely different distribution of renin and aldosterone patterns than normal people and that the distribution is in part a function of their different blood pressure. We now know that the fall in renin with age, at least in our hands in a large series of normal people, is blood pressure-related because if you don't get a rise in blood pressure with age you don't get a low renin with age. It has operationally proven useful to separate low, normal, and high because the world agrees that the low patients respond uniquely to diuretics and the high respond uniquely to drugs, whose actions have been debated here: propranolol, captopril and saralasin. Moreover, we have been able to show a lot of other different things about low-renin patients. They have a lower blood viscosity, they have lower cortisols and high renins have higher cortisols. In other words, the separation of the groups operationally allows us to examine seriously for the first time the question of heterogeneity and we well know there is heterogeneity of drug response. There are patients that respond only to propranolol and are normotensive and the opposite with a diuretic. In this setting of heterogeneity I believe that the pharmacology of these agents isn't so crucial as it seems to be and I just close by saying that indomethacin lowers the antihypertensive action of propranolol and diuretics and I don't accept that as meaning anything in particular because it blocks all of these agents and the acute drop in blood pressure with captopril my well be due to bradykinin release.

Brunner: I base my evidence on what I have seen the last 8 years working with different inhibitors of the renin system. Obviously, one has to keep one's mind open concerning specificity of these agents. Also, I would say all information coming out needs to be digested. In this context, I could answer Dr. Lever that we have done the same experiment and we didn't find the same results. I think it would be easy for me to answer to Dr. Gross "yes". That's a safe way of answering. But I prefer to say that I believe that renin together with sodium plays an important role in maintaining blood pressure in hypertensive patients.

Gross: Thank you very much. I should like to thank the panelists and all of you, especially those who contributed to the discussion. We are not able to give a clear answer to this question. I think in some forms of human hypertension it is clear that the renin system is of some significance and in others it is not. But, on the other hand, we end up with another question and this is I think one in honour of Peter Wolff who many years ago asked the question "Is essential hypertension a clinical entity?" And I think this is what John just said, it is doubtful that it is. So we have next time perhaps another question to answer or not to answer.

Renal Hormones

Renal Vasodepressor Hormones: The Kallikrein-Kinin and Prostaglandin Systems

O. A. CARRETERO[1], A. G. SCICLI

Although the primary function of the kidney is to regulate the volume and ionic composition of body fluids, the kidney is also an important endocrine organ. Through these two general functions it plays a major role in the regulation of blood pressure. It produces both vasopressor (antinatriuretic and vasoconstrictor) and vasodepressor (natriuretic and vasodilator) hormones. The role of the renin-angiotensin system (vasopressor) in the regulation of blood pressure and in the pathogenesis of hypertension has been established. On the other hand, the role of vasodepressor renal hormones, such as the kallikrein-kinin and prostaglandin systems, in the regulation of blood pressure and in the pathogenesis of hypertension is less well defined.

Kallikreins are enzymes which generates kinins, potent vasodilator peptides, from plasma substrates called kinogens. There are two main classes of kallikrein: plasma and glandular.

The plasma kallikrein system differs from the glandular kallikrein system not only in its biochemical and immunological characteristics, but also in its functions. Table 1 shows some of the differences between these two systems.

Glandular kallikreins are found in the urine, kidney, pancreas, salivary, and sweat glands, and in the intestine. Figure 1 shows the mechanism of kinins generation and destruction in the kidney.

In the kidney, the kallikrein-kinin system is located in the distal nephron [1, 2, 3]. The proximal tubules contain high amounts of kininase which destroys any filtered plasma kinins [4], thus limiting the intrarenal action of the kallikrein-kinin system to the distal part of the nephron where kinins are formed (Fig. 2). The collecting duct, interstitial cells of the medulla, and the renal papilla are very rich in prostaglandin synthetase [5]. In addition, it has recently been reported that the renal arterioles can also synthesize prostaglandin and prostacyclin [6]. PGE_2 appears to be the primary urinary prostaglandin, and it is incorporated into the urine in Henle's loop [7]. Prostaglandin synthesis in the kidney is partially controlled by the intrarenal formation of kinins [5, 8]. Since

---

1 This work was done during the tenure of an Established Investigatorship of the American Heart Association. Supported in part by a Michigan Heart Association Grand and N.I.H. Grant # HL 15839 and # HL 24650

Table 1. Characteristics of plasma and glandular kallikrein

	Plasma Kallikrein	Glandular Kallikrein
Molecular Weight:	100.000	24.000-44.000
Substrate:	HMWK	LMWK and HMWK
Kinin Released:	Bradykinin	Lys-bradykinin
Inhibited by SBTI:	Yes	No
Function:	a) Coagulation	a) Regulation of organ blood flow?
	b) Fibinolysis	b) Water and electrolytes excretion?
	c) Inflammation?	c) Blood pressure homeostasis?
	d) Complement activation?	
	d) Blood pressure homeostasis?	

LMWK = Low Molecular Weight Kininogen; HMWK = High Molecular Weight Kininogen; SBTI = Soya Bean Trypsin Inhibitor

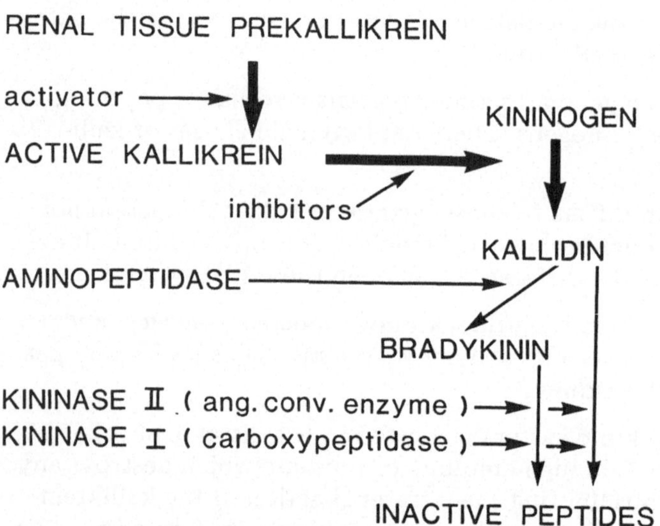

Fig. 1. The renal kallikrein-kinin system

intrarenal kinins are formed in the distal nephron, they probably stimulate prostaglandine synthesis mainly in the collecting duct, medulla, and papilla. An increase in intrarenal endogenous kinin concentration, either by stimulation of its production or by inhibition of its destruction, produces an increase in inner cortical renal blood flow, natriuresis, diuresis, and PGE_2 excretion [8, 9, 10]. Blockade of endogenous kinin formation with aprotinin and inhibition of their effect with antibodies against kinins have been reported to decrease natriuresis

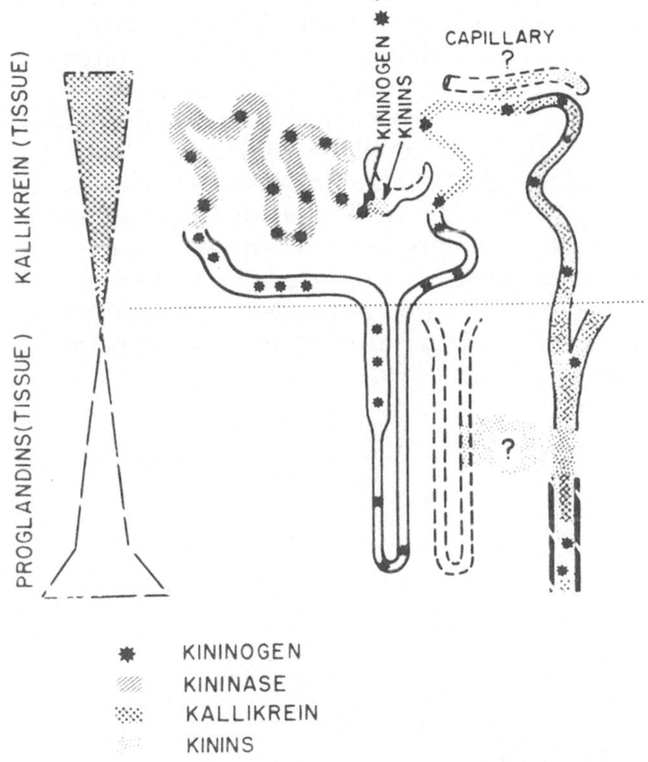

Fig. 2. Localization of the kallikrein-kinin system in the nephron. Renal kallikrein is formed and released by the distal tubule; kinin is generated in this part of the nephron, collecting duct, and papilla. Both kallikreins and kinins may pass to the interstitial and vascular space of the kidney. Intrarenal generated kinins can induce release of prostaglandin E_2 from the collecting duct, and interstitial cells of the medulla and papilla. The kininogen necessary for the formation of kinin may be plasma kininogen filtered by the glomeruli or produced by the nephron itself

in saltloaded rats [11, 12]. These data suggest that the intrarenal formation of kinins, either directly or through the release of prostaglandins, plays an important role in the regulation of renal blood flow distribution and sodium excretion.

Urinary kallikrein excretion has frequently been assumed to be an indicator of the intrarenal activity of the kallikrein-kinin system; however, this assumption has yet to be validated. This consideration must be kept in mind when interpreting urinary kallikrein excretion data [13]. Urinary kallikrein excretion has been reported to be both directly and inversely correlated to sodium and water excretion [14, 15]. There is no satisfactory explanation for these contradictory results.

143

Urinary kallikrein excretion is decreased in some patients with essential hypertension (Fig. 3) and in different models of experimental hypertension [16].
Kallikrein excretion is increased only in mineralocorticoid-induced hypertension [17]. Rats bred to be susceptible to the hypertensive effect of salt have
conspicuously low urinary kallikrein excretion even before they develop hypertension [18]. A deficiency in the activity of the kallikrein-kinin system may alter sodium and water excretion in susceptible rats and may thereby promote
hypertension during high salt intake [19]. It is even possible that similar defects
occur in a subclass of patients with essential hypertension and very low urinary
kallikrein excretion [16]. Furthermore, it has been reported that patients with
essential hypertension and low kallikrein excretion responded to the oral administration of glandular kallikrein with a greater decrease in blood pressure
than patients with normal kallikrein excretion [20].

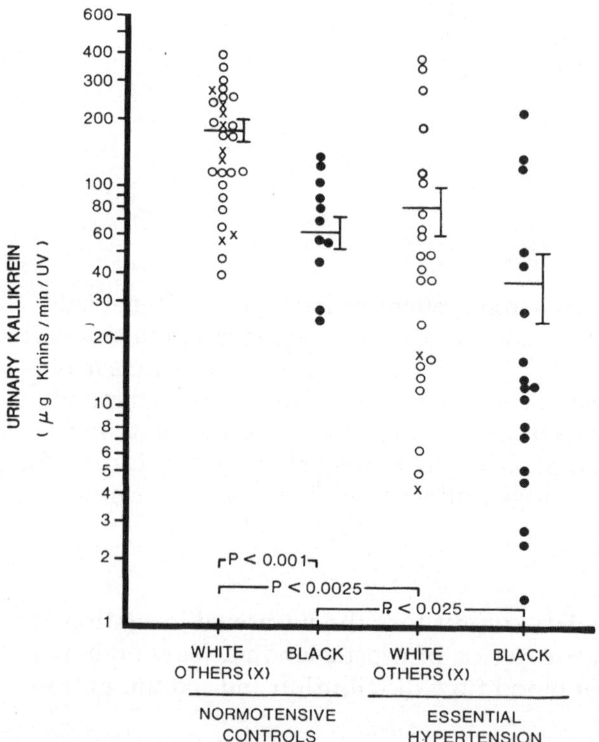

Fig. 3. Urinary kallikrein excretion in white and black normotensive controls
and in patients with essential hypertension (X in the white group indicates
race other than white or black). Horizontal and vertical bars indicate mean and
standard error, respectively. Scale in ordinate is in log

144

An increase in the activity of the renal kallikrein and prostaglandin systems
may contribute to the mechanisms of action of some antihypertensive drugs.
Diuretics have been reported to stimulate the excretion of kallikrein and prostaglandins; and hydralazine has been reported to stimulate the excretion of
kallikrein [16]. It has recently been reported that antibodies against kinins
block part of the acute anithypertensive effect of converting enzyme inhibitor
(Captopril or SQ 14.225) in spontaneous hypertensive rats and in two-kidney,
one-clip Goldblatt hypertensive rats [21]. Figure 4 shows changes in blood pressure after acute administration of Captopril in two-kidney, one-clip Goldblatt
hypertensive rats. Half of the rats were pretreated with antibodies against kinins
while the other half were pretreated with normal rabbit serum.

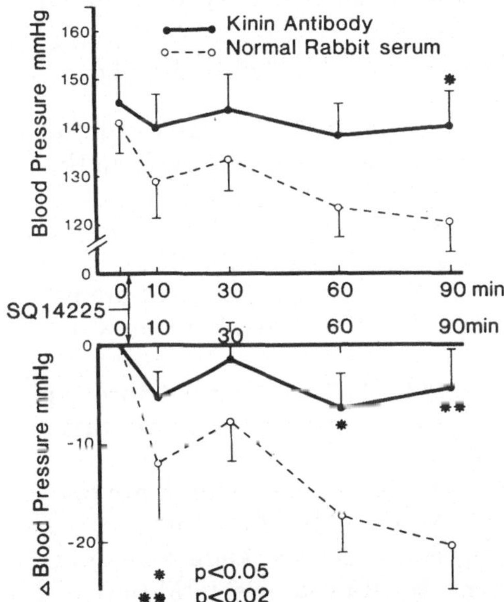

Fig. 4. Mean blood pressure (top) and delta blood pressure (bottom) in two-
kidney, one-clip Goldblatt hypertensive rats after the acute administration of
converting enzyme inhibitor (SQ 14.225, 100 mg/kg). Continuous line indicates rats pretreated with normal rabbit serum

In conclusion, the definite role of the renal kallikrein-kinin and prostaglandin
systems in the regulation of blood pressure and in the pathogenesis of hypertension is not completely understood. However, there is evidence which suggests
that they could play an important role in the regulation of blood volume and
vascular resistance, and consequently, in the regulation of blood pressure.

References

1. Scicli AG, Carretero OA, Hampton A, Cortes P, Oza NB (1976) Site of kininogenase secretion in the dog nephron. Am J Physiol 239 : 533-536
2. Ørstavik TB, Nustad K, Brandtzaeg P, Pierce JV (1976) Cellular origin of urinary kallikreins. J Histochem Cytochem 24 : 1037-1039
3. Scicli AG, Gandolfi R, Carretero OA (1978) Site of formation of kinins in the dog nephron. Am J Physiol 234 : F36-F40
4. Ward PW, Gedney CD, Dowben RM, Erdös EG (1975) Isolation of membrane bound renal kallikrein and kininase. Biochem J 15 : 755-758
5. McGiff JC, Wong PYK (1978) Prostaglandins and renal function. In: Proceedings of the 7th International Congress of Nephrology. Montreal, University of Montreal Press, pp 83-91
6. Terragno NA, McGiff JC, Terragno A (1977) Prostacyclin (PGI_2) production by renal blood vessels: Relationship to endogenous prostaglandin synthesis inhibitor (EPSI). Clin Res 26 : 545A
7. Williams WM, Frolich JC, Hies AS, Oates JA (1977) Origin of urinary prostaglandins. Kidney Int 11 : 256-260
8. Colina-Chourio J, Miller MP, McGiff JC, Nasjletti A (1976) Possible influence of intrarenal generation of kinins on prostaglandins release from the rabbit perfused kidney. Br J Pharmacol 58 : 165-172
9. Bailie MD, Barbour JA (1975) Effect of inhibition of peptidase activity on distribution of intrarenal blood flow. Am J Physiol 228 : 850-853
10. Nasjletti A, Colina-Chourio J, McGiff JC (1975) Disappearance of bradykinin in the renal circulation of dogs: Effects of kininase inhibition. Circ Res 37 : 59-65
11. Kramer HJ, Moch T, Sicherer L von, Dusing R (1979) Effects of aprotinin on renal function and urinary prostaglandins excretion in conscious rats after acute salt loading. Clin Sci 56 : 546-553
12. Marin-Grez M (1974) The influence of antibodies against bradykinin on isotonic saline diuresis in the rat. Pflugers Archiv 350 : 231-239
13. Carretero OA, Scicli AG, Nasjletti A (in press) Glandular kallikrein-kinin system: Methodology for its measurement. In: Radzialowski FM (ed) Hypertension research: methods and models
14. Carretero OA, Scicli AG (1976) Renal kallikrein: Its localization and possible role in renal function. Fed Proc 35(2) : 194-198
15. Margolius HS, Horwitz D, Pisano JJ, Keiser HR (1976) Relationship among urinary kallikrein, mineralocorticoids, and human hypertensive disease. Fed Proc 35(2) 203;206
16. Carretero OA, Scicli AG (1978) The renal kallikrein-kinin system in human and in experimental hypertension. Klin Wochenschr Suppl 1 56 : 113-125
17. Margolius HS, Horwitz D, Geller RG, Alexander RW, Gill JR, Pisano JJ, Keiser HR (1974) Urinary excretion in hypertension: Relationships to sodium intake and sodium-retaining steroids. Circ Res 35 : 820-829
18. Carretero OA, Scicli AG, Piwonska A, Koch J (1977) Urinary kallikrein in rats bred for their susceptibility and resistance to the hypertensive effect of salt and in New Zealand genetically hypertensive rats. Mayo Clin Proc 52 : 465-467

19. Carretero OA, Amin VM, Ocholik T, Scicli AG, Koch J (1978) Urinary
    kallikrein in rats bred for their susceptibility and resistance to the hyper-
    tensive effect of salt. A new radioimmunoassay for its direct determina-
    tion. Circ Res 42(5) : 727-731
20. Overlack A, Stumpe KO, Zywzok W, Ressel C, Krück F (1978) Defect in the
    kallikrein-kinin system in essential hypertension and reduction of blood
    pressure by orally given kallikrein. In: Kinin 78 Tokyo, Program Ab-
    stracts of International Symposium on Kinins. Plenum, New York, 94
21. Miyazaki S, Scicli AG, Polomski C, Carretero OA (1979) Role of kinins
    in the antihypertensive effects of converting enzyme inhibitor. Circ 60 :
    II-228

Plasma Kallikrein as an Activator of Inactive Renin ("Prorenin") – Studies In-Vitro and In-Vivo

F. H. M. DERKX, B. N. BOUMA, H. L. TAN-TJIONG, A. J. MAN IN
'T VELD, J. H. B. DE BRUYN, G. J. WENTING, M. A. D. H. SCHALEKAMP

Renin and Prorenin

Most proteolytic enzymes in plasma circulate as inactive precursors. These pro-enzymes are activated by limited proteolysis during physiological processes such as coagulation, fibrinolysis and complement-mediated reactions [1, 2]. For a long time most physiologists and clinicians were interested in renin as a classical circulating hormone [3], despite the well-known fact that renin is a proteolytic enzyme [4, 5]. The traditional endocrinologist's view, however, seems too limited. Recently it has become clear that renin circulates in plasma largely as an inactive form, which might be a proenzyme, prorenin, comparable to other proenzymes in plasma [6-10].

Inactive renin can be converted *in-vitro* into its active counterpart by treatment of plasma with acid [6, 8, 10]. This so-called acid-activation of renin is a two-stage process. Acidification itself has little or no effect on renin acitivity; the actual activation process occurs after pH has been restored to ncutral [11]. This activation at neutral pH can be blocked by serine protease inhibitors, thereby indicating that one or more endogenous serine proteases are involved in the *in-vitro* activation of inactive renin [11-14].

Figure 1 shows a typical experiment. Two ml human plasma, which contained disodium EDTA (5 mmol/l) as the anticoagulant, was dialysed at 4°C for 24 hours against a glycine-HCl buffer of pH 3,3 followed by dialysis against phosphate buffer of pH 7,5 again for 24 hours. Renin was determined by its ability to generate angiotensin I during incubation with an excess of purified sheep renin-substrate [8]. The incubate (pH 7,5) contained the following protease (angiotensinase) inhibitors: disodium-EDTA (1 mmol/l), 8-hydroxyquinoline sulphate (3,4 mmol/l), phenylmethylsulfonylfluoride (2,87 mmol/l) and aprotinin (Trasylol, Bayer) (100 kallikrein-inhibiting units/ml). After incubation for three hours at 37°C, the reaction was stopped by heating in a boiling waterbath. The quantity of angiotensin I that was formed during incubation was measured by radioimmunoassay, and compared with the quantity generated by standard human kidney renin (MRC standard 68/356). Results are expressed as micro-units of the standard per ml plasma (μU/ml) [8, 15-17].

In the experiment shown in Figure 1 the serine protease inhibitor, benzamidine-HCl, was added to normal plasma after the pH 3,3-dialysis step in a final con-

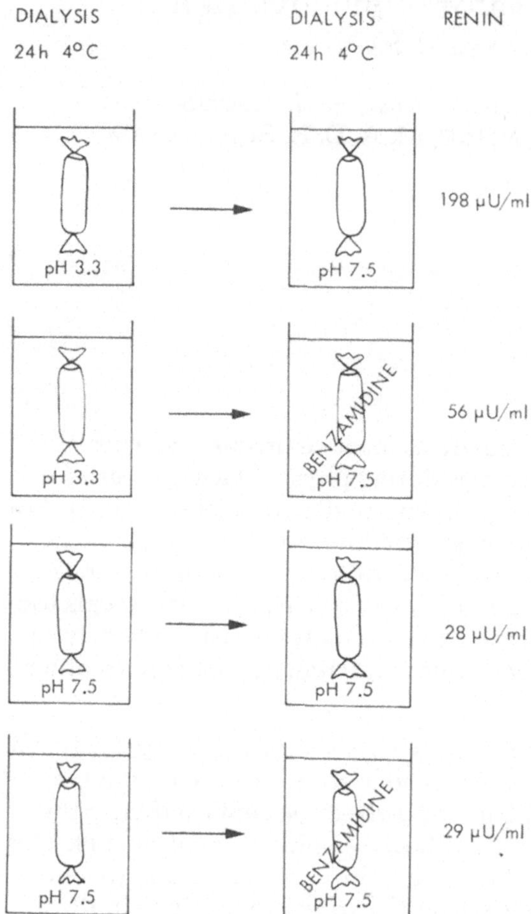

Fig. 1. Effect of the serine protease inhibitor benzamidine-HCl (10 mmol/l) on the activation of inactive renin in acid-pretreated normal plasma. Plasma was dialysed in two steps; the inhibitor was added to the second dialysis buffer. Note that the inhibitor had no effect on renin acitivity, when added to unacidified plasma. See text for details

centration of 10 mmol/l. This caused marked inhibition of the activation of inactive renin in the neutral phase. We have tested other protease inhibitors in this way, and the results are shown in Table 1. Among the substances tested, aprotinin (Trasylol), soya-bena trypsin inhibitor and benzamidine-HCl had the greatest effect. The inhibitor spectrum for renin activation is similar to that reported for plasma kallikrein [17]. None of the protease inhibitors interfered with the reaction between active renin and its substrate. This was demonstrated by adding the inhibitors to known amounts of human renin (MRC standard 68/356) before incubation with sheep renin-substrate.

Table 1. Effects of protease inhibitors on the activation of inactive renin

The same plasma pool was used in all experiments. The quantity of renin that
was activated in whole plasma after dialysis for 24 hours at pH 3,3 with subsequent dialysis for 24 hours at pH 7,5 without serine protease inhibitors was
taken as 100%. Acid-activitable renin in the plasma pool was 170 μU/ml.
Further details see text.

Protease inhibitor	Percentege inhibition of renin activation after pH 3,3-treatment (M ± SEM)
Aprotinin	
1250 inhibitor units/ml	89 ± 9 (n = 16)
125 inhibitor units/ml	30 ± 5 (n = 16)
Soya-bean trypsin inhibitor	
1250 inhibitor units/ml	83 ± 11 (n = 16)
125 inhibitor units/ml	74 ± 8 (n = 16)
Benzamidine-HCl	
0.01 mol/l	80 ± 7 (n = 4)
Lima-bean trypsin inhibitor	
1250 inhibitor units/ml	13 ± 3 (n = 4)
125 inhibitor units/ml	5 ± 2 (n = 4)
"Ovomucoid"	
1250 inhibitor units/ml	19 ± 3 (n = 4)
125 inhibitor units/ml	0 ± 5 (n = 4)

One inhibitor unit inhibits a quantity of trypsin that will produce an absorb-
ance at 253 nm of 0.001/min at pII 7.6 and 25°C with α-N-benzoyl-L-Arg-ethyl
ester (BAEE) as substrate (1 cm light-path)

Parallel Activation of 'Prorenin' and Plasma Prekallikrein In-Vitro

The enzymatic pathways of activating the systems of coagulation, fibrinolysis
and complement-mediated reactions are very complex, the more so since the
initiation of one sequence of enzymes may trigger the cascade-like activation of
a second system. Such cross-links between the various proteolytic systems depend on special key-enzymes. Plasma kallinkrein is an example, because it participates in the contact-activation of the intrinsic coagulation pathway, as well
as in fibrinolysis, complement activation, inflammatory reactions and kinin
generation [12].

Evidence is accumulating that kallikrein is also involved in the activation of the
renin-angiotensin system. We have already mentioned that substances known to
inhibit plasma kallikrein also interfere with activation of inactive renin, whereas

151

substances with less inhibitory effect on plasma kallikrein, such as lima-bean
trypsin inhibitor and the protease inhibitor from ovomucoid, which are known
to inhibit glandular kallikrein, have also less effect on the activation of inactive
renin.

To explore this further, we made parallel measurements of kallikrein, prekallikrein and renin in acid-pretreated plasma. For this purpose EDTA-plasma was
dialysed at 4°C for 24 hours against buffers of various pH. Glycine-HCl buffers
were used for the pH 1.5-4.0 range, and citric acid-phosphate buffers were used
for the pH 4.0-7.5 range [15-17]. After dialysis the pH was rapidly restored to
7.5 with NaOH solution (1 mol/l) followed by dialysis for 24 hours against
phsophate buffer of Ph 7.5. The method for measuring kallikrein is based on
the amidolytic action of this enzyme on the chromogenic substrate H-D-Pro-L-
Phe-L-Arg-p-nitroanilide (PPAN, Kabi) [18]. The linear relase of p-nitroaniline
was followed at 405 nm for 1-2 min in a 1-cm semimicrocuvette at 37°C and
pH 7.5. Results are expressed as nanokatals per ml (nkat/ml), one katal being
the quantity of enzyme that catalyses the conversion of one mole of substrate per second under the conditions of the assay. Plasma prekallikrein was
measured after its conversion to kallikrein by dextran sulphate [19] 100 μl
EDTA-plasma was mixed with 100 μl dextran sulphate (molecular weight approximately 500.00 daltons) (Pharmacia) dissolved in H_2O at a concentration
of 25 mg/l. The mixture was incubated for 7 min at 4°C, and kallikrein was
measured as described above. It should be noted that kallikrein retains its amidolytic action on low-molecular weight substrates, when it is bound to α_2-
macroglobulin. The kallikrein-α_2-macroglobulin complex, however, does not
act on high-molecular weight protein substrates [20]. Since we were interested
in the possibility that kallikrein acts on renin, it was important to design a
method for distinguishing between free kallikrein and α_2-macroglobulin-bound
kallikrein, which probably cannot attack protein-substrates . The method we
have developed is based on the fact that the amidolytic action of the kallikrein-
α_2-macroglobulin complex on the synthetic substrate PPAN cannot be inhibited by soya-bean trypsin inhibitor. This inhibitor was therefore added to acid-
pretreated plasma in a concentration sufficiently high (5.000 BAEE units/ml)
to cause complete inhibition of free kallikrein. The remaining amidolytic activity is therefore a measure of the kallikrein α_2-macroglobulin complex, and was
determined with PPAN as the substrate, as described above.

The results obtained in normal plasma are shown in Figure 2. It can be seen
that dextran sulphate-activatable prekallikrein was lowered in plasma that was
treated at pH below 5.0, and after treatment at pH 4.0 it could not be detected
anymore. The decrease of prekallikrein was associated with the appearance of
kallikrein-α_2-macroglobulin complex. At pH 4.0-pretreatment virtually all the
kallikrein, which was derived from prekallikrein, was bound to α_2-macroglob-
ulin. This complex was dissociated after treatment at pH below 4.0; free kallikrein appeared in the solution, and inactive renin was activated. This is compatible with the view that kallikrein is involved in the conversion of inactive
to active renin.

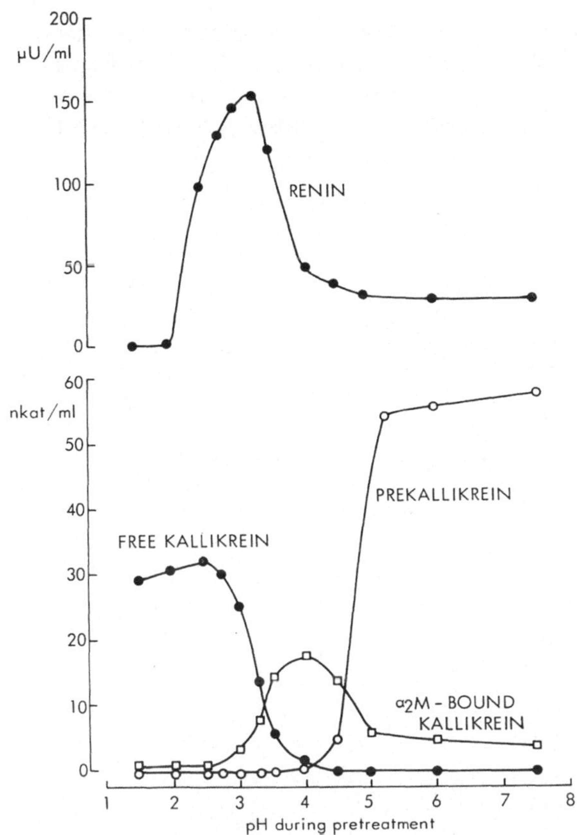

Fig. 2. Activation of inactive renin and prekallikrein in normal plasma (mean, $n = 3$). Plasma was first dialysed for 24 hours at various pH-values, as indicated on the horizontal axis. This was followed by dialysis again for 24 hours at pH 7,5. The plasma was then assayed for renin and kallikrein (amidolytic) activities. Kallikrein activity that was bound to α_2-macroglobulin was measured separately from free kallikrein. Upper part of figure: Renin. Lower part of figure: prekallikrein (○——○), α_2-macroglobulin-bound kallikrein (□——□), and free kallikrein (●——●). Note that the increase of renin activity at pH <4.0 coincides with the appearance of free kallikrein. See text for details

Proteolytic cleavage of plasma prekallikrein into 52.000 and 33.000 dalton fragments, which is known to be associated with the appearance of kallikrein activity, was followed in acid-pretreated plasma by SDS-polyacrylamide gel electrophoresis of added radioactive purified plasma prekallikrein [21]. ^{125}I-prekallikrein (approximately 27 μCi in 15 μl) was added to 600 μl normal plasma. The mixture was dialysed at pH 3.3 for 24 hours. At various time intervals after restoration of pH to 7.5, the mixture was analysed for the presence of cleavage fragments of ^{125}I-prekallikrein and for kallikrein and renin activities. After reduction by β-mercaptoethanol, the reaction mixture was subjected to

153

SDS-polyacrylamide gel (7.5%) electrophoresis at pH 7.2. The gels were sliced, and the radioactivity in each slide (1.2 mm) was counted. As shown in Figure 3, the appearance of cleavage products with an apparent molecular weight of 52.000 daltons was associated with the generation of kallikrein (amidolytic) and renin activities.

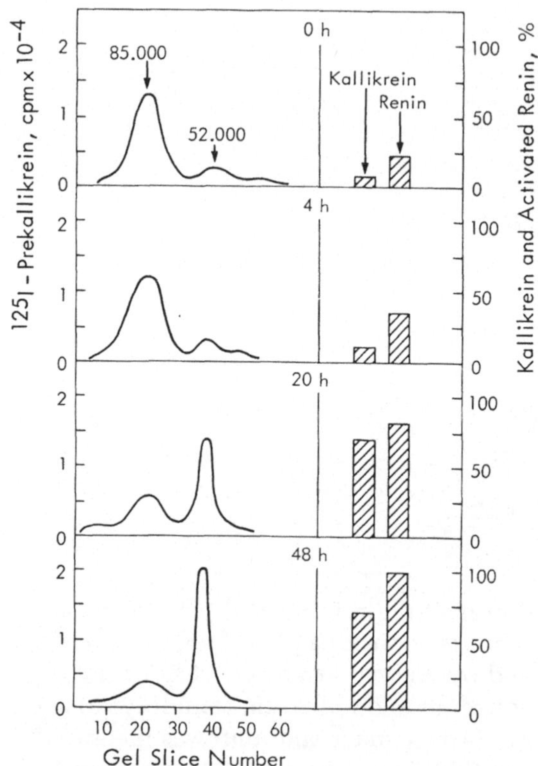

Fig. 3. Cleavage of ^{125}I-prekallikrein in acid-pretreated normal plasma. The radioactive prekallikrein was added to the plasma prior to acidification. After dialysis at pH 3.3 for 24 hours, the pH was restored to pH 7.5, and 4-48 hours later the reaction mixtures were analysed for the presence of cleavange products of ^{125}I-prekallikrein by SDS-polyacrylamide gel electrophoresis and for kallikrein (amidolytic) and renin activities. The appearance of cleavage products with an apparent molecular weight of 52.000 daltons indicates activation of prekallikrein. See text for details (From Derkx et al. [16], by courtesy of the publisher

A Factor XII-Prekallikrein-Dependent Pathway for Activating 'Prerenin' In-Vitro

More direct evidence that kallikrein is involved in the activation of inactive renin came from experiments in which the results of acid-treatment and trypsin-treatment of normal and factor XII (Hageman-factor)-and prekallikrein-(Fletcher-factor)-deficient plasmas were compared. The plasmas were dialysed at pH 3.3 for 24 hours, and after this the pH was rapidly restored to 7.5. The trypsin, 12.000 α-N-benzoyl-L-Arg-ethylester (BAEE)-units per mg protein (Sigma) was covalently bound to CNBr-activated Sepharose 4B in a concentration of 30 mg protein per gram dry Sepharose. The immobilized trypsin was added to the plasma in a final concentration of approximately 2000 BAEE-units/ml. The suspensions were slowly shaken at 4°C and the trypsin was removed by centrifugation [16, 17].

The results are shown in Figure 4. In normal plasma, identical renin activities were attained with acid and with trypsin. The rate of activation differed with the two procedures but the same plateau was reached, which indicated that all the renin that could be activated by serine protease was indeed activated.

Lineweaver-Burk plots of the reactions of naturally occurring active plasma renin, acid-activated plasma renin, trypsin-activated plasma renin and human kidney renin (MRC standard 68/356) with sheep-renin substrate gave identical Km-values. Thus, the increase in renin activity after acidification and with trypsin is caused by a parallel change in the number of active renin molecules rather than by changes in the enzymatic activity per molecule of active renin.

Factor XII-deficient and prekallikrein-deficient plasmas had much lower renin activity after pH 3.3-treatment than with trypsin-treatment. In fact, renin activity did not increase in the neutral phase after acid-dialysis. This demonstrates that the activation of inactive renin after acid-treatment depends on both factor XII and prekallikrein, whereas the activation with trypsin does not depend on these endogenous factors.

Identification of Kallikrein as the Major Activator of 'Prorenin' in the Factor XII-Prekallikrein-Dependent Pathway

Active factor XII fragment, factor β-XIIa (600 μg/ml), a gift from Dr. John Griffin, La Jolla, USA, gave a single band on SDS-polyacrylamide gel electrophoresis with an apparent molecular weight of 28.000 Kallikrein (200 μg/ml) was prepared by activation of purified plasma prekallikrein by factor β-XIIa, and was separated from factor β-XIIa by DEAE-Sephadex chromatography at pH 8.25 [22]. Factor β-XIIa (final concentration 10 μg/ml) was added to prekallikrein-deficient plasma after dialysis of the plasma at pH 3.3 for 24 hours and subsequent restoration of pH to 7.5. Plasma kallikrein (final concentration 32 μg/ml) was added to factor XII-deficient plasma, again after acid-dialysis and subsequent restoration of pH. As shown in Table 2, factor β-XIIa, in a physiological concentration, was not capable of generating active renin in pre-

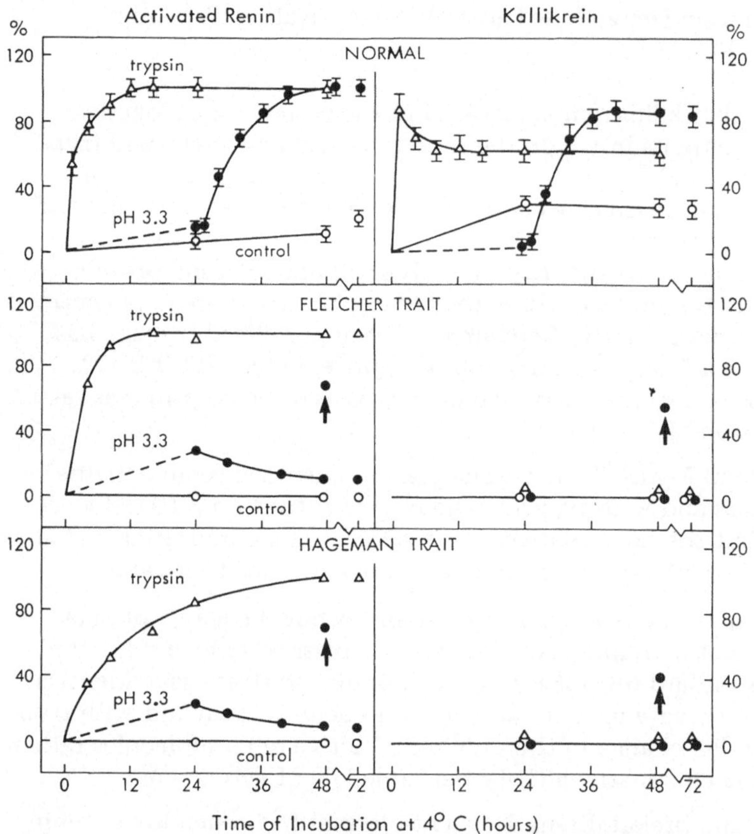

Fig. 4. Activation of inactive renin and prekallikrein in normal plasma (mean ± SEM, n = 10), prekallikrein (Fletcher factor)-deficient plasma and factor XII (Hageman factor)-deficient plasma. Two procedures were used: acidification and addition of trypsin. The generation of renin and kallikrein (amidolytic) activities was followed in acidified plasma after pH had been restored to 7.5 with NaOH (●——●), or after addition of immobilized trypsin (△——△). The increment of renin after 48 hours exposure to trypsin, and the kallikrein activity obtained after optimal activation of prekallikrein with dextran sulphate were taken as 100 percent activation. Plasma that was kept at 4°C without any other from of treatment served as a control (○—○). Note that renin did not increase in the deficient plasmas. This abnormality was partly restored by the addition of purified plasma prekallikrein (50 μg/ml) and factor XII (28 μg/ml) to respectively the pellikallikrein- and factor XII-deficient plasmas prior to acidification (results are indicated by arrows). See text for details. ———: pH 3.3. ———: pH 7.5 (From: Derkx et al [16], by courtesy of the publisher)

kallikrein-deficient plasma. In contrast, active kallikrein, again in a physiological concentration, caused complete activation of inactive renin in the absence of factor XII. This indicates that in the factor XII-dependent pathway, plasma

156

Table 2. Activation of inactive renin with plasma kallikrein and factor XII

		not treatment	Renin (μU/ml) pH 3.3-treatment	trypsin treatment	Active renin (percentage of total)
Normal ($n = 14$)	mean ± SEM	20 ± 1	116 ± 8	120 ± 9	18.6 ± 1.2
	range	13 − 26	81 − 160	80 − 170	11.3 − 25.6
Anephric ($n = 17$)	Mean ± SEM	5.2 ± 0.7	32 ± 7	34 = 8	17.3 ± 3.5
	range	0.4 − 10	6.9 − 100	8.0 − 104	0 − 41.0
Plasma-prekallikrein (Fletcher-factor)-deficiency	patient A 39		122	406	9.6
	patient B 10		28	247	4.0
	patient C 9.5		28	326	4.0
	patient D 8.4		80	510	1.6
— with added plasma prekallikrein (50 μg/ml)*	patient D 8.6		363	528	1.6
— with added factor β-XIIa (10 μg/ml)**	patient D —		82	—	—
Factor XII (Hagemann-factor)-deficiency	patient E 17		33	186	9.1
	patient F 22		42	206	10.6
— with added factor XII (28 μg/ml)*	patient F 15		112	186	8.1
— with added plasma kallikrein (32 μg/ml)**	patient F —		193	—	—

pH 3.3-treatment = dialysis for 24 hours at pH 3.3 with subsequent restoration of pH to 7.5 and dialysis for 24 hours at pH 7.5. Trypsin-treatment = incubation for 24 hours at pH 7.5 with Sepharose bound trypsin. * The proenzymes were added before pH 3.3-dialysis. ** The active enzymes were added to pH 3.3-treated plasma after restoration of pH to 7.5, and the mixtures were incubated at 4°C for 24 hours. See methods section for further details

kallikrein is the major, i.e. more direct, activator of inactive renin. The factor XII-dependency can be explained by the capacity of this factor to convert plasma prekallikrein to kallikrein.

Evidence that Plasma Kallikrein is Important for the Activation of "Prorenin" In-Vivo

The first evidence came from measurements of naturally occurring active renin and trypsin-activatable inactive renin in four subjects with prekallikrein-deficiency (Fletcher trait) (Table 2). The percentage of plasma renin that was active was abnormally low in each case. Three subjects had levels of active renin that were as low as in anephrics, and all subjects had abnormally high levels of inactive renin. In two subjects with factor XII-deficiency (Hageman trait) the abnormalities were less clear-cut; active renin was normal, and inactive renin was just above normal.

The second piece of evidence came from measurements of angiotensin-converting enzyme, renin and prekallikrein in the plasma of eight hypertensive subjects before and after a single dose of the orally active angiotensin-converting enzyme inhibitor, Captopril (50 mg). Converting enzyme was determined with a sensitive spectrophotometric assay [23]. It measures the rate of production of hippuric acid from the substrate hippuryl-L-His-Leu at 37°C and pH 8.3. Results are expressed as nanokatals per ml (nkat/ml), one katal being the quantity of enzyme that catalyses the conversion of one mole of substrate under the conditions of the assay.

As shown in Figure 5, Captopril caused a rapid fall of angiotensin-converting enzyme activity. This was accompanied with an equally rapid fall of blood pressure, a sharp rise of active renin, and a fall of dextran sulphate activatable prekallikrein. Sixteen hours after the gift of Captopril these parameters had more or less returned to their inital values.

Conclusion

The data demonstrate that plasma kallikrein can mediate activation of inactive renin *in-vitro*. They further provide circumstantial evidence that plasma kallikrein may also participate in the activation of inactive renin *in-vivo*. Besides trypsin and kallikrein, there are other proteolytic enzymes, such as plasmin [24, 25], pepsin [26] and cathepsin D [27] that are capable of activating inactive renin. At a first glance this seems to indicate that the activation process is rather unspecific, but the activation of other physiologically important proenzymes shows the same kind of "unspecifity". In fact, one now begins to realize that this apparent lack of specifity is the biochemical basis for linking the diverse functions of different proteolytic systems. Such a linkage is probably essential for establishing a fine homeostatic balance, for instance between the coagulation and fibrinolytic systems with their opposite effects on hemostasis,

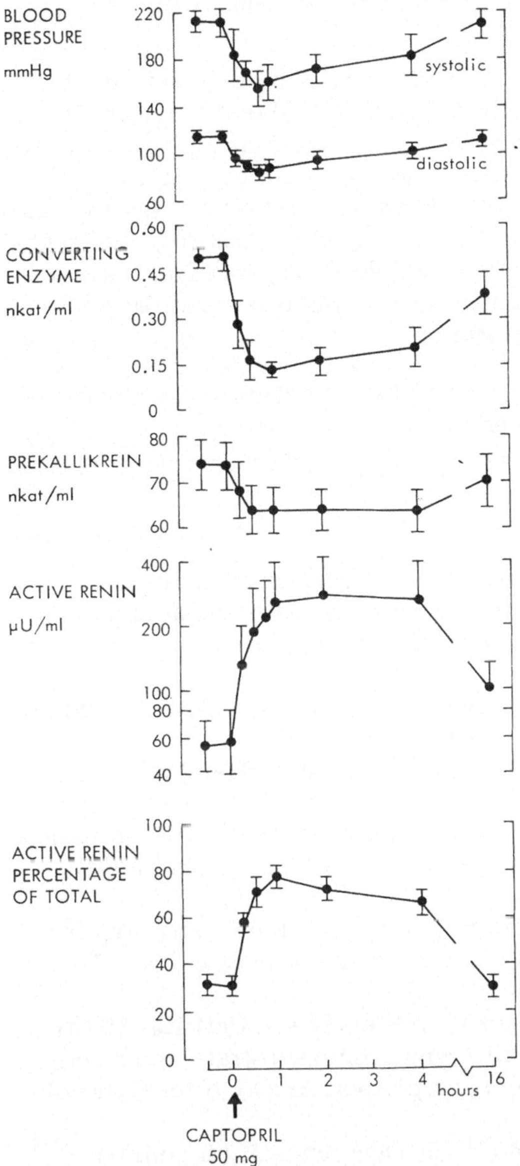

Fig. 5. Effects of the angiotensin-converting enzyme inhibitor, Captopril (50 mg orally), in hypertensive subjects (mean ± SEM, n = 8). The changes in arterial pressure, converting enzyme activity and active renin one hour after Captopril were significant at a P-value of less than 0.001 (paired t test). The change in plasma prekallikrein at that time was significant at a P-value of less than 0.05

and between the renin-angiotensin and kallikrein-kinin systems with their opposite effects on blood pressure.

There are other intriguing analogies. The cascade of proteolytic reactions that ultimately lead to coagulation can be activated by plasma-bound factors (intrinsic pathway) but tissue factors can also participate in some activation steps (extrinsic pathway). The same is true for the fibrinolytic process. It is therefore interesting that inactive plasma renin can be activated *in-vitro* not only by plasma kallikrein but also by glandular (renal) kallikrein, which is clearly different from plasma kallikrein [28, 29]. Thus, plasma kallikrein is part of an intrinsic pathway for activating the renin-angiotensin system, whereas glandular kallikrein might be involved in extrinsic activation.

Acknowledgement. This research was supported by a grant from the Organization of Health Research TNO, The Netherlands.

References

1. Kaplan AP, Austen KF (1975) Activation and control mechanisms of Hageman factordependent pathways of coagulation, fibrinolysis and kinin generation and their contribution to the inflammatory response. J Allergy Clin Immunol 56 : 491
2. Ogston D, Bennett B (1978) Surface-mediated reactions in the formation of thrombin, plasmin and kallikrein. Br Med Bull 34 : 107
3. Tigerstedt R, Bergmann PA (1898) Niere und Kreislauf. Skand Arch Physiol 8 : 223
4. Braun-Menendez E, Fasciolo JC, Leoir LF, Munou JM (1939) La substancia hipertensora de la sangre del rinon isquemiado. Rev Soc Argent Biol 15 : 420
5. Page IH, Helmer OM (1940) A crystalline pressor substance (angiotensin) resulting from the reaction between renin and renin activator. J Exp Med 71 : 29
6. Skinner SL, Cran EJ, Gibson R, Taylor R, Walters WAW, Catt KJ (1975) Angiotensin I and II, active and inactive renin, renin substrate, renin activity and angiotensinase in liquor amnii and plasma. Am J Obstet Gynecol 121 : 626
7. Day RP, Leutscher JA, Gonzales CM (1975) Occurence of big renin in human plasma, amniotic fluid and kidney extracts. J Clin Endocrinol Metab 40 : 1078
8. Derkx FHM, Wenting GJ, Mean in 't Veld AJ, Gool JMG van, Verhoeven RP, Schalekamp MADH (1976) Inactive renin in human plasma. Lancet II: 496
9. Sealey JE, Moon C, Laragh JH, Alderman M (1976) Plasma prorenin: cryoactivation and relationship to renin substrate in normal subjects. Am J Med 61 : 731
10. Leckie BJ, Mc Connel A, Morton JJ, Tree M, Brown JJ (1977) An inactive renin in human plasma. Circ Res 40 (Suppl) : 46

11. Atlas SA, Laragh JH, Sealey JE (1978) Activation of inactive plasma renin: evidence that both cryoactivation and acid activation work by liberating a neutral serine protease from endogenous inhibitors. Clin Sci Mol Med 55 (supp). 135s

12. Derkx FHM, Tan Tjiong HL, Schalekamp MADH (1978) Endogenous activator of plasma inactive renin. Lancet II : 218

13. Leckie BJ (1978) An endogenous protease activating plasma inactive renin. Clin Sci Mol Med 55 (suppl): 133s

14. Osmond DH, Loh AY (1978) Protease as endogenous activator of inactive renin. Lancet I: 102

15. Derkx FHM, Wenting GJ, Man in 't Veld AJ, Verhoeven RP, Schalekamp MADH (1978) Control of enzymatically inactive renin in man under various pathological conditions: implications for the interpretation of renin measurements in peripheral and renal venous plasma. Clin Sci Mol Med 42 : 529

16. Derkx FHM, Bouma BN, Schalekamp MPA, Schalekamp MADH (1979) An intrinsic factor XII-prekallikrein-dependent pathway activates the human plasma renin-angiotensin system. Nature 280 : 315

17. Derkx FHM, Tan Tjiong HL, Man in 't Veld AJ, Schalekamp MPA, Schalekamp MADH (1979) Activation of inactive renin by plasma and tissue kallikreins. Clin Sci 57 : 351

18. Claeson G, Friberger P, Knös M, Eriksson E (1978) Methods for determination of prekallikrein in plasma, glandular kallikrein and urokinase. Haemostasis 7 : 76

19. Kluft C (1973) Determination of prekallikrein in human plasma: optimal conditions for activating prekallikrein. J Lab Clin Med 91 : 83

20. Harpel PC (1973) Studies on human plasma α_2-macroglobulin-enzyme interaction. J Exp Med 138 : 508

21. Bouma BN, Miles LA, Beretta G, Griffin JH (in press) Human plasma prekallikrein; studies of its activation by activated factor XII and of its inactivation by diisoprophylphosphofluoridate.

22. Griffin JH, Cochrane CG (1976) Human factor XII (Hageman factor). Meth Enzym 45 : 56

23. Cushman DW, Cheung HS (1971) Spectrophotometric assay and properties of the angiotensin-converting enzyme of the rabbit lung. Biochem Pharmacol 20 : 1637

24. Derkx FHM, Tan Tjiong HL, Schalekamp MADH (1979) An activator of inactive renin in human plasma: its connection with kinin formation, coagulation and fibrinolysis (abstr). Proceedings of the sixth scientific meeting of the international society of hypertension, Göteborg, 29

25. Sealey JE, Atlas SA, Laragh JH, Silverberg M, Kaplan AL (1979) Plasma prorenin activation by plasmin, Hageman factor fragments, and plasma kallikrein (abstr). Proceedings of the sixth scientific meeting of the international society of hypertension, Göteborg, 56

26. Morris NG, Lumbers ER (1972) The activation of renin in human amniotic fluid by proteolytic enzymes. Biochim Biophys Acta 289 : 385

27. Morris BJ (1979) Activation of human inactive ("Pro") renin by cathepsin and pepsin. J Clin Endocrinol Metab 46 : 153
28. Sealey JE, Atlas SA, Laragh JH, Oza NB, Ryan JW (1978) Human urinary kallikrein converts inactive to active renin and is a possible physiological activator of renin. Nature 275 : 144
29. Derkx FHM, Tan Tjiong HL, Man in 't Veld AJ, Schalekamp MPA, Schalekamp MADH (1979) Activation of inactive renin by tissue kallikrein. J Endocrinol Metab 49 : 765

Urinary Kallikrein Activity in Rats with Renovascular Hypertension

G. BÖNNER, W. RASCHER, M. MARIN-GREZ, B. RASTETTER, F. GROSS

Summary

Renovascular hypertension in rats was induced by two different methods, the two kidney, one clip renal hypertension and the ligature of the aorta between the origins of both renal arteries. After unilateral renal artery stenosis no correlation was found between blood pressure and urinary kallikrein activity during the development of hypertension, but urinary kallikrein activity was reduced after hypertension was established.

Urinary kallikrein activity was lower in rats with severe hypertension than in rats with the mild form of hypertension (9.85 ± 2.2 μg bradykinin (BK) min^{-1}/d vs.25.0 ± 3.4; p < 0.001). After ligation of the aorta, the urinary kallikrein activity fell more rapidly than after unilateral renal artery stenosis. Unilateral nephrectomy also reduced urinary kallikrein activitiy, but less than in rats with severe renal hypertension. It is concluded [1] that renal kallikrein is probably not involved in the development of renovascular hypertension and [2] that in severe renal hypertension renal kallikrein activity is not only reduced in urine of the ischaemic kidney, but also in urine of the contralateral one.

Introduction

In various types of experimental and of clinical hypertension a decreased kallikrein activity in urine has been reported. In spontaneously hypertensive rats and in rats with renovascular hypertension excretion of kallikrein in urine is reduced [2, 3, 6, 7] and similar observations have been made in patients with essential or renal hypertension [4, 10, 12]. On the basis of these findings, is has been presumed that a diminished activity of the renal kallikrein-kinin system could be related to the increase in blood pressure [4]. However, the significance of that system for the development of high blood pressure is not clear at all. In order to obtain further information how changes in the activity of the renal kallikrein-kinin system might be related to the pathogenesis of renal hypertension we studied the excretion of kallikrein in the two kidneys, one clip model of renal hypertension and in the accelerated hypertension developing after ligation of the aorta between the origins of the two renal arteries.

Material and Methods

For unilateral nephrectomy, the left kidney was removed under ether anaesthesia in male Sprague-Dawley rats weighing 200 g. Weight-matched control rats were sham-operated. Seven days after unilateral nephrectomy urine was collected over 24 hours in metabolic cages.

In male Sprague-Dawley rats weighing 150 g, hypertension was induced by putting a silver clip of 0.19 mm internal diameter on the left renal artery leaving the contralateral kidney untouched. Sham operated rats were used as controls. For measurement of kallikrein activity urine was collected 2, 10 and 35 days after surgery over 24 hours in metabolic cages. At the end of each collection period, systolic blood pressure was measured by tail plethysmography.

In addition, rats of the same strain and weight were made hypertensive by ligation of the aorta between the origin of both renal arteries. The control rats were sham operated. Eight days after surgery, 24-hours-urine was collected for the measurement of kallikrein, sodium and potassium excretion. At the end of the collection period intraarterial blood pressure, kidney and body weight were determined.

Kallikrein activity was measured by two different methods: (1) the generation of kinins released from dog kininogen was determined by bradykinin radioimmunoassay as reported previously [12]; (2) urine was incubated with the chromogenic tripeptide H-D-Val-Leu-Arg-pNA in a modification of the method reported by Amundson [1]. The cleaved p-nitroaniline was measured by photometry and kallikrein activity was expressed in enzymatic units (U). In serial measurements, the kallikrein activity of one urine sample was determined simultaneously by those two methods, a good correlation ($r = 0.9454$; $p < 0.001$) of the values was found. Urinary sodium and potassium concentrations were determined by flame photometry. All values are given as means ± sem. The significance of differences between mean values was calculated by Student's t-test.

Results

One week after unilateral nephrectomy, urinary kallikrein activity was reduced to 58% of the excretion rate in intact rats (11.8 ± 0.8 μg BK min^{-1}/d vs. 20.3 ± 3.3; $p < 0.005$). Water, sodium and potassium excretions remained unchanged.

In the two kidneys, one clip renal hypertension (Table 1), blood pressure was slightly increased after only two days clamping, while kallikrein activity in the urine was unaltered. Ten days after surgery, blood pressure had increased to 150.0 ± 3.1 mm Hg ($p < 0.001$), but kallikrein activity remained unaffected. There was no difference in sodium and potassium excretion between hypertensive and normotensive rats. Five weeks after clamping, urinary kallikrein activity was lower in the hypertensive rats compared to the normotensive control

164

Table 1. Blood pressure, urinary volume and urinary kallikrein activity in male Sprague Dawley rats 2, 10 and 35 days after clamping of the left renal artery

Day after clamping	Blood pressure (mm Hg)		Urinary volume (ml)		Urinary kallikrein activity (μg BK min^{-1}/d)	
2	119.7 ± 2.1	+ 128.4 ± 2.3	13.1 ± 1.3	++ 22.3 ± 1.7	24.0 ± 1.6	21.7 ± 1.4
10	117.9 ± 2.9	++ 150.0 ± 3.1	13.4 ± 1.4	+ 17.7 ± 1.2	21.1 ± 2.1	18.1 ± 2.4
35	107.4 ± 2.7	++ 200.2 ± 7.1	14.3 ± 2.3	++ 43.1 ± 8.5	35.6 ± 1.5	++ 16.9 ± 2.9
group	control (n = 10)	hypertensive (n = 20)	control	hypertensive	control	hypertensive

+ $p < 0.05$ ++ $p < 0.005$

Table 2. Urinary kallikrein activity (UKAL), sodium and potassium excretion in 24 hours urine (U[Na$^+$] V, U[K$^+$]V), arterial blood pressure (ABP) and kidney weight in male Sprague Dawley rats 8 days after ligation of the aorta between the origin of both renal arteries

group	U KAL (U/d)	U [Na$^+$]V (mmol/d)	U[K$^+$]V (mmol/d)	right kidney (mg)	left kidney (mg)	ABP (mm Hg)
controls (n = 7)	0.87 ± 0.07	5.73 ± 0.25	3.83 ± 0.48	1155 ± 46	1087 ± 31	109.3 ± 3.5
	++	++	+	ns	++	++
aortic ligation (n = 6)	0.13 ± 0.04	3.06 ± 0.69	2.04 ± 0.34	1095 ± 55	552 ± 49	160.6 ± 8.8

+ $p < 0.05$ ++ $p < 0.005$

rats. When renal hypertensive rats were divided into two groups according to
the degree of hypertension, those with the severe course (group A) had a marked fall of kallikrein activity (9.85 ± 2.2 μg BK min^{-1}/d; p < 0.001). In rats with
the mild course of hypertension (group B) only a small reduction of kallikrein
activity (25.0 ± 3.4; p < 0.05), was observed compared to the normotensive
control rats (35.6 ± 1.5 μg BK min^{-1}/d). Thus, only 35 days after clamping,
blood pressure is inversly correlated to urinary kallikrein activity (r = 0.6285;
p < 0.01). At this time, the rats with severe hypertension had a small, but statistically not significant increase in electrolyte excretion (Na$^+$: A: 2.9 ± 0.8
mmol/d vs. C: 2.3 ± 0.2; K$^+$: A: 2.8 ± 0.5 mmol/d vs. C: 2.2 ± 0.1).

Eight days after aortic ligature kallikrein activity had decreased both in the renal
hypertensive rats (Table 2) and in the rats with total necrosis of the left kidney
and only a small increase in blood pressure (kallikrein activity: 0.44 ± 0.01
U/d, p < 0.001; blood pressure: 127 ± 4 mm Hg, p < 0.05). The daily excretion
of sodium and potassium was reduced significantly in the hypertensive rats as
compared to the normotensive rats. This was caused by the lower daily food
intake of the hypertensive rats (11.6 ± 1.1; vs. 22.7 ± 0.6 g; p < 0.001). Kidneys below the ligature were small and had an atrophic cortex, while the contralateral kidneys showed no detectable weight gain (Table 2). So, these findings resulted in a reduced total kidney mass.

Discussion

In renal hypertension both reduced [2, 12] and increased [11] kallikrein activity has been reported. In our experiments only in established hypertension a
diminished kallikrein activity was found, but not during the developmental
phase, when compared to the normotensive control rats, which showed the
normal increase of urinary kallikrein activity with age and weight gain (unpublished observations). Hence no correlation existed between the increase in blood
pressure and the reduction of urinary kallikrein activity. In contrast to the delayed decrease in kallikrein excretion after unilateral renal artery stenosis, a
prompt fall occurred after ligation of the aorta between the origins of the renal
arteries. Since, under these experimental conditions, the kidney distal to the
ligation became atrophic within one week, it might be possible that the diminished kallikrein activity in the urine is caused rather by the reduction of renal
mass than by the increase in blood pressure.

The significance of renal mass for the exretion of kallikrein is obvious by the
reduced excretion after unilateral nephrectomy where a decrease by 42% was
found. This dimination is in the same order as that seen in rats with total necrosis of the kidney behind the ligature of the aorta (49%).

In severe course of both forms of renovascular hypertension the excretion of
kallikrein falls by 65% if compared with the sham operated control rats. Hence
it may be concluded that kallikrein release is not only diminshed in the ischaemic kidney but also in the contralateral organ. No satisfactory explanation for

this more pronounced fall of kallikrein activity in the urine can be given, but several possibilities may be mentioned. Firstly, in the severe form of hypertension a greater excretion rate of plasma protein is known [5]. In the case of increased proteinuria, more plasmatic kallikrein inhibitors could be present in the urine. They may provoke a decrease of enzymatic activity of urinary kallikrein, while the enzyme content may remain unchanged. Secondly, there might also be a damage in the contralateral kidney caused by the prolonged influence of a markedly elevated blood pressure (8) with the consequence of a diminution of kallikrein release from the kidney. Thirdly the reduction of extracellular fluid volume or intravascular volume (7) or the decreased excretion of sodium and potassium might induce a diminished kallikrein excretion. However, as long as we dont know the physiological stimulus responsible for the release of kallikrein from the kidney it will not be possible to get more precise information in the factor(s) responsible for the diminished kallikrein activity in urine. On the other hand it may be stated that the results obtained do not indicate a direct relationship between the height of blood pressure and the excretion of renal kallikrein.

Acknowledgement: The synthetic chromogenic substrate (S 2266) was kindly supplied by Kabi Chemie, F.R.G. These studies were supported by the German Research Foundation within the SFB 90 "Cardiovaskuläres System". G. Bönner is recipient of a German Research Foundation fellowship, M. Marin-Grez of a Alexander von Humboldt Foundation fellowship.

References

1. Amundsen E, Pütter J, Friberger P, Knös M, Larsbraten M, Claeson G (1979) Methods for the determination of glandular kallikreins by means of a chromogenic tripeptide substrate. Plenum Press, New York
2. Carretero OA, Oza NB, Scicli AG, Schork A (1974) Renal tissue kallikrein, plasma renin and plasma aldosterone in renal hypertension. Acta Physiol Lat Am 24 : 448
3. Carretero OA, Amin HM, Ocholik T, Scicli AG, Koch G (1978) Urinary kallikrein in rats bred for their susceptibility and resistance to the hypertensive effect of salt. Circ Res 42 : 727
4. Carretero OA, Scicli AG (1978) The renal kallikrein-kinin system in human and in experimental hypertension. Klin Wochenschr Suppl I 56 : 113
5. Cottier P (1968) Die Gefäßerkrankung der Niere. In: Schwiegk H (ed) Nierenkrankheiten (Handbuch der Inneren Medizin 8/II). Springer, Berlin Heidelberg New York, p 513
6. Croxatto HR, Martin MS (1970) Kallikrein-like activity in the urine of renal hypertensive rats. Experientia 26 : 1216
7. Geller RG, Margolius HS, Pisano JJ, Keiser HR (1975) Urinary kallikrein excretion in spontaneously hypertensive rats. Circ Res Suppl I 36 : 103
8. Gross F, Dietz R, Mast GJ, Szokol M (1975) Salt loss as a possible mechanism eliciting an acute malignant phase in renal hypertensive rats. Clin Exp Pharmacol Physiol 2 : 323

9. Heptinstall RH (1966) Hypertension. In: Pathology of the Kidney. Churchill, London, p 119
10. Hulthin UL, Lecerof H, Hökfelt B (1977) Renal venous output of kinins in patients with hypertension and unilateral renal artery stenosis. Acta Med Scan 202 : 189
11. Johnston CJ, Matthews PG, Dax E (1976) Renin-angiotensin and kallikrein-kinin systems in sodium homeostasis and hypertension in rats. Clin Sci Mol Med 51 : 283s
12. Lechi A, Covi G, Lechi C, Corgnati A, Arosio E, Zatti M, Scuro LA (1978) Urinary kallikrein excretion and plasma renin activity in patients with essential hypertension and primary aldosteronism. Clin Sci Mol Med 55 : 51
13. Stocker M, Hornung J (1978) Application of bradykinin radio-immunoassay for the measurement of urinary kallikrein activity in rats. Klin Wochenschr Suppl I 56 : 127

Enhanced Parotid Kallikrein Secretion in Essential, Adrenal Hypertension and in Advanced Renal Failure – Inverse Relationship to Sodium Excretion[1]

A. RÖCKEL, G. STÜRMER, G. SCHMID, A. HEIDLAND

There are several lines of evidence that the renal kallikrein-kinin system (KKS) is altered in various forms of hypertension, probably indicating a defective vasodepressor system as a pathogenetic factor in blood pressure regulation. Urinary kallikrein excretion was found to be decreased in patients with essential [9, 15, 18, 19, 35], renovascular [13] and renoparenchymal hypertension [25, 27] and elevated in primary aldosteronism [18, 27]. Furthermore, a dependence of the activity of the renal KKS on factors involved in the pathogenesis of hypertension (extracellular volume [21], sodium- and potassium balance [1, 10, 19, 22, 26, 36], and mineralocorticoids [19]), was established.

The impact of the reduced kallikrein-excretion is limited by the possible dependence of urinary kallikrein excretion from the effective renal mass, which might be reduced in various forms of hypertension due to nephrosclerosis and/or the underlying vascular or inflammatory kidney disease. Therefore investigations of the KKS in other kallikrein-containing tissues might be of interest.

The major salivary glands seems suitable as an appropriate test model, since these glands as well as their secretions contain large amounts of kallikrein. The kallikrein containing striated duct cells of the parotis morphologically resemble that of the distale renal tubule, known to be the major target cells for mineralocorticoids, involved in the distal tubular sodium- and potassium handling. The structural conformity of these cells and the localization of kallikrein at the luminal border of the duct cells implies that its secretion might be linked with the local electrolyte transport, that means sodium reabsorption and potassium-secretion.

The present study was designed to investigate the salivary kallikrein excretion and to elucidate if there is a generalized disturbance of the kallikrein-kinin system in various forms of hypertension. Furthermore it was of interest to discover if there is an interaction between kallikrein-, sodium- and potassium handling in the parotid gland.

---

1 Supported by the "Deutsche Forschungsgemeinschaft" SFB Biomund

Methods

The studies were carried out at rest and by fasting between 8.00 a.m. and 11.00 a.m. in five groups of patients. Consent was obtained from each subject. Patients with cardiac arrhythmias, cardiac insufficiency or with hypertension classified as belonging to WHO grade III and malignant hypertension were excluded. All patients and probands were on a sodium diet with an average of 5-10 g NaCl/die.

Controls

30 subjects aged 34.7 ± 1.27 years with normal renal function and no history of renal disease were studied. Their plasma creatinine ($P_{creat.}$) was below 1.3 mg/dl and their blood pressure $121.4/81.1 \pm 1.97/1.83$ mm Hg.

Essential Hypertension

13 patients aged 31.3 ± 2.16 years with a $P_{creat.} < 1.3$ mg/dl and no history and signs of renal disease were studied. Their blood pressure was $156.8/107.6 \pm 2.80/1.66$ mm Hg. Eight of them were classified as belonging to WHO grade I and five to WHO grade II. Antihypertensive drugs (β-receptor-blocking agents and thiazides) were discontinued at least 14 days before the experiment.

Reno-parenchymal Hypertension

All patients with renal hypertension had chronic glomerulonephritis. Thirteen of the patients were classified as belonging to WHO grade II and seven patients to WHO grade I. The $P_{creat.}$ was less than 3 mg/dl in ten patients (group I), and higher than 3.0 mg/dl (group II) in ten patients.

Group I: The mean age of the patients was 37.7 ± 4.64 years and their blood pressure was $161.4/108.6 \pm 4.84/2.82$ mm Hg. The antihypertensive therapy (thiazides, loop diuretics, dihydralazine, clonidine) was discontinued at least 8 days prior to the study. These patients had no restriction of dietary protein.

Group II: The 10 patients aged 44.0 ± 4.91 years with a blood pressure of $162.0/110.0 \pm 11.21/5.94$ mm Hg were treated antihypertensively with loop diuretics, β-receptor-blockers, hydralazine and/or clonidine. Antihypertensive drugs were omitted at least 8 days before the experiment. Beside their sodium restriction, they received a mixed low protein diet (20-40 g/day) combined in 5 patients ($P_{creat.} > 8$ mg/dl) with essential amino acids (7.5 g/d).

Haemodialysis

Six uraemic hypertensive patients (blood pressure: $171/106 \pm 6.0/14.7$ mm Hg) on regular haemodialysis for 27.0 ± 25.2 months were studied. Their ages averaged 44.2 ± 11.9 years, and their GFR ranged from 0 to 4 ml/min. The hypertensive patients were treated with clonidine (450 μg/d;n = 2), guanfacine (4 mg/d;n = 2) and phenoxybenzamine (2 mg/d;n = 1), respectively. Antihypertensive therapy was discontinued at least 24 hours before experiment. Seven patients had glomerulonephritis, two had pyelonephritis, and one had polycystic kidney disease. Patients were dialysed for 6 hrs, three times weekly using either RP 5 (Rhone Poulene, medical) or Gambro Optimal (Gambro Lundia) dialysers. A dietary protein intake of 1 g/kg/day was advised and supplements of vitamin B 6 (15 mg/day) were given.

Phaeochromocytoma

A 13 year old boy with a norepinephrine producing phaeochromocytoma was investigated (using citrate for stimulation of salivary flow rate) before therapy (blood pressure: 180/130 mm Hg) and three weeks after (blood pressure: 130/90 mm Hg) ectomy of the tumor.

Collection of Saliva

The main excretory duct of the parotid gland was cannulated unilaterally with a polyvinyl ethylene tubing. Stimulation of the flow rate was obtained by subcutaneous injection of pilocarpine (0.06 mg/kg b.w.) or by citrate. Only the data from individuals with flow rates increasing higher than 1.0 ml/min were used for statistical analysis. For methods see Kreusser et al. (1972) (14).

Kallikrein measurements were performed as described by Amundsen et al. (1978) using the chromogenic substrate S 2266 of Kabi, Stockholm. Salivary sodium and potassium concentrations were analysed by flame photometry.

Statistical Analysis

The results are given as mean values ± SEM. Differences between the various groups of patients were examined by the non-paired student-test.

Results

Control subjects (black areas: mean value ± SEM):

The salivary kallikrein- (r = 0.36; Fig. 1) and potassium-concentration (r = 0.40; Fig. 2) is inversely correlated to the flow rate, whereas the sodium-concentration is directly correlated to the flow rate (r = 0.64; Fig. 3). A direct correlation was established between the parotid kallikrein concentration (pKC) and the potassium concentration (r = 0.46; Fig. 4) and an inverse one with the sodium concentration (r = 0.56;Fig. 5). Between potassium and sodium concentration an inverse relationship could be demonstrated (Fig. 6).

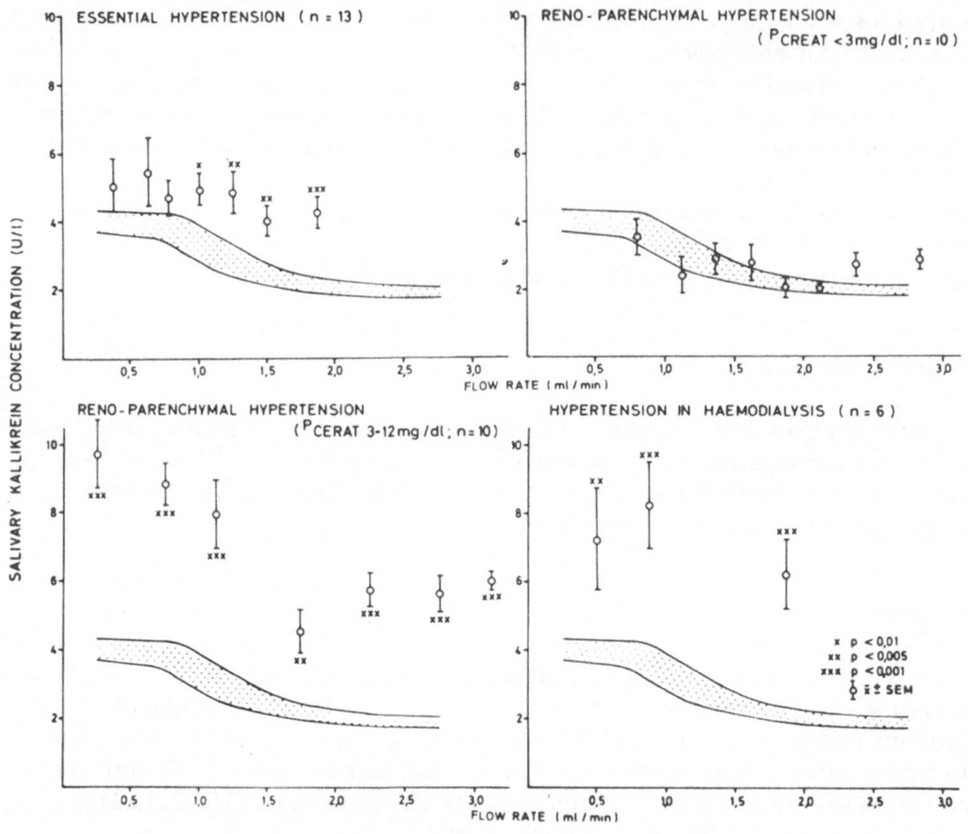

Fig. 1. Flow dependent salivary kallikrein concentration in controls (n = 13; striated area : $\overline{x}$ ± SEM) and in patients with essential and renoparenchymal hypertension. Salivary kallikrein concentration is significantly enhanced in essential hypertension and renal failure ($P_{creat.}$ > 3 mg/dl), but normal in renoparenchymal hypertension ($P_{creat.}$ < 3 mg/dl)

Under pilocarpine stimulation (flow rate (f.r.): 1.5-2.0 ml/min) the kallikrein- and potassium-concentration was nearly constant with 2.0 ± 0.4 U/l, and 10.0 ± 0.50 mval/l, respectively, whereas sodium concentration increased linearly up to 85.8 ± 5.0 mval/l; (f.r. : 2.0 ml/min). The kallikrein concentration was found to be higher with lower f.r. (− 0.75 ml/min : 4.0 ± 0.3 U/l) and during the first 2-3 min following pilocarpine stimulation (3.6 ± 1.4 U/l). These data were therefore not taken for statistical analysis. On the average, the f.r. increased to 1.5 ± 0.6 ml/min after pilocarpine stimulation.

Under stimulation with citrate (f.r.: 1.0 ml/min) the kallikrein- and potassium concentration was 3.8 ± 0.6 U/l and 12.0 ± 2.3 mval/l, respectively. The parotid sodium concentration increased up to 85.0 ± 2.8 mval/l (f.r. : 2.0 ml/min). The mean parotid flow rate was 1.2 ± 0.8 ml/min.

172

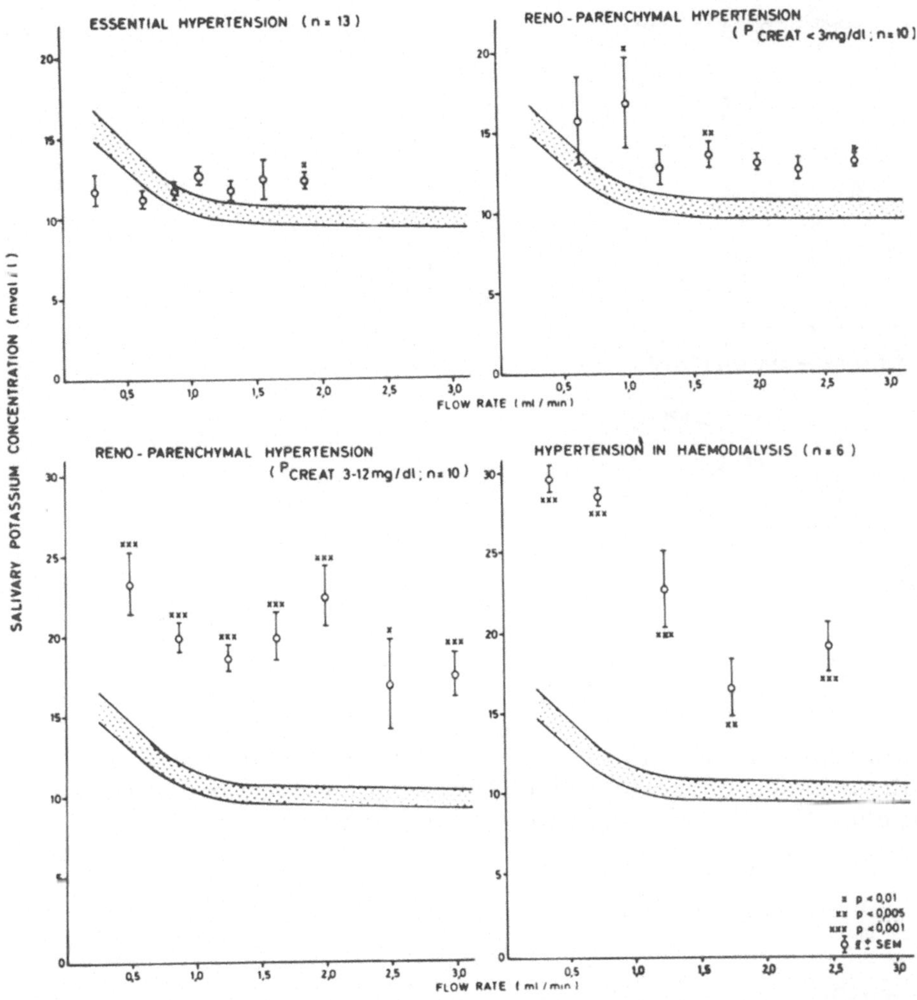

Fig. 2. Flow dependent salivary potassium concentration in controls and in patients with essential and renoparenchymal hypertension. Potassium concentration is significantly increased in the four hypertensive collectives

Essential Hypertension

At a f.r. > 1.0 ml/min parotid kallikrein concentration is significantly elevated (f.r. : 1.9 ml/min : 4.3 ± 0.45 U/l (p < 0.001)). Parotid potassium concentration was slightly elevated at a f.r. between 1.0 and 1.8 ml/min; at a f.r. > 1.8 ml/min a significant increase to 12.4 ± 0.6 mval/l (p < 0.01) was established. Sodium concentration decreased to 52.0 ± 3.0 mval/l (f.r. : 1.8 ml/min; p < 0.001; control value (c.v.) : 76.0 ± 3.0 mval/l). Parasympathetically stimulated f.r. was significantly decreased to 1.1 ± 0.3 ml/min.

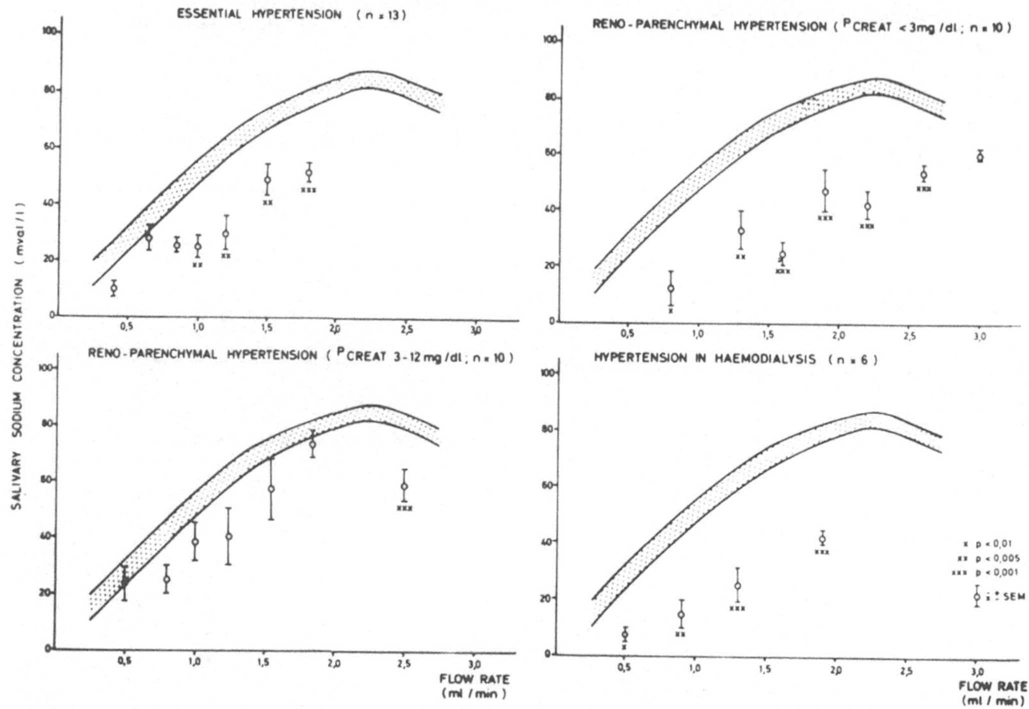

Fig. 3. Flow dependent salivary sodium concentration in controls and in patients with essential and renoparenchymal hypertension. Sodium concentration is significantly reduced in these forms of hypertension

Renoparenchymal Hypertension

Group I

Parotid sodium concentration significantly decreased to 47.5 ± 7.5 mval/l (f.r. : 1.9 ml/min, p < 0.001; v.c. : 74.0 ± 3.0 mval/l), whereas potassium concentration was elevated to 13.5 ± 0.9 mval/l (f.r. : 1.6 ml/min; p < 0.05). Kallikrein concentration was not significantly altered.

Group II

Parotid kallikrein- and potassium concentration significantly increased to 5.75 ± 0.50 U/l (f.r. : 2.25 ml/min; p < 0.001) and 22.5 ± 1.90 mval/l (p < 0.001), whereas sodium concentration was lowered to 58.0 ± 5.5 mval/l (f.r. : 2.5 ml/min; p < 0.01; c.v. : 82.0 ± 2.5 mval/l).

Hypertension in Haemodialysis

Kallikrein and potassium concentration in parotid saliva was significantly elevated to 6.25 ± 1.0 U/l (f.r. : 1.9 ml/min; p < 0.01) and 19.0 ± 1.50 mval/l

174

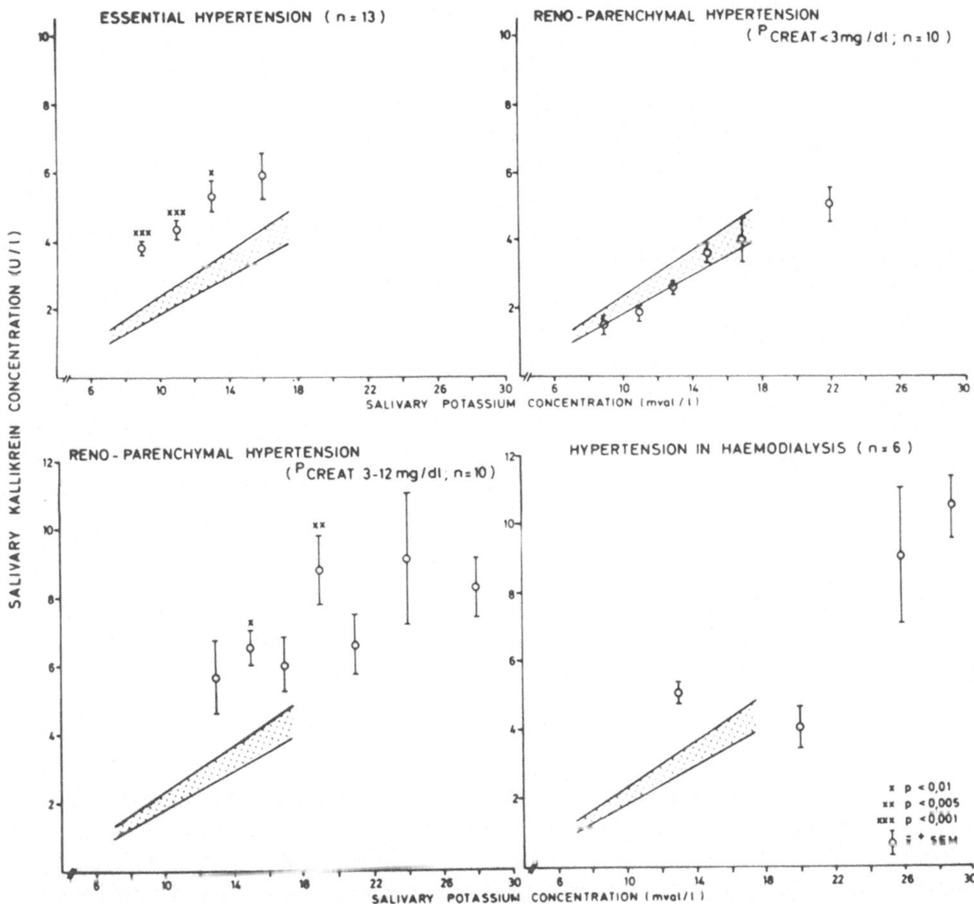

Fig. 4. Relationship between salivary kallikrein- and potassium concentration in controls and patients with essential and renoparenchymal hypertension. Salivary kallikrein concentration is prevalently elevated in essential hypertension. In advanced renal failure kallikrein- and potassium concentration is comparably increased, whereas in renoparenchymal hypertension ($P_{creat.}$ < 3 mg dl) the values were in the normal range

(f.r. : 2.5 ml/min; p < 0.001), respectively. The sodium concentration was lowered to 42.5 ± 2.5 mval/l (f.r. : 1.9; p < 0.001; c.v. : 79.0 ± 3.0 mval/l).

Renal-medullary Hypertension

In a 13 year old boy with phaechromocytoma and a blood pressure of 180/130 mm Hg salivary kallikrein- and potassium concentration was elevated after citrate stimulation to 12.6 U/l, (f.r. : 1.0 ml/min; c.v. : 4.0 ± 0.6 U/l) and 34.4

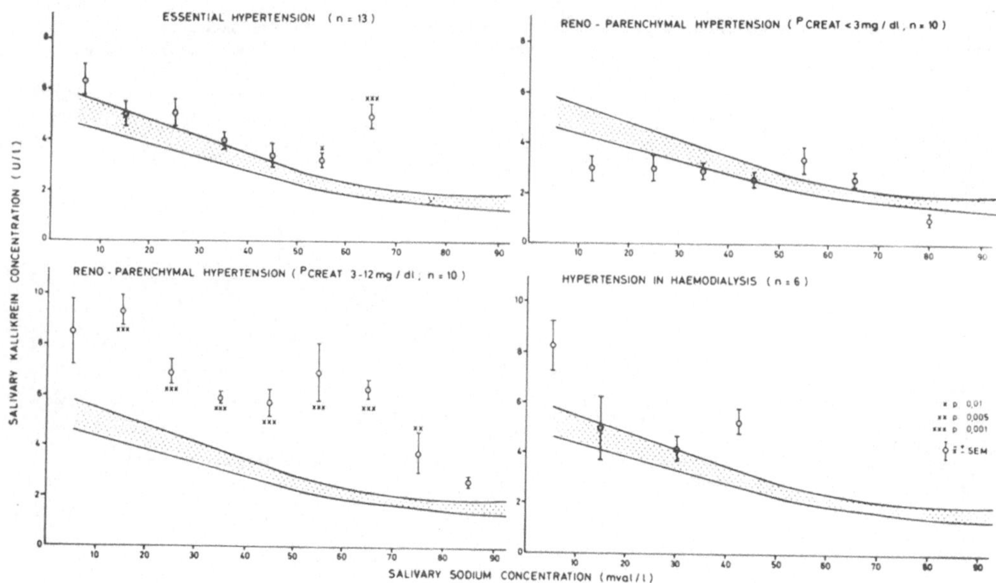

Fig. 5. Relationship between salivary kallikrein- and sodium concentration in controls and in patients with essential and renoparenchymal hypertension. Salivary kallikrein is prevalently excreted in essential hypertension and advanced renal failure

mval/l (f.r. . 1.0 ml/min; c.v. 12.0 ± 2.3 mval/l). Parotid sodium concentration was 20.2 mval/l (f.r. : 1.0 ml/min; c.v. : 50.0 ± 5.0 mval/l). After ectomy of the tumor, blood pressure was normalized. At a comparable f.r. the salivary concentration of kallikrein and potassium were lowered to 5.52 U/l and 22.0 mval/l, respectively, whereas sodium concentration remained constantly.

Discussion

In normal subjects in the parasympathetic stimulated parotid saliva the kallikrein concentration was lower than that published by Eichner et al. [8]. This may be due to the different methods used for the determination; the BAEE-esterase activity might be partly influenced by other esterolytic active proteases, whereas the amidolytic assay utilizing a chromogenic peptide substrate seems to be more specific. Furthermore, differences in the analytical procedure (for instance incubation time) should be taken into account when comparing the results.

In human hypertension Wotman et al. (1969) were the first who investigated the kallikrein activity (BAEE-esterase-activity) in parotid saliva. The results obtained showed no significant difference in the controls and hypertensive subjects. However, the investigations were limited to patients with renoparenchymal hypertension.

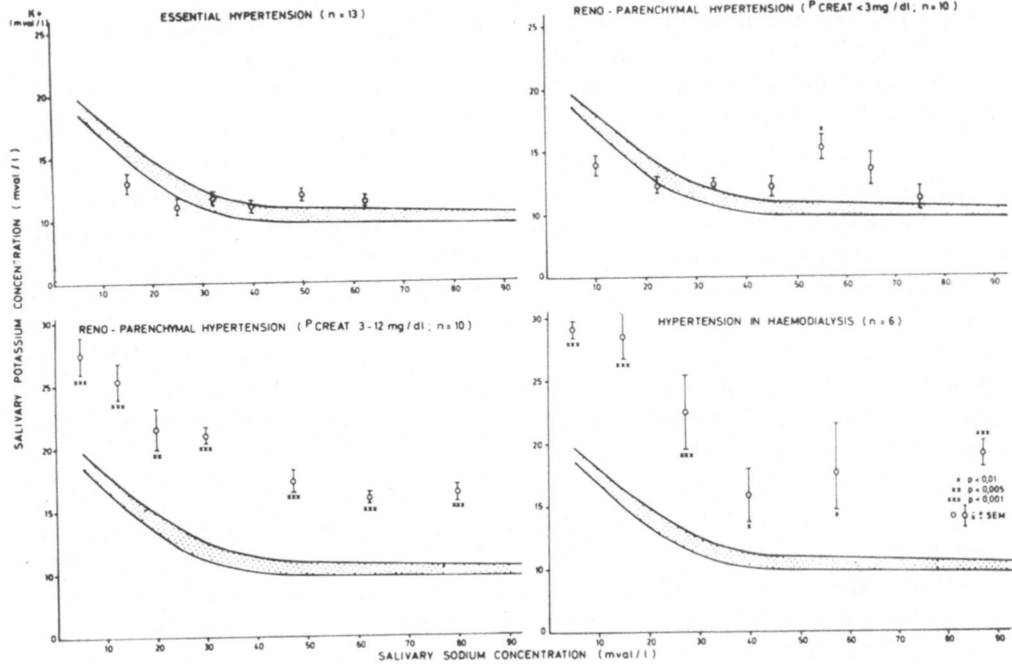

Fig. 6. Relationship between salivary potassium and sodium concentration in controls and in patients with essential and renoparenchymal hypertension. Salivary potassium is prevalently excreted in renoparenchymal hypertension

In essential hypertension as well as in advanced renal failure parotid kallikrein concentration was found to be enhanced. Insofar it can be stated, that the kallikrein secretion of the parotid gland differs markedly from the renal kallikrein secretion. Whether the enhanced kallikrein secretion has some physiological implications such as an increased formation of bradykinin cannot be answered as yet. It is conceivable that in hypertension an inhibitor of the kallikrein activity prevents the formation of kinins similar to the observations made in patients with cystic fibrosis of the pancreas [16].

Concerning the pathogenesis causing in increased salivary kallikrein secretion several mechanisms might be involved. A counterregulatory kallikrein stimulation (due to the elevated blood pressure) can not be proved, since in renoparenchymal hypertension (P $_{creat.}$ < 3 mg/dl) the kallikrein output was not enhanced. Furthermore, a significant relationship between blood pressure and kallikrein concentration — as in experimental hypertension [34] was not established. This indicates that the elevation of blood pressure per se cannot be the single cause of the enhanced kallikrein secretion.

Moreover the increase in salivary kallikrein secretion does not seem to be linked to the activity of the renin angiotensin system. Two patients with a high-renin essential hypertension, and four with a low-renin hypertension showed a comparable pattern of kallikrein output. This agrees with the results obtained in 1-clip-2-kidney- and in DOCTMA salt hypertension [34]. In both models parotid kallikrein concentration is enhanced, even though opposite effects on plasma renin activity are known.

The renal kallikrein excretion is partly controlled by the effective level of circulating, sodium-retaining steroids. This has been shown in man and rats on low sodium diet as well as after administration of mineralocorticoids which enhanced the urinary kallikrein excretion. The observed effects could be suppressed by adrenalectomy in rats and by administration of spironolactone in man [18, 27]. Subnormal plasma-levels and/or a hyporesponsiveness of the KKS to mineralocorticoids could be possible explanations for the low urinary kallikrein excretion in essential hypertension. But in spontaneous hypertensive rats and in human essential hypertension the blood concentrations of the mineralocorticoid hormone were normal.

Increased plasma catecholamine concentrations were found in patients with essential hypertension [5, 7, 11, 17, 32] and in patients receiving regular dialysis treatment [4, 24], at least temporarily, implying an enhanced overall sympathetic activity. Moreover in hypertension an enhanced reagibility of the vascular system [31] as well as of the salivary glands measured by the salivary cAMP output [33] in response to catecholamines is suggested. In the patients with renoparenchymal hypertension (with normal or only slightly impaired kidney function) the plasma catecholamine concentration seems to be unchanged [6].

α-adrenergic drugs and in a minor degree parasympathetic and β-adrenergic stimulation cause a degranulation of granular and striated duct cells and an enhanced salivary kallikrein excretion [23, 29, 30]. The assumption of an activated adrenergic system as the cause of the increased kallikrein secretion in parotid saliva is further supported by the observation of an enhanced secretion of α-amylase [12] and cyclic AMP [33] in the parotid saliva of patients with essential hypertension as well as in rats with experimental hypertension. The enhanced salivary kallikrein excretion of the patient with phaeochromocytoma and the normalization after ectomy of the tumor confirms the suspicion. The hypothesis of an adrenergic induced rise of kallikrein output in hypertension has finally to be proven by administration of both α- and β-adrenergic blocking agents in hypertension.

A direct correlation between kallikrein concentration in parotid saliva and the grade of renal insufficiency (as measured by plasma creatinine level) was established. The enhanced kallikrein output in advanced renal failure was independent of the blood pressure level. Thus, in four normotensive patients on regular dialysis treatment the kallikrein excretion was elevated, too. An enhanced catecholamine release and/or a reduced inactivation in uraemia might cause the increase of kallikrein output.

In the final saliva of the major salivary glands the kallikrein activity is inversely related to sodium concentration: The lower the sodium concentration, the higher the kallikrein-activity and vice versa. Thus, the salivary kallikrein concentration in submandibular gland (rat, cat) is highest, whereas the flow dependent sodium concentration is the lowest of the major salivary glands. On the other hand in the secretion of the lacrimal glands which contains a plasma-like sodium concentration, there is no kallikrein activity detectable.

The inverse relationship between kallikrein and sodium concentration in final saliva is also present after administration of both α- and β-adrenergic drugs, which enhance the reabsorption of sodium and stimulate the secretion of kallikrein and potassium in the duct system [28, 38].

Even under pathophysiological conditions, the inverse relationship between kallikrein and sodium in the saliva can be demonstrated: Thus in patients with essential hypertension and endstage kidney disease there is a markedly reduced concentration of sodium in the parotid saliva and an enhanced secretion of kallikrein. A similar pattern was obtained by Schmid et al. (1979) in the parotid saliva of rats with genetic, DOCTMA-salt and renovascular hypertension.

According to these physiological and pathophysiological relationships, one could assume that there is a link between sodium transport and kallikrein secretion. This link could be present in two fashions: On the one hand it could be possible, that an enhanced sodium reabsorption in the duct system increases the intracellular sodium concentration and thereby releases calcium ions from the intracellular reservoirs, which may serve to trigger zymogen granular exocytosis in conjunction with a release of cyclic AMP. This increased formation of cyclic AMP may favour the secretion of kallikrein [2]. In the distal tubule of the kidney, too, there is some evidence for such a link between sodium reabsorption and kallikrein secretion. Thus after application of amiloride, which blocks the sodium channels of the collecting duct system, there is a simultaneous decrease of kallikrein secretion [20].

On the other hand it might be conceivable that in the various forms of hypertension an enhanced exocytosis of kallikrein into the saliva induces an increased permeability of the luminal plasma membrane of the striated ducts which enhance the sodium reabsorption.

Summary

There are several lines of evidence that the renal kallikrein-kinin system is altered in various forms of hypertension. The impact of these results is limited by the possible dependence of urinary kallikrein excretion from the effective renal mass, which might be reduced in hypertension due to nephrosclerosis and/or the underlying inflammatory kidney disease. Therefore investigations of the kallikrein-kinin system in other kallikrein containing tissues might be of interest.

In normal subjects the kallikrein excretion of parotid saliva is inversely related to flow rate and sodium concentration. An increased salivary kallikrein concentration is found in human essential, adreno-medullary and renoparenchymal hypertension associated with impaired kidney function. In contrast to the kallikrein secretion the flow dependent sodium concentration of parotid saliva is reduced in human essential and renoparenchymal hypertension, which indicates an enhanced sodium reabsorption in the glandular duct system. Furthermore in most forms of hypertension, there is a tendency of higher potassium levels in the saliva.

The pathogenesis of the enhanced glandular kallikrein secretion in hypertension is discussed with regard to a counterregulatory mechanism in hypertension as well as to a sympathetico-adrenergic activation. The enhanced sodium reabsorption in the duct system in the various forms of hypertension could be the cause as well as the consequence of the high blood pressure.

Key words

parotid saliva — kallikrein-human essential, adreno-medullary and renoparenchymal hypertension — sympathetic activity — sodium- and potassium transport

References

1. Adetuyibi A, Mills IH (1972) Relation between urinary kallikrein and renal function, hypertension and excretion of sodium and water in man. Lancet II : 203-207
2. Albano J, Bhoola KD, Heap PF, Lemon MJC (1976) Stimulus-secretion coupling: Role of cyclic AMP, cyclic GMP and calcium in mediating enzyme (kallikrein) secretion. J Physiol 258 : 631-658
3. Amundsen E, Pütter J, Friberger P, Knös M, Larsbraten M, Claeson G (1979) Methods for the determination of glandular kallikrein by means of a chromogenic tripeptide substrate. Plenum Press, New York
4. Brecht HM, Ernst W, Koch KM (1976) Plasma noradrenaline levels in regular haemodialysis patients. Dialysis Transplantation Nephrology 12 : 281-289
5. Brecht HM, Banthien F, Ernst W, Schoeppe W (1976) Increased plasma noradrenaline levels in essential hypertension and their decrease following long-term treatment with a β-blocking agent (Pindolol). Clin Sci 51 : 485-488
6. Brecht HM (1978) Untersuchungen zur pathophysiologischen Bedeutung des sympathischen Nervensystems, des Renin-Angiotensin-Systems und der Natrium-Bilanz bei der essentiellen und renoparenchymalen Hypertonie. Habilitationsschrift, Frankfurt
7. Dargie HJ, Franklin SS, Reid JL (1977) Plasma noradrenaline concentrations in experimental renovascular hypertension in the rat. Clin Sci Mol Med 52 : 477-483
8. Eichner H, Eichner V, Friedler F, Hochstrasser K (1976) Zum Sekretionsverhalten der BAEE-Esterase (Kallikrein) im gesunden menschlichen Parotissekret unter fraktionierter Abnahme bei Ruhe und Reiz. Laryng Rhinol 55 : 239-244

9. Elliot AH, Nuzum FR (1934) The urinary excretion of a depressor substance (kallikrein of Frey and Kraut) in arterial hypertension. Endocrinology 18 : 462-474

10. Geller RG, Margolius HS, Pisano JJ, Keiser HR (1972) Effects of mineralocorticoids, altered sodium intake, and adrenalectomy on urinary kallikrein in rats. Circ Res 31 : 857-861

11. Grobecker H, Saavedra JM, Roizen MF, Weise V, Kopin IJ, Axelrod J (1976) Peripheral and central catecholaminergic neurons in genetic and experimental hypertension in rats. Clin Sci Mol Med Suppl 3 51 : 377-380

12. Heidland A, Hennemann H, Lenhart FP, Kreusser W, Wigand ME (1974) Ional and enzymatic compositon of parotid saliva in arterial hypertension. In: pp 162-174 Distler A, Wolff H-P (eds) Hypertension, current problems Thieme, Stuttgart

13. Keiser HR, Margolius HS, Brown R, Rhamey R, Foster J (1976) Urinary kallikrein in patients with renovascular hypertension. In: Pisano JH, Austen KF (eds) Chemistry and biology of the kallikrein-kinin-system in health and disease. Fogarty Center Proceeding 27 : 423-426

14. Kreusser W, Heidland A, Hennemann H, Wigand ME, Knauf H (1972) Mono- and divalent electrolyte patterns, pCO_2 and pH in relation to flow rate in normal human parotid saliva. Eur J Clin Invest 2 : 398-406

15. Lechi A, Covi G, Lechi C, Corgnati A, Arosio E, Zatti M, Scuro LA (1978) Urinary kallikrein excretion and plasma renin activity in patients with essential hypertension and primary aldosteronism. Clin Sci Mol Med 55 : 51-55

16. Lieberman J, Littenberg GD (1969) Increased kallikrein content of saliva from patients with cystic fibrosis of the pancreas. Pediat Res 3 : 571-578

17. Louis WJ, Doyle AE, Anavekar S (1973) Plasma norepinephrine levels in essential hypertension. N Engl J Med 288 : 599-601

18. Margolius HS, Geller R, Pisano JJ, Sjoerdsma A (1971) Altered urinary kallikrein excretion in human hypertension. Lancet II : 1063-1067

19. Margolius HS, Horwitz D, Pisano JJ, Keiser HR (1974) Urinary kallikrein excretion in hypertensive man. Relationship to sodium intake and sodium-retaining steroids. Circ Res 35 : 82-825

20. Margolius HS (1979) Kallikrein, renal function and hypertensive diseases. 8th Workshop conference Hoechst, Enzymatic Release of Vasoactive Peptides, Schloß Heinsheim

21. Marin-Grez M, Cottone P, Carretero OA (1972) Evidence for an involvement of kinins in regulation of sodium excretion. Am J Physiol 223 : 794-796

22. Marin-Grez M, Carretero OA (1973) The relationship between urinary kallikrein and natriuresis. In: Haberland GL, Rohen JW (eds) p 113-122 Kininogenases (Kallikreins). Schattauer, Stuttgart

23. Matthews RW (1974) The effects of autonomic stimulation upon the rat submandibular gland. Arch Oral Biol 19 : 989-994

24. McGrath BP, Ledingham JGG, Bendict CR (1978) Catecholamines in peripheral venous plasma in patients on chronic haemodialysis. Clin Sci Mol Med 55 : 89-96

25. Milas JA, Levy SB, Holle R, Frigon RP, Stone RA (1978) Urinary kallikrein (UKa): Relationship to hypertension in renal parenchymal disease (RPD). Clin Res 26 : 366 A
26. Mills IH, MacFarlane, NAA, Ward PE, Obika LFO (1976) The renal kallikrein-kinin system and the regulation of salt and water excretion. Fed Proc 35 : 181-188
27. Miyashita A (1971) Urinary kallikrein determination and its physical role in human kidney. Jap J Urol 62 : 507-518
28. Orstavik TB, Nustad K, Brandtzaeg P, Pierce JV (1976) Cellular origin of urinary kallikreins. J Histochem Cytochem 24 : 1037-1039
29. Orstavik TB, Gautvik KM (1977) Regulation of salivary kallikrein secretion in the rat submandibular gland. Acta Physiol Scand 100 : 33-44
30. Orstavik TB (1978) The distribution and secretion of kallikrein in some exocrine organs of the rat. Acta Physiol Scand 104 : 431-442
31. Philipp T, Distler A, Cordes U (1978) Sympathetic nervous system and blood pressure control in essential hypertension. Lancet II : 959-963
32. Reid JL, Zivin JA, Kopin IJ (1975) Central and peripheral adrenergic mechanisms in the development of deoxycorticosterone — saline hypertension in rats. Circ Res 37 : 569-579
33. Schmid G, Hempel K, Fricke L, Wernze H, Heidland A (1976) Cyclic AMP content of human parotid saliva in arterial hypertension and its correlation with plasma renin activity. In: Heidland A, Hennemann H, Kult J (eds) Renal insufficiency. pp 32-36 Thieme, Stuttgart
34. Schmid G, Röckel A, Heidland A (in press) BAEE-esterase (kallikrein-like) acticity in parotid saliva of normal rats and rats with various forms of experimental hypertension (genuine, reno-vascular and DOCA-salt hypertension). Eur J Pharmacol
35. Werle E, Korsten H (1938) Der Kallikreingehalt des Harns, des Speichels und des Blutes bei Gesunden und Kranken. Z Ges Exp Med 103 : 153
36. Wong PY, Talamo RC, Williams GH, Coleman RW (1975) Response of the kallikrein-kinin and renin-angiotensin systems to saline infusion and upright posture. J Clin Invest 55 : 691-698
37. Wotman S, Mandel ID, Greenbaum K (1969) Studies on human salivary kallikrein. Biochem Pharmacol 18 : 1261-1264
38. Young JA, Martin CJ (1971) The effect of a sympatho- and a parasympathomimetic drug on the electrolyte concentration of primary and final saliva in the rat submaxillary gland. Arch Ges Physiol 327 : 285-289

Identification of Angiotensin II- and Kinin-Dependent Mechanisms in Essential Hypertension

A. Overlack, K. O. Stumpe, I. Heck, C. Ressel, M. Kühnert, F. Krück

Introduction

Recently, pharmacologic tools have been used to assess the specific contributions of the renin-angiotensin system to the pathogenesis of essential hypertension [1-3]. One agent, SQ 14.225, and orally active inhibitor of the angiotensin-converting enzyme [4] has been shown to lower pressure in patients with both essential and renovascular hypertension [5-8]. It has been postulated that the blood pressure changes with converting enzyme inhibition are mediated by a fall in angiotensin II concentration [1-3]. However, interpretation of pressure responses to converting-enzyme inhibition has been complicated, since the angiotensin-converting enzyme is identical to the kininase II [9]. Therefore, the fall in blood pressure with converting enzyme inhibition could also be due to diminished degradation of bradykinin [10-12].

The present study was designed to determine whether changes in renin-angiotensin- and/or kallikrein kinin system activity are responsible for blood pressure responses to SQ 14.225. The kallikrein inhibitor aprotinin was used as a tool to seperate the specific contributions of the kallikrein-kinin system to blood pressure changes with converting enzyme inhibition.

Patients and Methods

The study population comprised 26 patients with essential hypertension. All patients had a diastolic pressure greater than 100 mm Hg and had not taken antihypertensive drugs, previously.

Plasma renin activity, plasma aldosterone- and plasma angiotensin II-concentrations were measured by radioimmuno-assay. Plasma converting enzyme was measured by its ability to release dipeptides from acylated tripeptides. Data were analyzed by the Student's paired t-test.

Results

The acute effect of a single oral dose of 100 mg of SQ 14.225 on supine blood pressure was studied in a group of nine patients (Fig. 1). The enzyme inhibitor

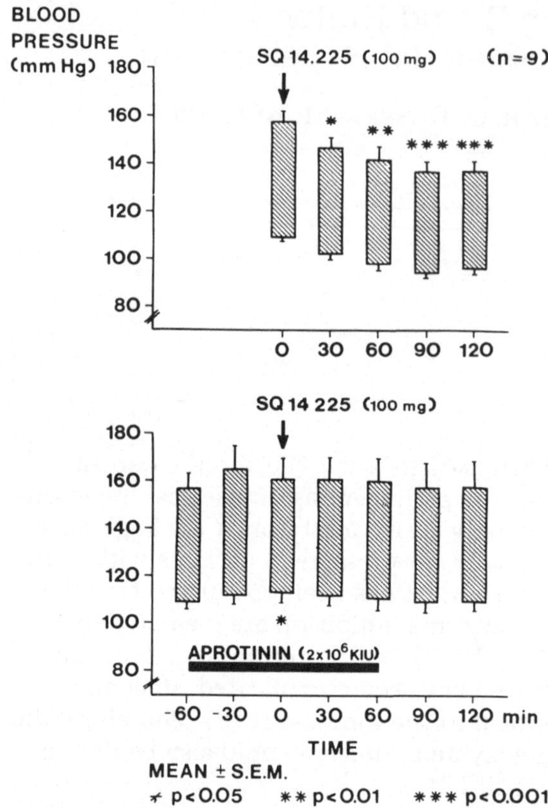

Fig. 1. Blood pressure responses to SQ 14.225 alone (upper part) and in combination with aprotinin (lower part) in untreated essential hypertensive patients

induced a prompt and striking fall in both systolic and diastolic pressure within
60 to 120 min after its administration. Two days later the same group of patients was studied again. The kallikrein inhibitor aprotinin was then infused in
a dose of 2 000 000 kallikrein-inhibitor-units (KIU) within two hours. Aprotinin
caused a slight but not significant rise in blood pressure, and prevented the expected fall in pressure with administration of SQ 14.225. When the nine patients were classified according to their plasma renin activity, it became evident,
that two patients had markedly elevated renin levels. In these patients blood
pressure decreased significantly with SQ 14.225 despite aprotinin induced kal-
likrein-inhibition (Fig. 2).

Conversely, SQ 14.225 did not reduce blood pressure in the kallikrein-blocked
patients with low- and normal-renin activity. It is interesting to note that these
latter patients had markedly low urinary kallikrein excretion rates, whereas
the two high-renin patients had urinary kallikrein activities within the normal
range.

184

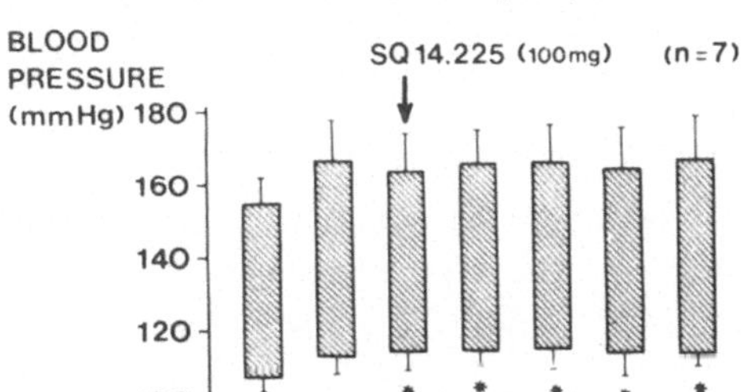

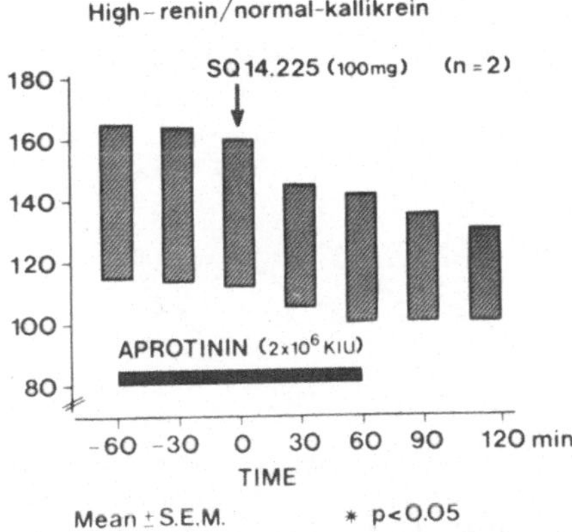

Fig. 2. Blood pressure responses to aprotinin in combination with SQ 14.225 in untreated essential hypertensive patients with low- and normal-renin (upper part) and high-renin (lower part)

In a second group of seven patients plasma renin activity was stimulated by four weeks treatment with hydrochlorothiazide. Administration of a single 100 mg dose of SQ 14.225 resulted in a significant decrease in both systolic and diastolic pressure (Fig. 3). When these patients were infused with aprotinin, it became evident that blockade of kallikrein did not prevent the marked fall in blood pressure caused by the converting-enzyme inhibitor.

Figure 4 demonstrates the responses of plasma renin activity, angiotensin II, converting enzyme activity, and plasma aldosterone to a single dose of SQ 14.225 in the nine patients of the first study group. Plasma renin activity rose significantly within 60 min. On the contrary, plasma concentrations of angiotensin II and of aldosterone as well as angiotensin converting enzyme activity showed the expected declines. Infusion of aprotinin was associated with a significant fall in plasma renin activity and a blunted response of renin to converting enzyme inhibition. These data are in keeping with the idea that kallikrein

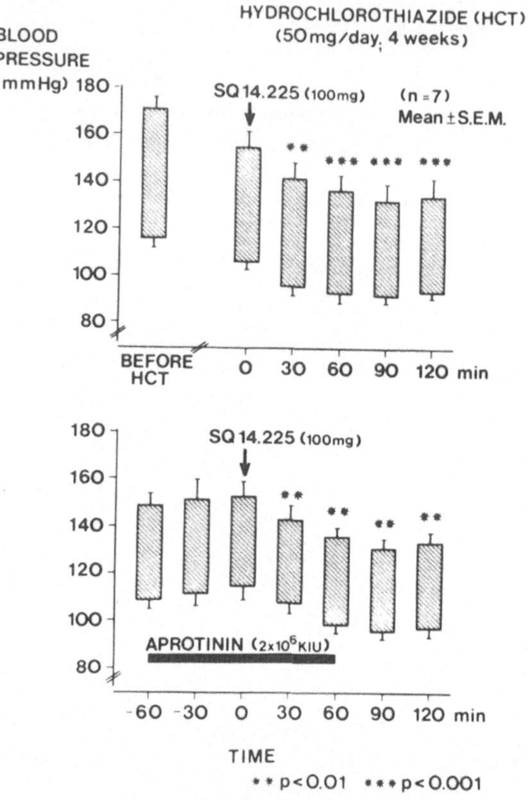

Fig. 3. Blood pressure responses to SQ 14.225 alone (upper part) and in combination with aprotinin (lower part) in hydrocholorothiazide-treated patients

may be involved in the in-vivo activation of renin [13, 14]. The responses of plasma angiotensin II, aldosterone and converting enzyme activity to the combined administration of SQ 14.225 and aprotinin were similar to those observed with converting enzyme inhibition alone.

Patients pretreated with hydrochlorothiazide for four weeks, showed an increase in plasma renin activity as well as in plasma concentration of angiotensin II and aldosterone (Fig. 5). Administration of SQ 14.225 was followed by a pronounced, almost six-fold rise in renin activity and a decrease in angiotensin II, plasma aldosterone and converting enzyme. Infusion of aprotinin reduced thiazide-stimulated renin, but in contrast to the group without diuretic therapy, it did not prevent the marked rise in renin with SQ 14.225. The long-term effect of SQ 14.225 was evaluated in a group of ten patients, who were treated with a daily dose of 450 mg for at least four weeks. In six patients blood pressure was normalized with the enzyme inhibitor alone; the others needed additional diuretic therapy in order to achieve blood pressure control (Fig. 6).

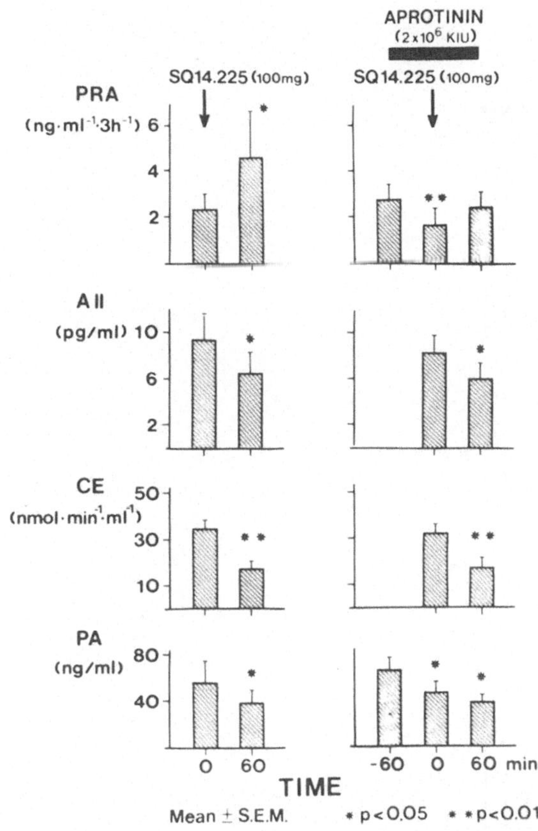

Fig. 4. Effect of SQ 14.225 and aprotinin on plasma renin activity (PRA), angiotensin II concentration (A II), converting enzyme activity (CE) and plasma aldosterone concentration (PA) in untreated essential hypertensive patients

Aprotinin-induced kallikrein inhibition resulted in a gradual but small rise in systolic and diastolic pressure, which became significant two hours after starting aprotinin infusion. With long-term converting enzyme inhibition a significant rise in plasma renin activity and a decrease in angiotensin II, aldosterone, and converting enzyme activity were observed (Fig. 7). Infusion of aprotinin reduced significantly SQ 14.225-stimulated renin activity, but did not influence the other parameters.

Discussion

Angiotensin converting-enzyme inhibition lowers arterial blood pressure in patients with high-, normal- and low-renin essential hypertension. In normal- and low-, but not in high-renin patients the acute blood pressure response to a single dose of SQ 14.225 is blocked by aprotinin-induced kallikrein inhibition.

187

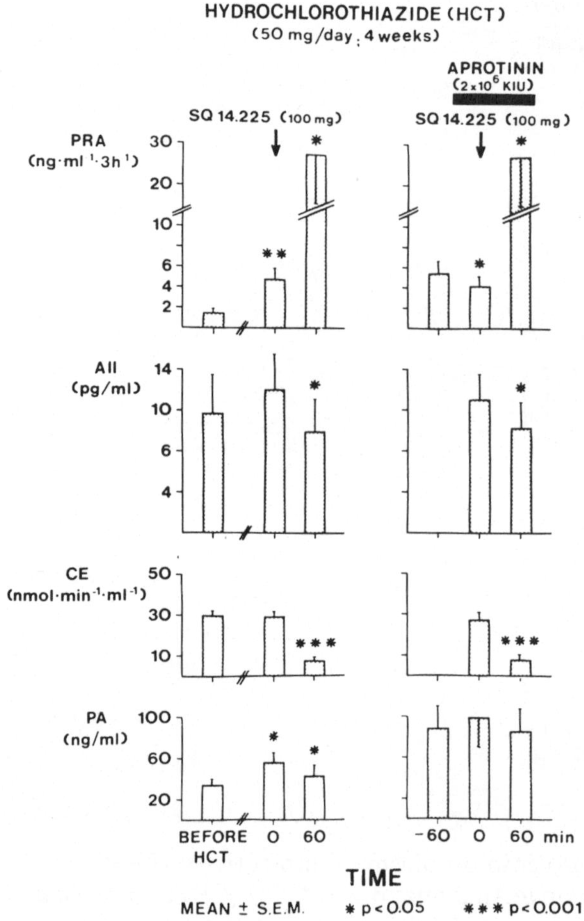

Fig. 5. Effect of SQ 14.225 and aprotinin on hydrochlorothiazide-induced changes in PRA, A II, CE and PA

On the other hand, blood pressure reduction with long-term converting-enzyme inhibition can be overcome only in part by blockade of kallikrein. Inhibition of kallikrein with aprotinin lowers basal and stimulated renin activity and blocks SQ 14.225-induced increases in renin in untreated patients, but not in those treated with diuretics.

It may be concluded, that the acute blood pressure lowering effect of SQ 14.225 observed in patients with low- and normal-renin hypertension is mainly due to kallikrein-kinin system activation. On the contrary, in high-renin patients the acute pressure response to converting-enzyme inhibition appears to be mediated predominently by a fall in angiotensin II concentration. With long-term converting-enzyme inhibition, kallikrein-kinin system activation seems to play a minor role in blood pressure reduction. Interpretation of these latter

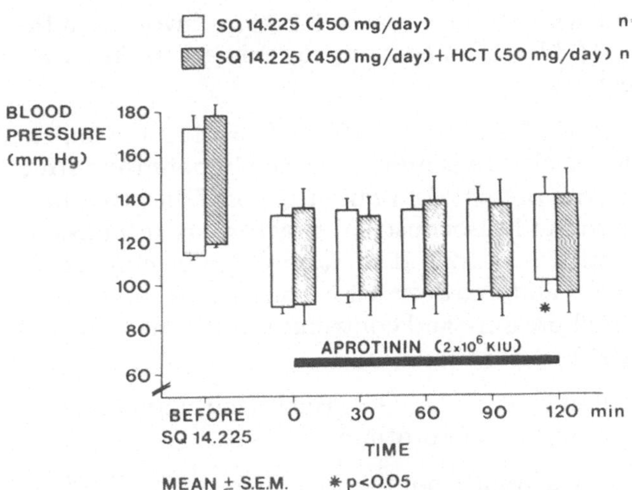

Fig. 6. Effect of aprotinin infusion on blood pressure after long-term treatment with SQ 14.225 alone or in combination with hydrochlorothiazide

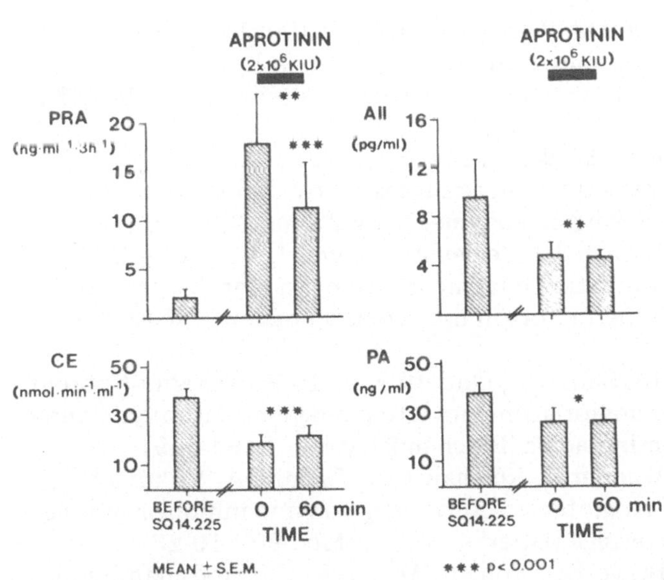

Fig. 7. Effect of aprotinin on SQ 14.225-induced changes in PRA, A II, CE and PA

results, however, is tempered by the fact that aprotinin was infused only for two hours and that blood pressure was not continuously recorded after the infusion had been stopped.

189

The present results are consistent with the idea that kallikrein is involved in the in-vivo activation of renin [13, 14]. Measurements of pro-renin are in progress to settle this question more precisely.

Although it is clear that on the basis of a clinical study such as this, it is impossible to define with precision the mechanisms underlying the hypotensive effect of converting-enzyme inhibition, the present data raise the possibility that the concomitant changes of vasodilator and vasoconstrictor factors are responsible for the hemodynamic changes with SQ 14.225. If so, it may also be concluded that an increase in renin-angiotensin- and/or a decrease in kallikrein-kinin-system activity affect regulation of arterial pressure and contribute to the maintenance of high blood pressure in essential hypertension.

Acknowledgement. We are indebted to Prof. Dr. G.L. Haberland, Bayer AG, Leverkusen F.R.G., for generous supplies of aprotinin.

This work was supported in part by a grant from the Land Nordrhein-Westfalen (No. II B 5 — FA 8052).

References

1. Case DB, Wallace JM, Keim HJ, Weber MA, Drayer JIM, White RP, Sealey JE, Laragh JH (1976) Estimating renin participation in hypertension: Superiority of converting enzyme inhibitor over saralasin. Am J Med 61 : 790-796
2. Case DB, Wallace JM, Keim HJ, Weber MA, Sealey JE, Laragh JH (1977) Possible role of renin in hypertension as suggested by renin-sodium profiling and inhibition of converting-enzyme. N Engl J Med 296 : 641-646
3. Gavras H, Brunner HR, Laragh JH, Sealey JE, Gavras I, Vukovich RA (1974) An angiotensin converting-enzyme inhibitor to identify and treat vascoconstrictor and volume factors in hypertensive patients. N Engl J Med 291 : 817-821
4. Gushman DW, Cheung HS, Sabo EF, Ondetti MA (1977) Design of potent competitive inhibitors of angiotensin-converting enzyme. Carboxyalkanoyl and mercaptoalkanoyl amino acids. Biochemistry 16 : 5484-5491
5. Brunner HR, Gavras H, Waeber B, Kershaw GR, Turini GA, Vukovich RA, McKinstry DN, Gavras I Angiotensin-converting enzyme inhibitor in long-term treatment of hypertensive patients. Am Int Med 90 : 19-23
6. Cody jr RJ, Tarazi RC, Bravo EL, Fonad FM (1978) Haemodynamics of orally-active converting enzyme inhibitor (SQ 14.225) in hypertensive patients. Clin Sci Mol Med 55 : 453-459
7. Ferguson RK, Brunner HR, Turini GA, Gavras H, McKinstry DN (1977) A specific orally active inhibitor of angiotensin-converting enzyme in man. Lancet 1 : 775
8. Gavras H, Brunner HR, Turini GA, Kershaw GR, Tifft CP, Cuttelod S, Gavras I, Vukovich RA, McKinstry DN (1978) Antihypertensive effect of

the oral angiotensin converting-enzyme inhibitor SQ 14.225 in man. N Engl J Med 298 : 991-995

9. Erdös EG (1977) The angiotensin I converting enzyme. Fed Proc 36 : 1760-1765
10. Williams GH, Hollenberg NK (1977) Accentuated vascular and endocrine response to SQ 20881 in hypertension. N Engl J Med 297 : 184-188
11. Miurhead EE, Prewitt RL, Brooks jr B, Brosius jr WL (1978) Antihypertensive action of the orally active converting enzyme inhibitor (SQ 14.225) in spontaneously hypertensive rats. Circ Res Suppl I 43 : I-53-I-59
12. McCaa RE, Hall JE McCaa CS (1978) The effects of angiotensin I-converting enzyme inhibitors on arterial blood pressure and urinary sodium excretion. Role of the renal renin-angiotensin and kallikrein-kinin systems. Circ Res Suppl I 43 : I-32-I-39
13. Derkx FHM, Bouma BN, Schalekamp MPA, Schalekamp MADH (1979) An intrinsic factor XII-prekallikrein-dependent pathway activates the human plasma renin-angiotensin system. Nature 280 : 315-316
14. Sealey JE, Atlas SA, Laragh JH, Oza NB, Ryan JW (1978) Human urinary kallikrein converts inactive to active renin and is a possible physiological activator of renin. Nature 275 : 144-145

Free Communications

Interactions Between Angiotensin II and ACTH on the Human Adrenal Gland[1]

W. Oelkers, M. Schöneshöfer, G. Schultze,
R. Fuchs-Hammoser, F. Venema

1. Introduction

In several animal species and in man, ACTH and angiotensin II seem to be the
most important regulatory factors of corticosteroid secretion. Chronic overproduction of ACTH results in increased cortisol and adrenal androgen secretion
(Cushing's disease), while aldosterone levels are usually normal or suppressed
[1]. Chronic overproduction of angiotensin II, either physiologic (e.g. sodium
deficiency) or pathologic (e.g. renin-producing kidney tumor or renal artery
stenosis) leads to increased plasma and urinary aldosterone levels, but signs of
hypercortisolism are absent. Short-term administration of ACTH produces a
rise in plasma cortisol *and* aldosterone levels [2], while short-term infusions of
angiotensin II increase plasma aldosterone, but not plasma cortisol [3]. In adrenal cell suspensions derived from animals or man, ACTH stimulates cortisol as
well as aldosterone secretion, and even angiotensin II, besides its effect on aldosterone secretion, stimulates cortisol release [4-7].

Both peptides are obviously able to stimulate the release of cortisol from the
zona fasciculata and of aldosterone from the zona glomerulosa. The question
arises why chronic overproduction of ACTH does not lead to a rise in aldosterone, and why cortisol levels are not elevated in patients with high renin and
angiotensin II states.

In order to reproduce endocrine effects in the early phase of chronic elevations
of plasma angiotensin II or ACTH levels, we performed infusion studies with
low doeses of Ile^5-angiotensin II and of 1-24 ACTH of a few days duration in
normal man. Some results of these studies were published recently [8, 9]. Plasma steroid levels and urinary aldosterone excretion were measured by specific
radioimmunoassays after partial purification by paper chromatography [10,
11]. The methods for measuring plasma renin activity, plasma angiotensin II
and ACTH concentrations are described elsewhere [9].

---

1 Supported by a grant from the Deutsche Forschungsgemeinschaft (Oe 47/7)

2. Experimental Protocols and Results

2.1 Prolonged Infusions of Angiotensin II

Protocol I

Two normal young males, who ingested a constant diet containing 135 mM of sodium and 70 mM of potassium per day, received infusions of 3 ng/kg/min of angiotensin II for 132 hours (5 1/2 days).

Figure 1 shows the results in one of these subjects: plasma angiotensin II rose to levels similar to those observed in moderately sodium deficient normal subjects (40-80 pg/ml). Plasma aldosterone and the excretion rate of aldosterone-18-glucuronide (AER) were increased during the whole infusion period, despite significant sodium retention. Although plasma angiotensin II levels were rather constant during infusion, plasma aldosterone exhibited fluctuations between levels at 9:00 a.m. and 9:00 p.m., which were similar to those of plasma cortisol. In this subject, as well as in the second one, plasma cortisol levels at 9:00 a.m. were lower than on the control day during infusion day 1-4, but rose back to control on infusion days 5 and 6 (Fig. 2). As shown in the same figure, plasma levels of 18-0H-deoxycorticosterone at 9:00 a.m. exhibit changes similar to those of cortisol during angiotensin II infusion.

Protocol II

Four normal young males ingested a diet containing 150 mM of sodium and 70 mM of potassium per day for six says. Days 5 and 6 were the control days in the metabolic ward. On days 7, 8, and 9, 3 ng/kg/min angiotensin II were infused. In Figure 3, these days are referred to as days, 1, 2, and 3 of infusion. During angiotensin II infusion, sodium intake was gradually reduced in order to prevent gross sodium retention, as had occurred in the two subjects of protocol I, (see sodium balance data in Fig. 1!). In Figure 3, mean plasma levels of several steroids at 9:00 a.m. during angiotensin II infusion are shown as the percentage of steroid levels at 9:00 a.m. of the preinfusion control days. Aldosterone levels rose markedly, but cortisol levels were slightly, although significantly below control on days 1 and 2 of infusion. Cortisol levels on the third infusion day are no longer significantly different from control. The changes of other corticosteroids during angiotensin II infusion were not impressive. The slight fall of plasma cortisol levels during the first days of angiotensin II infusion is in accordance with our findings in protocol I. With respect to the cortisolstimulatory potency of angiotensin II *in vitro* (see introduction), these observations were quite unexpected.

Protocol III

Four normal young males received a diet containing 15 mM of sodium and 70 mM of potassium for eleven days. Days 7 and 8 were the control days in the metabolic ward. 6 ng/kg/min of angiotensin II were infused on days 9, 10 and 11. In Figure 4, which shows the percentage changes of plasma steroid levels during infusion, these days are referred to as days 1, 2 and 3 of infusion.

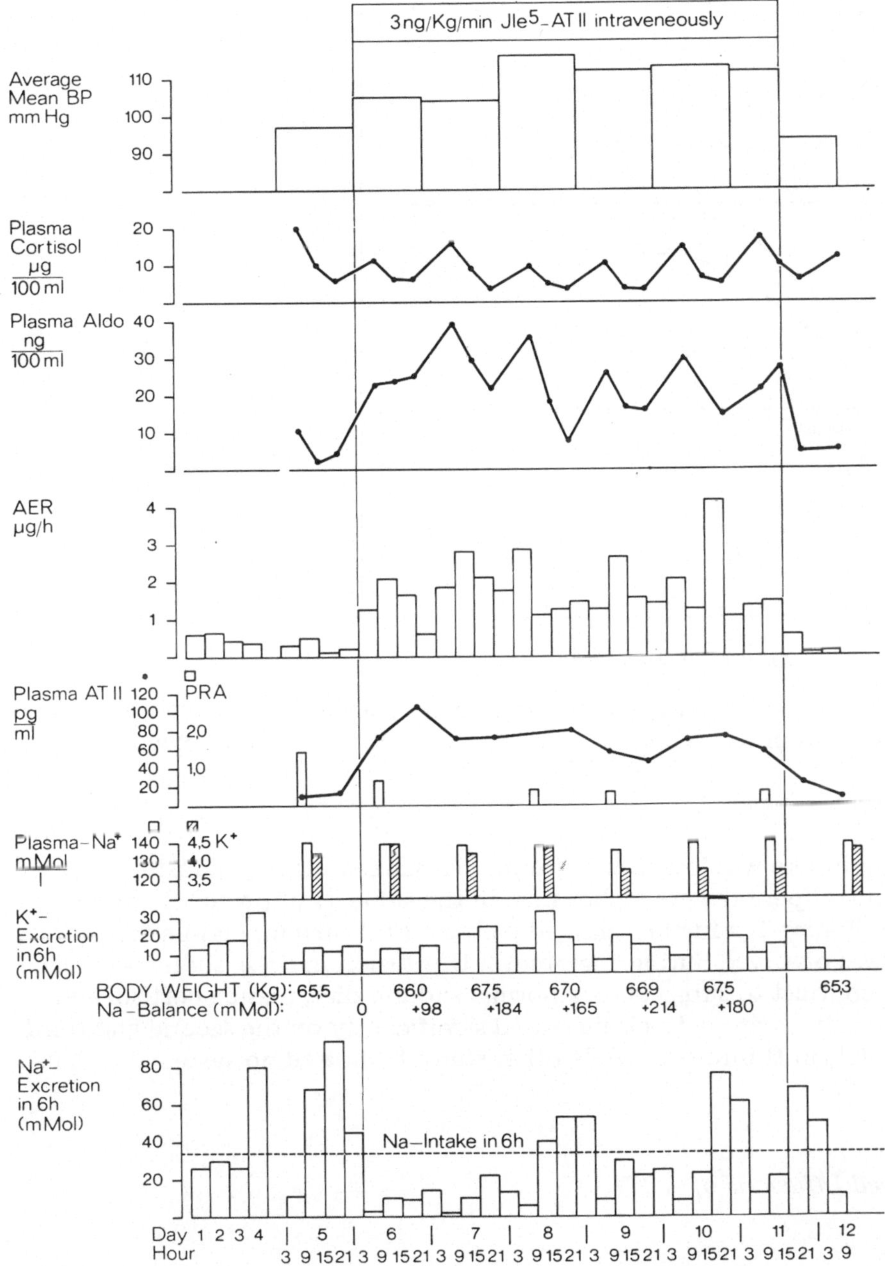

Fig. 1. Prolonged angiotensin II infusion in a subject of protocol I. BP = blood pressure; AER = excretion rate of aldosterone-18-glucuromide; ATII = angiotensin II; PRA = plasma renin activity. Sodium-intake and -excretion rates are shown for six-hour periods

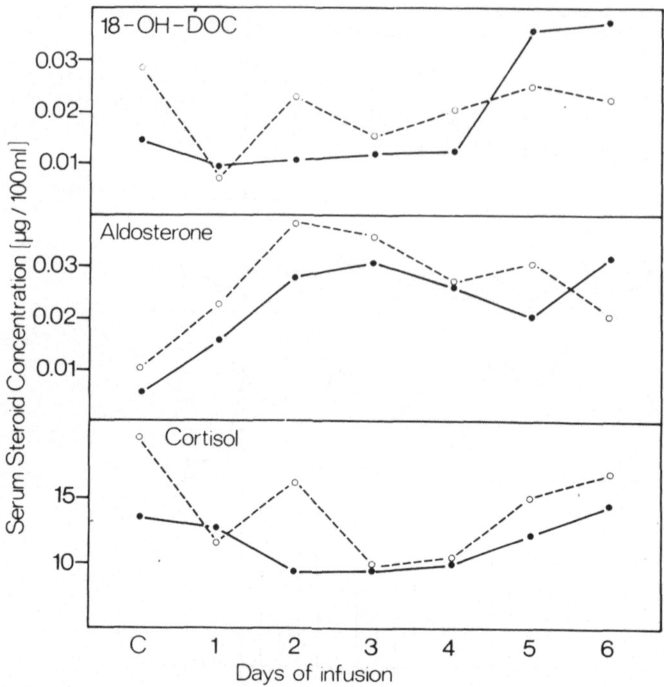

Fig. 2. Plasma steroid levels at 9 a.m. in the two subjects studied according to protocol I. C = preinfusion control day. 18-OH-DOC = 18-OH-deoxycortico-sterone

Since sodium intake was low in this group, plasma and urinary aldosterone levels in the control period were higher than in the subjects of protocol I and II. As shown in Figure 4, a further marked increase of 9:00 a.m. plasma aldosterone levels was observed during angiotensin II infusion in these sodium-deficient subjects. In contrast to subjects on a normal sodium diet, plasma cortisol and also plasma corticosterone levels increased significantly on the second and third day of angiotensin II infusion, while other steroids showed no systematic changes.

2.2 Prolonged Infusions of ACTH

Protocol IV

Two normal young males received a diet containing 150 mM of sodium per day and 70 mM of potassium per day, two others received 15 mM of sodium per day for ten days altogether. Days 5 and 10 were the pre- and post-infusion control days in the metabolic ward. From day 5 (9:00 p.m.) up to day 9 (9:00 p.m.) 5 U of ACTH per day were continuously infused intravenously. In Figure 5, days 6 to 9 of the protocol are referred to as days 1 to 4 of ACTH infusion.

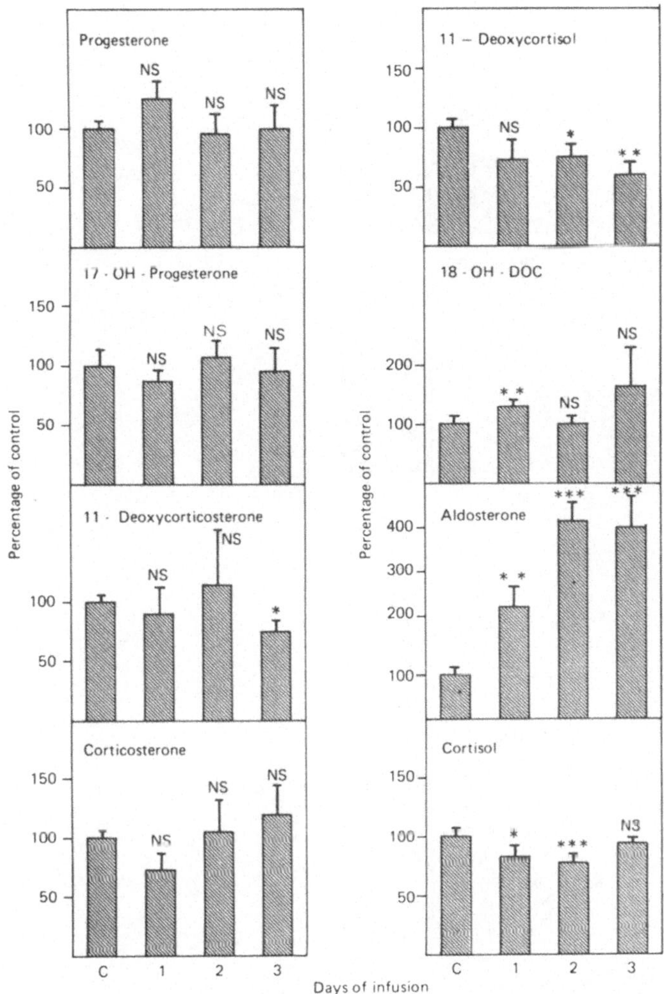

Fig. 3. Percentage changes of plasma steroid levels during angiotensin II infusion (3 ng/kg/min) in subjects on normal sodium diet (protocol II). NS = no significant change from control. ★ = p < 0.005; ★★ = p < 0.01; ★★★ = p < 0.001

This dosage of ACTH is slightly higher than the estimated secretion rate of ACTH during the early morning hours in normal man [12], but it must be emphasized that this rate of ACTH secretion was stimulated by infusion for four continuous days. Plasma cortisol (not shown in Fig. 5) in all subjects was continuously stimulated during ACTH infusion to levels between 30 and 70 µg/ 100 ml. The individual plateaus of plasma cortisol were higher than the 9:00 a.m. cortisol levels on the preinfusion control day. Figure 5 shows the effect of ACTH on plasma aldosterone levels and also on plasma renin activity (PRA). ACTH infusion stimulated plasma aldosterone in a transient manner. Plasma aldosterone, which was measured at 9:00 a.m. and at 9:00 p.m., was stimulated

199

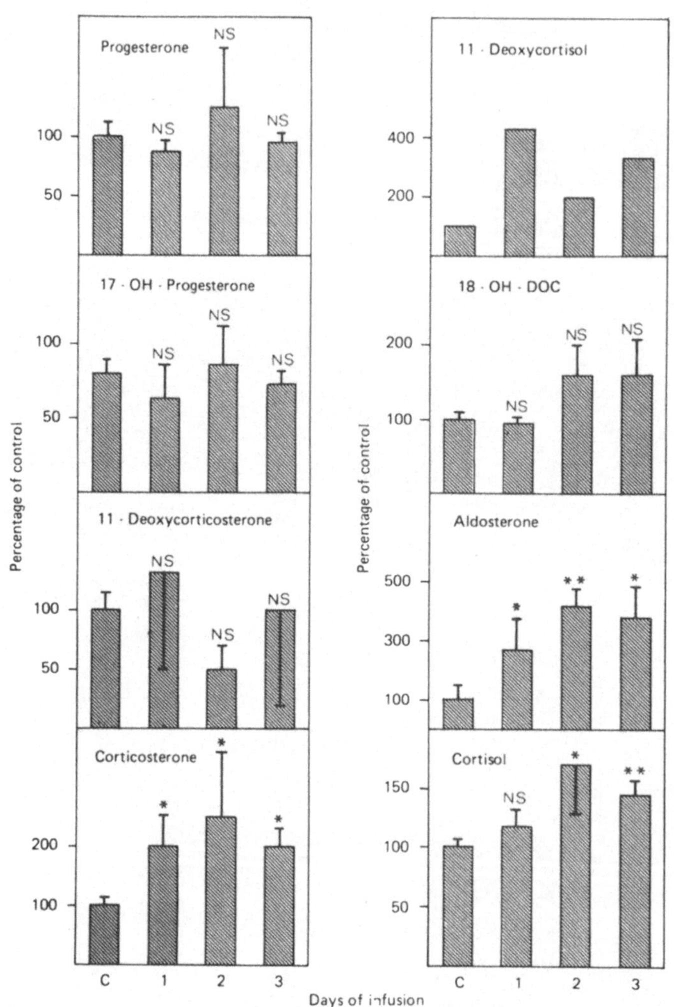

Fig. 4. Percentage changes of steroid levels during angiotensin II (6 ng/kg/min) in four subjects on a low sodium diet (protocol III). Symbols as in Figure 3. 11-deoxycortisol was measured in one subject only

during the first 24 to 36 hours of ACTH infusion, but fell to control levels or below control during the last two days of ACTH infusion. Surprisingly enough, PRA showed a pattern similar to plasma aldosterone in all four subjects. It rose initially and fell later on. The coefficient of correlation between al PRA and plasma aldosterone levels before, during and after ACTH infusion ($n = 52$) was significantly positive (r = 0.78; p < 0.001).

Although it is obvious that the effect of ACTH on aldosterone secretion from adrenal cells *in vitro* does not depend on changes in angiotensin II concentra-

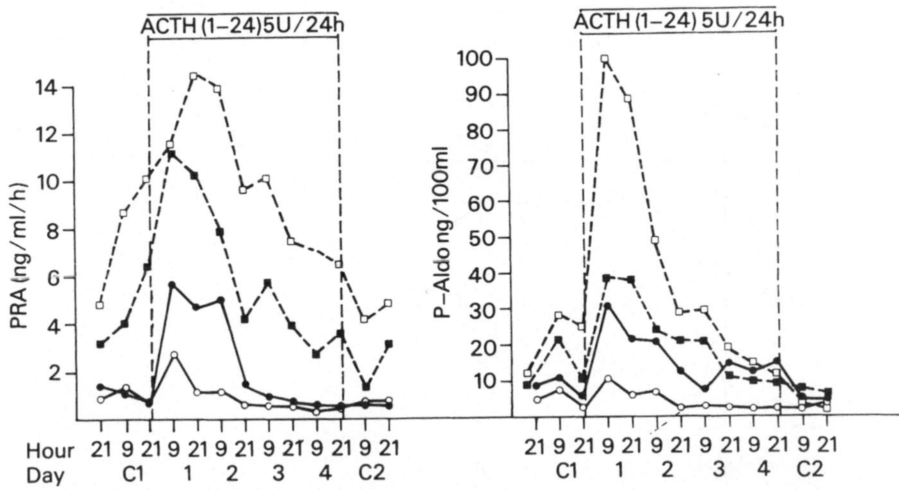

Fig. 5. Effect of low dose (5U/24 h) ACTH infusion for four days on plasma renin activity (PRA) and plasma aldosterone concentration in two subjects on a normal (○,●) and two subjects on a low sodium (□,■) diet (protocol IV). C_1, C_2 = pre- and post-infusion control days

tion, it appears possible according to our results that the effect of ACTH on aldosterone secretion *in vivo* is in part mediated by changes in renin and angiotensin levels.

Protocol V

In order to further elucidate the effect of ACTH on renin and aldosterone, we restudied the early phase of ACTH infusion using a new protocol with more frequent blood sampling for hormone measurements.

Three normal young males received a diet containing 150 mM of sodium for seven days. Day 5 was the control day in the metabolic ward, when plasma hormone measurements were performed in the recumbent position. From day 6 at 6:15 a.m. up to day 7 at 5:00 p.m. (referred to as day 2 and 3 in Figure 6), 10 U of ACTH per day were infused. Figure 6 shows the results in one subject. ACTH and cortisol levels were permanently elevated during ACTH infusion. Plasma aldosterone showed an initial rise after two hours of infusion. Thereafter, it fell to levels slightly above control. Plasma aldosterone started to rise. In the three subjects taken together, the coefficient of correlation between plasma ACTH and aldosterone levels during ACTH infusion was + 0.266, while that between PRA and aldosterone was + 0.522. These results support our working hypothesis that renin and angiotensin II, at least in part, mediate the effect of ACTH on aldosterone secretion.

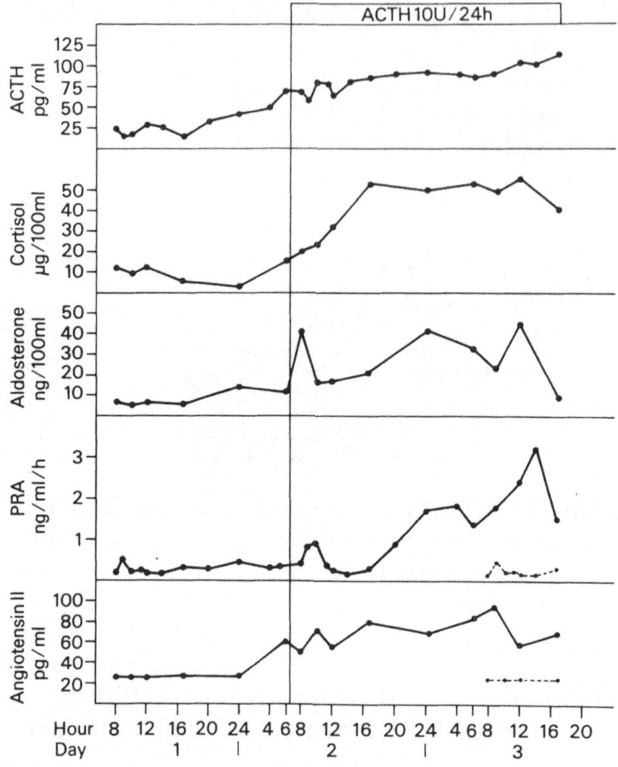

Fig. 6. Endocrine effects of 10 U of ACTH/24 h administered for 35 hours to a subject of protocol V. PRA = plasma renin activity. Dashed curves below the solid curves of PRA and angiotensin II represent measurements on the preinfusion control day 1

3. Discussion

Angiotensin II stimulates cortisol release from human [5, 6] and bovine [4, 7] adrenal cells *in vitro*. In our own bovine adrenal *in vitro* model, the threshold dose of angiotensin II (10^{-11} M) for the stimulation of cortisol and aldosterone release is identical and within the physiologic range of plasma angiotensin II concentration. In the study of McKenna et al [6], who incubated human adrenal cells with angiotensin II, the threshold dose for the stimulation of cortisol release was slightly higher. It is, therefore, likely, that normal or moderately elevated plasma angiotensin II levels in the intact human organism exert some stimulatory effect not only on the zona glomerulosa but also in the zona fasciculata. Our angiotensin II infusion studies in sodium repleted normal subjects, however, revealed a slight fall of 9:00 a.m. plasma cortisol levels during the first days of angiotensin II infusion. This is probably due to some kind of counterregulation by other factors influencing cortisol secretion. A recently published study by Semple et al. [13] may explain our findings: these authors performed

202

short-term low dose infusions of angiotensin II in man and measured plasma
ACTH levels. They observed a fall in plasma ACTH within a few minutes after
starting the angiotensin II infusion. It is not known for how long plasma ACTH
is suppressed by angiotensin II if the peptide is infused for a few days. If the
slight depression of plasma cortisol in our experiments was due to ACTH suppression, one might conclude that this effect is not maintained to the same extent during prolonged angiotensin II infusion, since in experiments of protocol
I and II, plasma cortisol rose back to control levels at the end of the infusion
periods of 5 1/2 days and three days duration respectively. It is likewise possible that a chronically elevated plasma angiotensin II level exerts some "trophic"
effect not only on the zona glomerulosa [9], but also on the zona fasciculata.
This latter effect, and perhaps a less pronounced depression of plasma ACTH
levels may be the reason for the slight elevation of 9:00 a.m. plasma cortisol
levels in sodium deficient normal subjects (protocol III) during angiotensin II
infusion. In this group, plasma angiotensin II levels were already increased during the preparatory period of 6 days duration, and the dose of angiotensin II
infused later on was higher than in the subjects studied according to protocols
I and II.

The view that changes in plasma ACTH levels during angiotensin II infusion
minimize changes in cortisol secretion is supported by data of Slater et al. [14]
obtained in hypophysectomized and nephrectomized dogs. In these animals,
very small doses of angiotensin II lead to increased cortisol secretion, and the
threshold doses of angiotensin II stimulating aldosterone and cortisol release
were identical.

Recent observations by David et al. [15] in patients with congenital aldosterone
deficiency and of Horner et al. [16] in patients with the salt losing form of
adrenal 21-hydroxylase deficiency have shown that in the state of severe sodium deficiency, elevated renin (and probably angiotensin) levels strongly stimulate the zona fasciculata and increase the cortisol production rate [15] or the
secretion of cortisol-precursors [16].

A transient increase of aldosterone secretion by ACTH, if administered for a
few days, as observed in subjects of protocol IV, was first described by Liddle
et al. [17]. The question why aldosterone secretion falls in the second phase of
the study in spite of continuous ACTH administration is unresolved so far. Our
study demonstrates for the first time a stimulation of renin secretion by chronic administration of ACTH in a slightly supraphysiologic dosage. As shown in
Figure 6 (protocol V) PRA does not rise immediately after starting the ACTH
infusion. There is a lag period of about ten hours. Thereafter, changes in plasma
aldosterone are better correlated with those of PRA than with those of plasma
ACTH concentrations. As shown in Figure 5, the decline of plasma aldosterone
during the last two days of ACTH infusion is paralleled by a decline in PRA.
These observations allow the following tentative explanation:

During chronic ACTH administration, aldosterone secretion is vigorously stimulated by increased conversion of cholesterol to pregnenolone during the first
few hours. Later on, the extent to which ACTH is able to stimulate aldosterone

output seems to be controlled by the actual plasma renin and angiotensin II concentration. High angiotensin II levels open the floodgate through which ACTH is pushing aldosterone precursors, low angiotensin levels create one or more bottlenecks in the biosynthetic pathway to aldosterone. It is likely that angiotensin II controls two steps of steroidogenesis, 1. the step between cholesterol and pregnenolone and 2. the step(s) between corticosterone and aldosterone [18]. The recent observation that ACTH stimulates the conversion of 11-deoxycortisol to cortisol [19] may explain why low angiotensin II levels do not restrict the effect of ACTH on cortisol secretion.

This view of an interaction of ACTH and angiotensin II on the adrenal level may also help to explain the observations by Ganong et al. in the dog [20] and by Kem et al. in man [21] that ACTH, in acute experiments, exerts a much stronger effect on aldosterone secretion in the sodium deplete than in the replete state. Angiotensin II levels are high in the former and low in the latter condition.

Wo do not yet know by which mechanism ACTH raises plasma renin activity. We have excluded the possibility that increased plasma renin substrate levels are the cause of the rise of PRA. The mechanism of action of ACTH on renin release is presently being investigated.

References

1. Biglieri EG, Hane S, Slaton PE, Forsham PH (1963) In vivo and in vitro studies of adrenal secretions in Cushing's syndrome andprimary aldosteron- J Clin Invest 42 : 516-524
2. Dluhy RG, Himathongkam T, Greenfield M (1974) Rapid ACTH test with plasma aldosterone levels. Improved diagnostic discrimination. Ann Int Med 80 : 693-696
3. Oelkers W, Brown JJ, Fraser R, Lever AF, Morton JJ, Robertson JIS (1974) Sensitization of the adrenal cortex to angiotensin II in sodium deplete man. Circ Res 34 : 69-77
4. Kaplan NM (1965) The biosynthesis of adrenal steroids: Effects of angiotensin II, adrenocorticotropin and potassium. J Clin Invest 12 : 2029-2039
5. Williams GH, Braley LM (1977) Effects of dietary sodium and potassium intake and acute stimulation on aldosterone output by isolated human adrenal cells. J Clin Endocrinol Metab 45 : 55-64
6. McKenna TJ, Island DP, Nicholson WE, Liddle GW (1978) Angiotensin stimulates cortisol biosynthesis in human adrenal cells *in vitro.* Steroids 33 : 127-136
7. Venema F, Oelkers W Unpublished observations
8. Oelkers W, Schöneshöfer M, Schultze G, Bauer B (1978) Effect of prolonged low-dose infusions of Ile^5-angiotensin II on blood pressure, aldosterone and electrolyte excretion in sodium replete man. Klin Wochenschr 56 : 37-41

9. Oelkers W, Schöneshöfer M, Schultze G, Wenzler M, Bauer B, L'age M, Fehm H (1978) Prolonged infusions of Ile^5-angiotensin II in sodium replete and deplete man: Effects on aldosterone, ACTH, cortisol, blood pressure and electrolyte balance. J Clin Endocrinol Metab 46 : 402-413
10. Schöneshöfer M (1977) Simultaneous determination of eight adrenal steroids in human serum by radioimmuno-assay. J Steroid Biochem 8 : 995-1009
11. Vecsei P, Penke B, Joumaah A (1972) Radioimmunoassay of free aldosterone and of its 18-oxo-glucuronide in human urine. Experientia 28 : 622-624
12. Nugent CA, Eik-Ness K, Samuels LT, Tyler FH (1959) Changes in plasma levels of 17-hydroxycorticosteroids during the intravenous administration of adrenocorticotropin (ACTH). IV. Response to prolonged infusions of small amounts of ACTH. J Clin Endocrinol Metab 19 : 334-343
13. Semple PF, Buckingham JC, Mason PA, Fraser R (1979) Suppression of plasma ACTH concentration by angiotensin II infusion in normal humans and in a subject with steroid 17 α hydroxylase defect. Clin Endocrinol 10 : 137-144
14. Slater JDH, Harbour BH, Henderson HH, Casper AGT, Bartter FC (1963) Influence of the pituitary and the renin-angiotensin system on the secretion of aldosterone, cortisol and cortisoterone. J Clin Invest 9 : 1504-1520
15. David RR, Asnis M, Drucker WD (1972) Disturbance of cortisol production in congenital aldosterone deficiency. J Clin Endocrinol Metab 35 : 604-608
16. Horner JM, Hintz RL, Luetscher JA (1979) The role of renin and angiotensin in salt-losing, 21-hydroxylase-deficient congenital adrenal hyperplasia. J Clin Endocrinol Metab 48 : 776-783
17. Liddle GW, Duncan LE, Bartter FC (1956) Dual mechanism regulating adrenocortical function in man. Am J Med 21 : 380-386
18. McKenna TJ, Island DP, Nicholson WE, Liddle GW (1978) Angiotensin stimulates both early and late steps in aldosterone biosynthesis in isolated bovine glomerulosa cells. J Steroid Biochem 9 : 967-972
19. McKenna TJ, Island DP, Nicheolson WE, Miller RB, Lacroix A, Liddle GW (1979) ACTH stimulates late steps in cortisol biosynthesis. Acta Endocr (Kbh) 90 : 122-132
20. Ganong WF, Biglieri EG, Mulrow PJ (1966) Mechanisms regulating adrenocortical secretion of aldosterone and glucocorticoids. Recent Prog Horm Res 22 : 381-414
21. Kem DC, Gomez-Sanchez C, Kramer NJ, Holland OB, Higgins JR (1975) Plasma aldosterone and renin activity response to ACTH infusion in dexamethanone-suppressed and sodium-depleted man. J Clin Endocrinol Metab 40 : 116-124

Disturbed Regulation of Aldosterone and Sodium Excretion in a Subgroup of Essential Hypertensives

A. HELBER, G. WAMBACH, W. HUMMERICH, G. BÖNNER,
K. A. MEURER, W. KAUFMANN

Introduction

The phenomenon of low plasma renin activity in approximately 25% of essential hypertensives has initiated a great deal of interest into investigating signs of mineralocorticoid excesss in these patients. The results obtained were highly controversial. However, several abnormalities in mineralocorticoid production in patients with essential hypertension have been reported by the groups of Melby [12] and Genest [5, 6] and Luetscher [2, 4] demonstrating an inappropriate suppression of aldosterone secretion in essential hypertensives by sodium loading.

These findings led us to study the excretion of aldosterone and other steroids in a larger group of essential hypertensives during different sodium intake and especially under conditions of sodium loading. In an additional series of experiments, blood pressure response to spironolactone in these patients was related to previously measured excretion of aldosterone during sodium loading. Finally the results obtained in essential hypertensives were compared to those in patients with primary hyperaldosteronism due to adrenal adenomas and due to adrenal hyperplasia.

Material and Methods

Urinary excretion rates of aldosterone, Na^+ and K^+ were determined in: 56 healthy controls, 143 patients with essential hypertension, 16 patients with primary hyperaldosteronism, 12 with adrenal adenoma and four with histologically proven bilateral adrenal micronodular hyperplasia. In 35 healthy controls, 90 patients with essential hypertension and 16 patients with primary hyperaldosteronism aldosterone, and the quantity of electrolytes excreted in the urine during a 24-hour period were measured under different conditions: during free Na^+ intake and after four days of Na^+ deprivation (50 meq/day Na^+) and finally after six days of Na^+ loading (260 meq/day Na^+). After four days of Na^+ deprivation and after six days of Na^+ loading under the conditions stated above, a steady state condition between Na^+ intake and Na^+ excretion was established. A total of 117 aldosterone-excretion determinations in controls were therefore compared to 290 determinations in patients with essential hypertension.

27 patients with essential hypertension and eight patients with primary hyperaldosteronism of adenoma origin were treated with 200 mg spironolactone/day over a period of four weeks after a two week placebo period. Blood pressure was followed on an outpatient basis.

Excretion of aldosterone (C-18-glucuronide) was measured radioimmunologically after 24 hours pH 1 — incubation of urine and chromatographic purification of the extract [8].

Other steroids referred to in the paper were measured radioimmunologically after chromatographic prepurification of the urinary or plasma extract.

Renin activity in plasma was measured radioimmunologically by the Haber (7) method with the angiotensin-I-J$_{125}$-radio-immunoassay (Squibb, USA). Values are given in ng AT · ml^{-1} · h^{-1}.

Results

In patients with essential hypertension ($n = 134$) there is a distinctly lower correlation ($r = 0.66$) between aldosterone excretion and log Na$^+$/K$^+$-ratio in urine compared to controls ($n = 56$, $r = 0.87$). The reason for this is a higher aldosterone excretion during high sodium intake in a substantial number of patients.

Figure 1 summarizes values of aldosterone excretion of healthy controls, patients with essential hypertension and patients with primary hyperaldosteronism during Na$^+$ loading (Na$^+$-excretion over 175 meq/day). The highest control value for aldosterone excretion under these conditions was 6 μg/day. In patients with essential hypertension there was a bimodal behaviour of aldosterone excretion. The majority of patients ($n = 64$) had a suppression of excretion of aldosterone by conditions of Na$^+$ loading below 6 μg/day with a mean value of 2.7 ± 1.4 (SD) μg/day (Group A), whereas a second smaller group of patients ($n = 36$) had aldosterone excretions above the highest control value with an average of 10.0 ± 3.0 (SD) μg/day despite forced Na$^+$ loading (Group B).

Four patients with primary hyperaldosteronism and histologically proven bilateral adrenal micronodular hyperplasia had an aldosterone-excretion during Na$^+$ loading in the same range as the above mentioned Group B-patients of essential hypertensives. Under similar conditions aldosterone-excretion in adenoma patients with primary hyperaldosteronism was distinctly higher.

The bimodal distribution of aldosterone excretion values during Na$^+$ loading suggests two seperate groups of essential hypertensives: Those with suppressible aldosterone excretion (Group A) and those with non suppressible aldosterone excretion during Na$^+$ loading (Group B). In order to demonstrate further differences between these two groups of essential hypertensives, the relationship between the excretion of aldosterone and the urinary Na$^+$/K$^+$ ratio under dif-

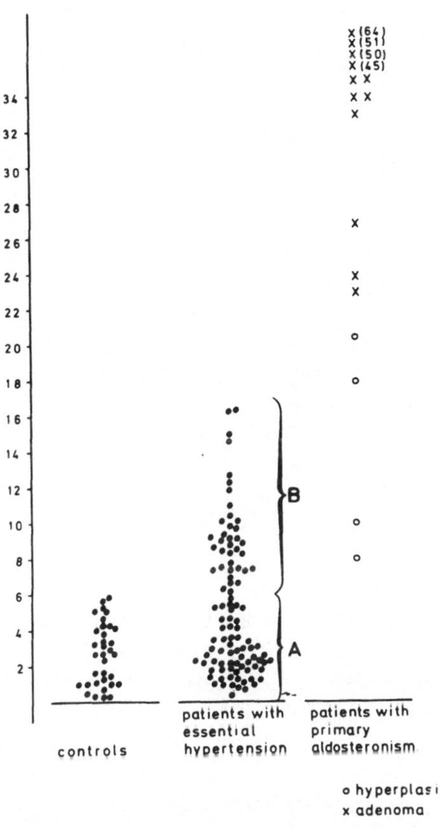

Fig. 1. Aldosterone-excretion during sodium loading (Na⁺-excretion above 175 meq/day) of controls, patients with essential hypertension and patients with histologically proven adrenal adenoma or adrenal hyperplasia and primary hyperaldosteronism

ferent Na⁺ intake, concentration of K⁺ in serum during Na⁺ loading, PRA after Na⁺ deprivation and blood pressure response on spironolactone treatment was studied in both groups.

Figure 2 demonstrates the relation between excretion of aldosterone to the Na+/K⁺ ratio in 24 hour urine collections in group A (left) and group B (right) essential hypertensives. Group A patients exactly follow the correlation range of the control group with a high coefficient of correlation (r = 0.71, aldosterone excretion to log Na⁺/K⁺ ratio). The aldosterone excretion of group B patients is similar to controls or group A patients during Na⁺ deprivation, already higher during normal Na⁺ intake but distinctly higher during Na⁺ loading. The correla-

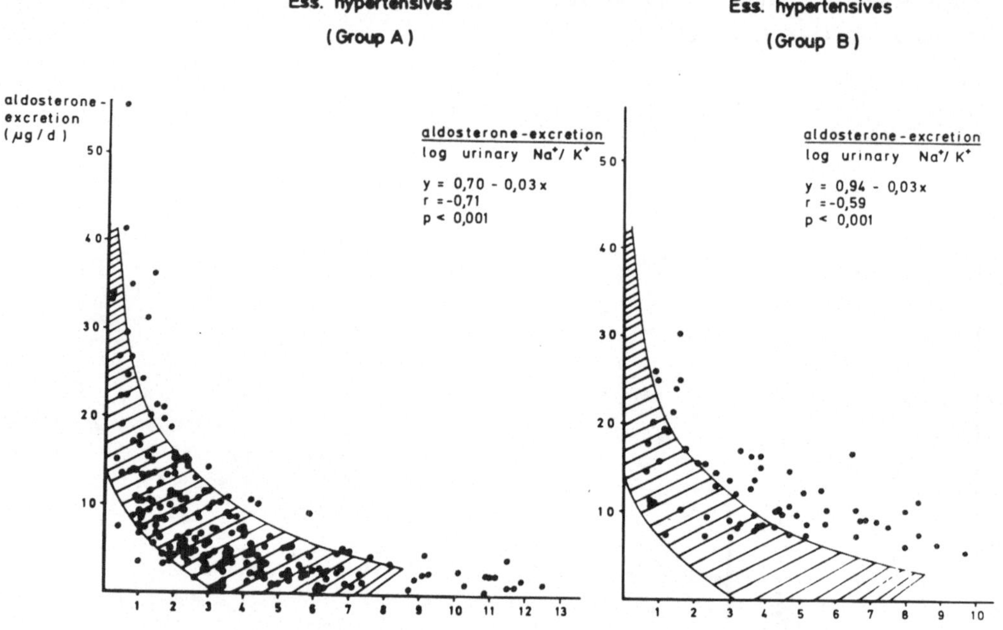

Fig. 2. Aldosterone-excretion in relation to Na^+/K^+-ratio in 24 hours-urine in patients with essential hypertension and under sodium loading suppressible aldosterone excretion (group A, left) and non suppressible aldosterone excretion (group B, right). Shadowed area stands for control region

tion coefficient between aldosterone excretion and log Na^+/K^+ ratio ($r = 0.56$) is markedly different from those of group A patients or controls.

Concentrations of K^+ in serum during Na^+ loading in group A and B essential hypertensives and patients with primary hyperaldosteronism are summarized in *Figure 3:* Concentration of K^+ in serum in group A patients was 4.26 ± 0.37 (SD) meq/l, in group B patients 3.81 ± 0.44 (SD) meq/l. The difference is ($p < 0.001$) statistically significant. The concentration of K^+ in the serum of four patients with histologically proven adrenal hyperplasia and primary hyperaldosteronism was in the same range as that in group B patients with essential hypertension. The concentration of K^+ in serum of adenoma patients with primary hyperaldosteronism was 2.6 ± 0.34 (SD) meq/l. In addition there is a significant correlation between the concentration of K^+ in serum and aldosterone excretion in essential hypertensives during Na^+ loading ($r = 0.47, p < 0.001$).

PRA after four days of Na^+ deprivation (50 meq Na^+ and 50 meq K^+ intake per day) in recumbent and upright position was evaluated in 33 patients with essential hypertension. There is no bimodal behaviour of PRA among these patients. Group B patients show a tendency towards lower PRA values (0.81 ± 1.09 (SD) ng AT $\cdot$ ml^{-1} $\cdot$ h^{-1} recumbent to 1.15 ± 1.56 (SD) ng AT $\cdot$ ml^{-1} $\cdot$ h^{-1}

210

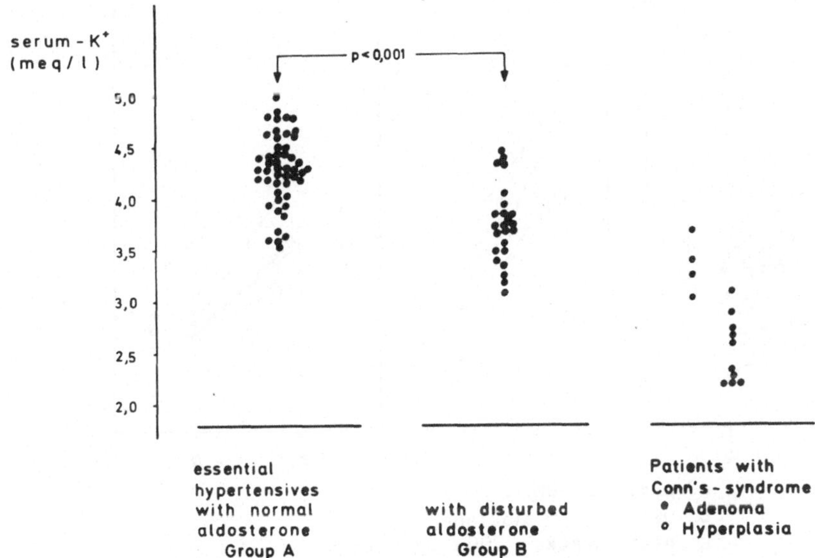

Fig. 3. Serum-K$^+$-concentration during sodium loading of essential hypertensives (group A : left, Group B: middle) and patients with primary hyperaldosteronism (● : adenoma patients, ○ : patients with adrenal hyperplasia

upright) compared to group A patients (1.07 ± 0.97 (SD) ng AT · ml^{-1} · h^{-1}
recumbent to 2.10 ± 1.75 (SD) ng AT · ml^{-1} · h^{-1} upright). There is however,
no significant difference in PRA between both groups.

Figure 4: summarizes the blood pressure response to spironolactone therapy
after four weeks of therapy with 200 mg spironolactone daily in 27 patients
with essential hypertension and eight patients with primary hyperaldosteronism and adrenal adenoma. The mean arterial blood pressure in 18 group A patients with essential hypertension fell from 127 ± 14 (SD) mm Hg before therapy to 118 ± 14 (SD) after therapy (— 9 mm Hg), in 9 group B essential hypertensives from 143 ± 18 (SD) mm Hg before therapy to 121 ± 14 (SD) mm Hg
after therapy (— 22 mm Hg) and from 130 ± 8 (SD) mm Hg to 109 ± 3 (SD)
mm Hg (— 21 mm Hg) in patients with primary hyperaldosteronism and adrenal
adenoma. The difference in blood pressure reduction between both groups of
essential hypertensives was significant (p < 0.05) despite of the relatively small
number of patients studied so far. In all 27 patients with essential hypertension studied, there was a significant correlation (r = 0.45, p < 0.01) between
excretion of aldosterone during Na$^+$ loading and Δ mean arterial blood pressure
before and after 4 weeks of therapy with 200 mg spironolactone.

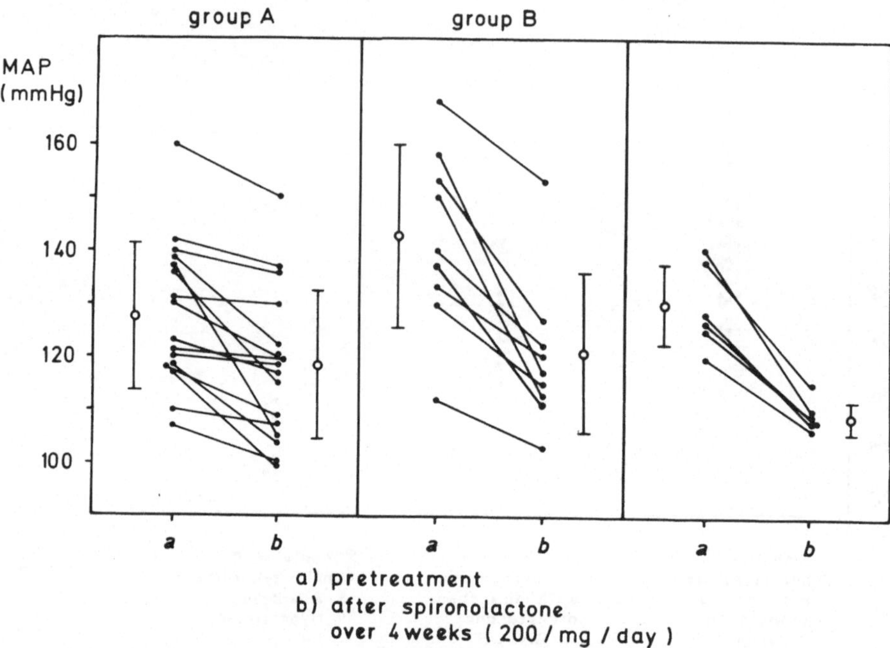

Fig. 4. Mean arterial blood-pressure-response (MAP) after 4 weeks treatment with 200 mg spironolactone/day in group A and group B essential hypertensives and patients with primary hyperaldosteronism due to an adrenal adenoma

There are minor differences also in age and duration of hypertension in both groups of patients with essential hypertension (Table 1). Group B-patients are heavier in body weight and have a tendency towards obesity, where-as group A-patients have a body weight, which is comparable to average peoples weight.

ACTH-dependent steroids are not significantly different in both groups of patients (Fig. 5). Cortisol-excretion is insignificantly lower in both groups of patients during sodium loading compared to a control-group with cortisol excretion of 37.7 ± 15.1 μg/day. Plasma-progesterone-levels as well as deoxycorticosterone-excretion in essential hypertensives were not significantly different from these in controls and no significant differences were found between both groups of patients during sodium loading.

Discussion

In patients with uncomplicated essential hypertension the relation between the excretion of aldosterone and sodium intake or Na$^+$-excretion is remarkably impaired compared to healthy controls. Luetscher et al. [11], Kloppenburg et

212

Table 1. Age, sex and risk factors in both groups of essential hypertensives

	Age (years)	*Sex*	*Body weight* real (kg)	in % of aver.	*Height* (cm)	Chole- sterol (mg%)	Tri- glycerides (mg%)	Uric acid (mg%)
Patients with <u>*normal*</u> *aldosterone–regul.*	37,2 ± 10,8	♀: 50,0% ♂: 50,0%	72,7 ± 13,6	105,2 ± 13,0	170,8 ± 8,6	233,3 ± 43,9	169,4 ± 80,3	4,51 ± 1,60
Patients with <u>*disturbed*</u> *aldosterone–regul.*	44,5 ± 11,5	♀: 61,5% ♂: 38,5%	78,9 ± 10,0	112,8 ±16,4	170,1 ± 6,3	225,8 ± 45,4	190,8 ± 84,3	5,46 ± 1,10

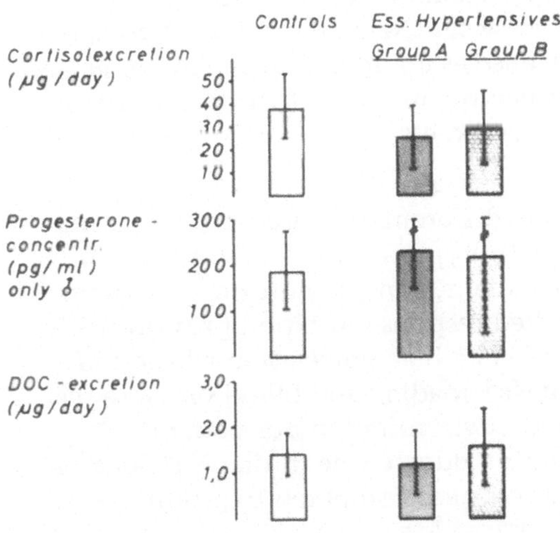

Fig. 5. ACTH-dependent steroids during sodium-loading in controls and patients of group A and B essential hypertensives

al. [10] and ourselves [9] reported an incomplete suppression of aldosterone after Na⁺ loading by measuring plasma aldosterone or aldosterone secretion or -excretion. The disturbed relation between aldosterone and Na⁺ in essential hypertensives is again reflected in our study by a distinctly lower coefficient of correlation between excretion of aldosterone and Na^+/K^+ ratio in urine-compared to controls.

In our study the difference in aldosterone regulation between controls and essential hypertensives however, is a consequence of an aldosterone regulation defect in only a smaller part of the patients group: During Na^+-loading a bimodal distribution of aldosterone excretion values was found. In the major group of essential hypertensives excretion of aldosterone and excretion of Na^+ and K^+ or Na^+/K^+ ratio in urine follow exactly the correlation range of controls. In a second smaller group of essential hypertensives (Group B) however, aldosterone excretion is not suppressible below the highest control value despite forced Na^+-loading. Correlation coefficient between aldosterone excretion and log Na^+/K^+ ratio in urine of this group of patients (Group B) is distinctly different compared to controls or to group A essential hypertensives.

The group of patients with essential hypertension and sustained aldosterone excretion during Na^+-loading exhibits some effects of mineralocorticoid excess: They do have a lower concentration of K^+ in serum during Na^+-loading and a better blood pressure response to spironolactone. PRA is not yet significantly different from the PRA in the other group of essential hypertensives, although a tendency towards lower PRA values was seen in the group of essential hypertensives with sustained excretion of aldosterone during Na^+ loading.

Group B-patients are heavier in body weight compared to group A-essential hypertensives. A significantly higher body weight was reported by Yeoman et al. (15) in hypervolemic essential hypertensives compared to the major group of hypovolemic essential hypertensives. Hypervolemic hypertension is diuretic responsive and possibly caused by a relative excess of salt and water induced by mineralocorticoid excess.

Blood pressure response to spironolactone differentiates primary, non-renin-mediated forms of hyperaldosteronism with hypertension from secondary, renin-mediated hyperaldosteronism (B). In fact, a major portion of patients with essential hypertension shows a marked response of blood pressure with spironolactone therapy. In a recent study [1] a high correlation was found between secretion of aldosterone during Na^+ loading and blood pressure response to spironolactone. A similar response was found in our patients. Patients (Group B) with sustained excretion of aldosterone during Na^+ loading had a significantly better blood pressure response compared to group A essential hypertensives.

There appears to be much confusion in literature about low renin essential hypertension being a specific subgroup of essential hypertension with hyper-mineralocorticoidism and better blood pressure response to spironolactone. Some authors have found a better blood pressure response in low renin hypertension to spironolactones, others have not confirmed these findings. Benraad et al. [1] found no correlation of blood pressure response to spironolactone and PRA, but did report a good correlation of aldosterone secretion during Na^+ loading to blood pressure response to spironolactone. Our experience is

214

similar. In our experiment low PRA is found in both groups of patients with essential hypertension; those with normal aldosterone — and those with sustained aldosterone excretion during Na^+ loading.

After six days of Na^+ loading we are not able to differentiate the group of essential hypertensives with sustained excretion of aldosterone from four histologically and biochemically proven patients with hyperaldosteronism and micronodular adrenal hyperplasia. They exhibit similar aldosterone excretion values and similar concentrations of K^+ in serum during Na^+ loading. A marked fluctuation of the concentration of K^+ in serum up to normal values in "hyperplasia — patients" with hyperaldosteronism was also reported by Ferriss et al. [3, 4]. In most reports on the subject, "hyperplasia — patients" with hyperaldosteronism had distinctly higher PRA values compared to adenoma patients [4], as it was the case in our group B patients.

We believe therefore, that our patient group with inadequate high aldosterone excretion during Na^+-loading may reflect qualitatively a similar pathogenetic defect in mineralocorticoid secretion as "hyperplasia — patients" with hypermineralocorticoidism. However, only those patients with complete and prominent features of mineralocorticoid excess were operated so far and so diagnosis was proven by histological examination of the adrenals only in a part of this group of patients.

Presently, there is only speculation concerning the possible mechanism for the above mentioned regulation defect of aldosterone in a group of essential hypertensives. There is no difference in ACTH-dependent steroids as cortisol and progesterone between these two groups of essential hypertensives. So ACTH most probably does not play a role in pathogenesis of sustained aldosterone secretion during sodium loading in our group B- essential hypertensives.

Summary

In patients with grade I and II essential hypertension, studied during sodium loading (Na^+-excretion above 175 meq/day), we found a bimodal behaviour of aldosterone excretion, separating two groups of patients: In the major part of essential hypertensives sodium loading led to a suppression of aldosterone excretion below 6 μg/day, which is the highest control value during sodium loading, with an average of 2.7 ± 1.4 (SD) μg/day. Aldosterone excretion of a second group of patients was not suppressible below 6 μg/day despite forced sodium loading, resulting in an average value of 10.0 ± 3.0 (SD) μg/day. During sodium deprivation or free sodium intake, aldosterone excretion of the first group of patients followed exactly the behavior of normotensive controls, whereas in the second group of essential hypertensives the correlation of aldosterone excretion and log. Na-excretion or log. Na^+/K^+-ratio in 24 hour urine (r = 0.59) was far below the control value of r = 0.87. Serum potassium concentration during sodium loading was significantly (p < 0.001) lower (3.81 ± 0.44 meq/l) in the essential hypertensives with non suppressible aldosterone excretion

compared to those with suppressible aldosterone excretion (4.26 ± 0.37 meq/l).
The blood pressure response on treatment with 200 mg spironolactone/day
was better (p < 0.05) in patients with non suppressible aldosterone excretion
compared to essential hypertensives with normalaldosterone regulation. The
plasma renin activity of both groups of patients was not significantly different,
however there was a tendency towards lower PRA — values in the patient group
with non suppressible aldosterone excreting during sodium loading.

References

1. Benraad H, Drayer J, Hoefnagels W, Kloppenburg P, Benraad T (1978)
   Role of aldosterone in antihypertensive effect of spironolactone in essential
   hypertension. Clin Pharmacol Ther 24 : 638
2. Collins RD, Weinberger MH, Dowdy AJ, Nokes GW, Gonzales CM,
   Luetscher JA (1970) Abnormally sustained aldosterone secretion during
   salt loading in patients with various forms of benign hypertension, relation
   to plasma renin activity. J Clin Invest 49 : 1415
3. Ferriss JB, Beevers DG, Brown JJ, Davies DL, Fraser R, Lever AF, Mason
   P, Neville AM, Robertson JIS (1978) Clinical, biochemical and pathological features of low-renin ("primary") hyperaldosteronism (Review). A
   Heart J 95 : 375
4. Ferriss JB, Beevers DG, Brown JJ, Fraser R, Lever AF, Padfield PL,
   Robertson JIS (1978) Low-renin ("primary") hyperaldosteronism.
   Differential diagnosis and distinction of subgroups within the syndrome
   (Review). Am Heart J 95 : 641
5. Genest J, Nowaczynski W, Kuchel O, Sasaki C (1972) Plasma progesterone
   levels and 18-Hydroxy-deoxycorticosterone secretion rate in benign essential hypertension in humans. In: Genest J, Koiw (eds) Hypertension 72.
   Springer, Berlin Heidelberg New York, p 293
6. Genest J, Nowaczynski W, Kuchel O, Sasaki C, Boucher R, Rojo-Ortega
   JM, Constantinopoulos G, Ganten D, Messerli F (1976) The adrenal cortex
   and essential hypertension. Recent Prog Horm Res 32 : 377
7. Haber E, Koerner T, Page LB, Kliman B, Purnode A (1969) Application of
   a radioimmunoassay for angiotensin I to the physiologic measurement of
   plasma renin activity in normal human subjects. J Clin Endocrin 29 : 1349
8. Helber A, Kaufmann W (1973) Radioimmunologische Methode zur Aldo-
   steronbestimmung im Urin. Klin Wochenschr 51 : 1164
9. Helber A, Meurer KA, Rosskamp E, Wambach G, Dickmans HA, Kaufmann
   W (1974) Aldosteronexkretion und Plasmareninaktivität von Patienten mit
   essentieller Hypertonie und mit reninsupprimiertem Hyperaldosteronis-
   mus. Klin Wochenschr 52 : 966
10. Kloppenburg PWC, Drayer JIM, Benraad HB, Benraad TJ (1974) Normal
    aldosterone versus supranormal aldosterone hypertension: An alternative
    to normal renin versus low renin hypertension. In: Distler A, Wolff HP,
    (eds) Current problems in hypertension. Thieme, Stuttgart, p 143

11. Luetscher JA, Beckerhoff R, Dowdy AJ, Wilkinson R (1972) Incomplete
    suppression of aldosterone secretion and plasma concentration in hyperten-
    sive patients on high sodium intake. In: Genest J, Koiw (eds) Hypertension
    72. Springer, Berlin Heidelberg New York, p 286
12. Melby JC, Dale SL, Wilson TE (1971) 18-Hydroxy-DOC in human hyper-
    tension. Circ Res Suppl II 28 : 143
13. Spark RF, Melby JC (1968) Aldosteronism in hypertension. Ann Intern
    Med 69 . 685
14. Spark RF, Melby JC (1971) Hypertension and low plasma renin activity:
    Presumptive evidence for mineralocorticoid excess. Ann Int Med 75 : 831
15. Yeoman GD, Dustan HP, Tarazi RC, Bravo EL (1976) Hypertension,
    obesity and blood volume. Abstract, Kidney I 10 : 538

Studies on the Influence of Salt and Water Balance and Blood Pressure Regulation in Hypertensive Patients

H. Liebau, M. Hilfenhaus, O. Schober, P. Mariss

One of the major paradoxes in the regulation of sodium excretion is that the patient or experimental animal with elevated blood pressure does not excrete more sodium than normotensives, although it has been known for almost a century that there is a correlation between renal perfusion pressure and sodium excretion (Cushny, 1971; Winton, 1951/52).

According to Guyton's concept of blood pressure regulation elevation of blood pressure in any case of hypertension is the consequence of a diminished capacity of the kidney to excrete sodium (Guyton and Coleman, 1969). In this context, however, the mechanism of *exaggerated* natriuresis observed in hypertensive patients following an acute saline load (Birchall, 1953; Farnsworth, 1946; Hanenson, 1959) is not well understood.

The present study was designed to get more information on factors controlling the urinary excretion of a saline load in normotensive and hypertensive man

Methods

Patients: 10 normotensives (9 male, 1 female), their ages ranging from 15 to 51 years and 11 patients with essential hypertension (8 male, 3 female), their ages ranging from 21 to 55 years, were investigated. All patients had a normal renal function as assessed by the endogenous creatinine clearance and were free of signs of heart failure. Antihypertensive or diuretic treatment was discontinued at least ten days prior to the study. The patients received a standard diet with a sodium content of 120-140 mmol/l and with unrestricted fluid intake. On the day of the study the patients remained supine from the night before.

Physiological Studies

Following a single shot injection of ^{24}Na and ^{82}Br and an injection of ^{51}Cr-labelled erythrocytes, small samples of blood were taken for the determination of the plasma disappearance rate of ^{24}Na and ^{82}Br to calculate the distribution coefficients according to a three compartment model. 30 min later blood was taken for the determination of PRA, plasma catecholamines and blood volume.

Two hours later at about 11.00 a.m. 2000 ml/1.73 m^2 of body surface area
of 0.9% saline warmed up to 37°C were infused within 30 min into a cubital
vein.

Urine was collected by spontaneous voiding during the periods: 24 hrs. before
the experiment, 3 hrs. before infusion and from 0-3 hrs, 3-5 hrs. and 5-21 hrs.
after the start of the infusion.

Before, during and after the infusion, the following parameters were measured:
Arterial blood pressure by sphygmomanometry; peripheral venous pressure in
the cubital vein, blood volume by ^{51}Cr-labelling of the patients' erythrocytes,
and changes of the blood volume by repeated measurements of the hematocrit;
plasma renin activity (PRA) by a radioimmunoassay of angiotensin I, generated
in vitro, plasma catecholamines by a radioenzymatic method; urinary electrolytes by flamephotometry. Net fluid load was calculated by substracting the
corresponding urine volume from the infused volume, and changes of the extravascular fluid volume were calculated by subtracting changes of blood volume
(BV) from the net fluid load.

All volumes and excretion rates were adjusted to 1.73 m^2 of body surface area.

Results

The values of the distribution of ^{82}Br and ^{24}Na at different time intervals are
given in Figure 1. There was no significant difference between the hypertensive
and the normotensive group at any time.

Effect of Saline Infusion on Blood Pressure and Body Fluid Volumes

Control values of heart rate, venous pressure and of BV were not significantly
different between the normotensive and the hypertensive group (Table 1).
Heart rate, venous pressure and BV were significantly increased and hemato-
crits were decreased during saline infusion in both groups. In the hypertensive
group the increase in BV was significantly smaller than in the normotensive
group. The increases in BV and in heart rates were not accompanied by an increase in mean arterial pressure (MAP), neither in the normotensive nor in the
hypertensive group; on the contrary, diastolic blood pressure slightly decreased
during the saline infusion.

Effect of Saline Infusion on Sodium Excretion

Urine volume and urinary sodium excretion were elevated after the saline infusion (Fig. 2). The maximum excretion rates, which were observed during the
first three hours after the infusion in both groups, were significantly higher in
the hypertensive than in the normotensive group. During the period of 5-21

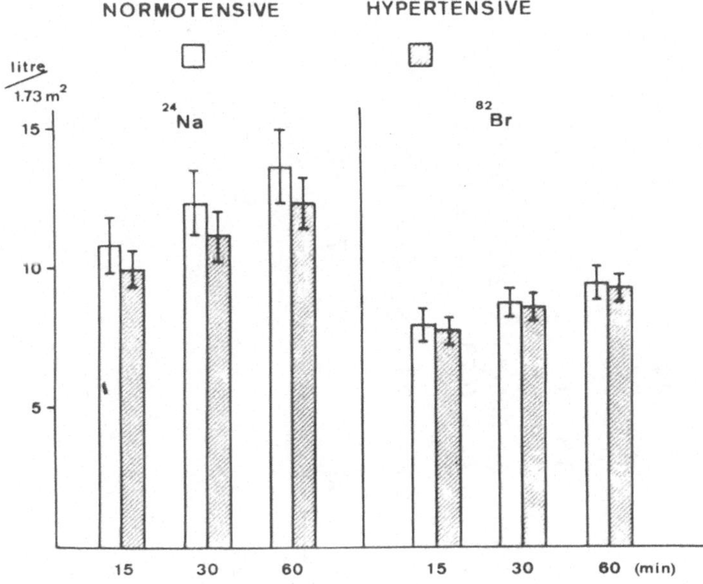

Fig. 1. Distribution space of ^{82}Br and ^{24}Na after a single shot injection after different time intervalls

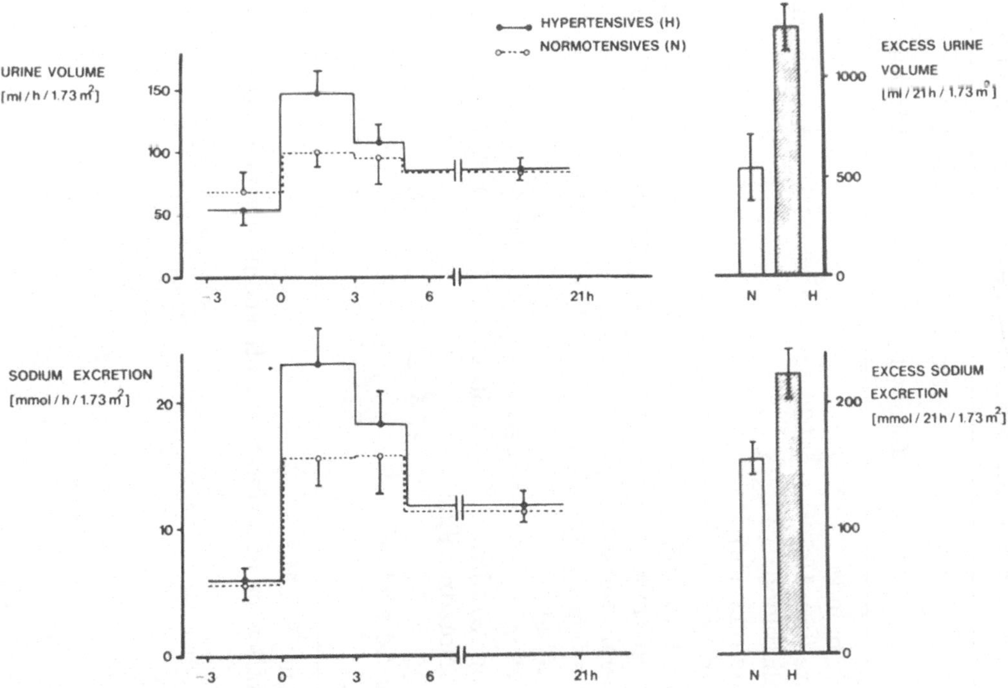

Fig. 2. Effect of saline infusion on urinary excretion of sodium and volume in hypertensive and normotensive man

Table 1. Effect of saline infusion on hemodynamic and hormonal factors on normotensive and in hypertensive patients

	Normotensives (n = 10)		Hypertensives (n = 11)	
	Control	End of Infusion	Control	End of Infusion
Systolic blood pressure (mm Hg)	129 ± 3a)	131 ± 4a n.s.b)	191 ± 8a)	193 ± 9a n.s.b)
Diastolic blood pressure (mm Hg)	83 ± 2	80 ± 2 n.s.	125 ± 250	119 ± 4 0.005
Mean arterial pressure (mm Hg)	98 ± 2	97 ± 2 n.s.	147 ± 5	144 ± 6 n.s.
Heart rate (min^{-1})	74 ± 4	79 ± 4 0.05	80 ± 3	86 ± 4 0.01
Peripheral venous pressure (cm H$_2$O)	9.2 ± 1.0	12.7 ± 1.0 0.001	9.3 ± 0.8	1.9 ± 1.1 0.005
Blood volume (ml/1.73 m^2)	4644 ± 268	5616 ± 365 0.001	4553 ± 250	5350 ± 282 0.001
PRA (ng AI/ml/h)	1.66 ± 0.31	0.87 ± 0.17 0.005	1.46 ± 0.34	0.78 ± 0.22 0.005
Plasma Noradrenaline (pg/ml)	195 ± 24	166 ± 23 n.s.	232 ± 20	176 ± 21 0.05
Plasma Adrenaline (pg/ml)	77 ± 10	54 ± 8 n.s.	102 ± 28	53 ± 7 n.s.

a) mean ± S.E.M.
b) Significance of differences to the control values analyzed by paired t-test

hrs. after the infusion the excretion rates were still elevated above control levels, but not different between both groups.

Effect of Saline Infusion on Plasma Renin and Plasma Catecholamines

PRA and plasma catecholamine values were not significantly different between the normotensive and the hypertensive group before, during and after the infusion. PRA decreased about 50% of the control values at the end of the infusion (Table 1). A statistically significant decrease of the plasma noradrenaline concentration was observed only in the hypertensive group at the end of the infusion (Table 1).

Relationship Between MAP, PRA, Sodium Excretion and Body Fluid Distribution after Saline Infusion

The ratio $\triangle BV/\triangle EVFV$ (blood volume/extravascular fluid volume) was calculated as an indicator of the intra- and extravascular distribution of the infused fluid volume. In the *normotensives* correlations existed between the sodium excretion rate and the control values of PRA. In the hypertensives $\triangle BV/\triangle EVFV$ and the sodium excretion rate after the load were significantly correlated to the control values of PRA and of MAP (Table 2). A significant correlation also existed between the factor $\triangle BV/\triangle EVFV$ and the sodium excretion after the load.

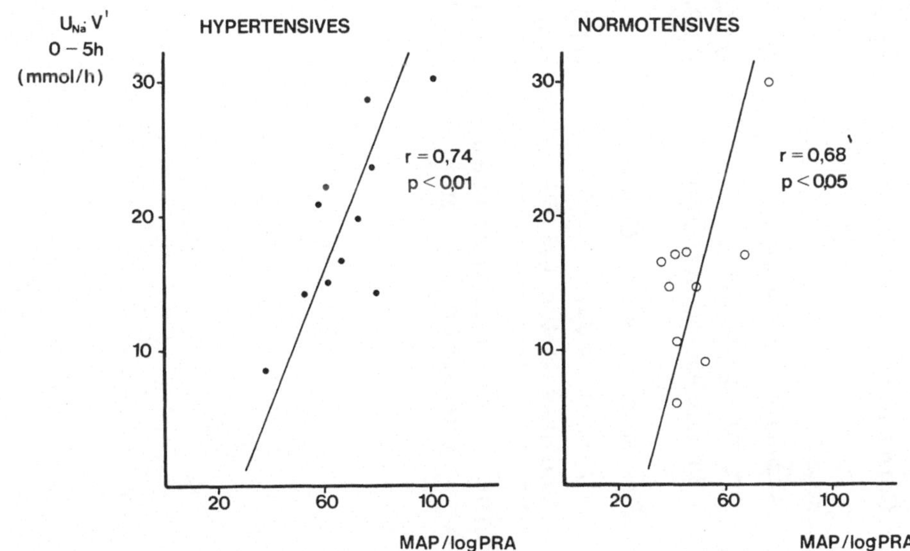

Fig. 3. Initial sodium excretion in relation to mean arterial blood pressure and PRA

Table 2. Relationship of blood pressure and PRA with sodium excretion and fluid distribution after saline infusion in normotensive and in hypertensive patients
IVFV = intravascular fluid volume; EVFV = extravascular fluid volume

Correlation	Normotensives			Hypertensives		
	r	p	n	r	p	n
Mean arterial pressure						
vs. $\triangle$ IVFV/$\triangle$ EVFV[a]	0.243	n.s.	10	−0.674	< 0.05	11
Sodium excretion 0-5 h[b]	0.030	n.s.	10	0.707	< 0.05	11
Plasma renin activity (Control)						
vs. $\triangle$IVFV/$\triangle$EVFV[a]	0.530	n.s.	10	0.891	< 0.001	11
Sodium excretion 0-5 h[b]	−0.657	< 0.05	10	−0.678	< 0.05	11

a) Changes from the control value at 60 min after start of infusion
b) Periods after start of infusion

Discussion

An acute expansion of the intravascular space by a saline infusion induces an
increase in cardiac output, which is supposed to be medeated by the Frank-
Starling-mechanism. Any increase in cardiac ouput is a consequence of an increase in BP or a decrease in TPR. In our experiments BP did not increase during the infusion, indicating that the TPR decreased. A decrease in TPR or renal
vascular resistance due to a saline infusion was observed by Schalekamp et al.,
1971. According to findings of Messmer et al, 1972 hemodilution, indicated
in our experiments by the decrease in the hematocrit, effects a marked decrease in blood viscosity and consequently according to Hagen-Poiseulle's law
in the TPR. Additionally an afferent arteriolar dilatation is induced in the kidney by a rise of the tubular pressure after a saline infusion (Kiil, 1975). Therefore, it must be taken into account, that the increase in CO due to volume expansion might be a consequence of the decrease of TPR, a view which is confirmed by observations of others (Ulrych et al, 1964), that in man the Frank-
Starling-mechanism is overrided by a reflex mechanism. The smaller increase
in blood volume in the hypertensives was not only due to an exaggerated urinary excretion, but also because the fluid was shifted more rapidly from the
intravascular to the extravascular space.

The plasma disappearance rate of ^{82} Br and of ^{24} Na before the infusion were
not different between both groups. This indicates that in the steady state condition the exchange of salt and fluid between the intravascular and the extravascular space is not different between hypertensives and normotensives.

The observation that the velocity of the urinary excretion and the shift of the
load to the extravascular space were correlated to each other as well as to the
level of blood pressure and of renin indicates that physical (BP) and hormonal
factors play an important role in the distribution and excretion of a saline
fluid load. In dogs, Raeder et al. (1974) could demonstrate, that the urinary
sodium excretion rate due to a load is proportional to the height of BP.

It is generally accepted, that a relationship exists between PRA and the sodium
balance. In any case of volume depletion (dietary sodium deficiency, saluret-
ics, hemorrhage) PRA is increased and vice versa. Therefore, it seems possible
to regard PRA as an indicator of the degree of volume expansion. If the absolute rate of sodium excreted depends not only on the height of BP but also on
the degree of extracellular volume expansion (Kiil, 1975), a correlation should
exist between the term BP/PRA and the initial sodium excretion rate; furthermore, no difference should exist between the hypertensive and the normotensive
group.

Figure 3 gives the result of the calculation. There existed a good correlation
between the rate of initial sodium excretion and the term MAP/log PRA in the
normotensive as well as in the hypertensive group with a similar slope and inter-
cept of the regression lines in both groups. This finding confirms the concept,
that the capacity of the kidney to excrete sodium is normal in essential hypertension. Variations of the sodium excretion rate can be explained by variations
of the degree of volume expansion and by the height of BP.

The more rapid shift of the fluid load from the intravascular to the extravascular space in the hypertensives may be explained by physical forces: The decrease in TPR by hemodilution effects an increased translation of the hydrostatic blood pressure to the capillary bed. Therefore, an increased amount of fluid might be squeezed off from the vascular bed.

Thus, the more rapid shift of the fluid load from the intravascular into the extravascular space and the exaggerated urinary excretion in hypertensives can be explained as a consequence of hemodilution and of the physical force of elevated blood pressure.

Summary

1. In ten normotensive control subjects and in eleven patients with benign essential hypertension isotonic saline was administrated intravenously. Determinations of blood pressure, blood volume, plasma renin activity, plasma noradrenaline concentration and urinary excretion of salt and fluid were carried out before, during and after the infusion.
2. No increments of blood pressure were observed, neither in the normotensive nor in the hypertensive patients, during the infusion and thereafter.
3. The expansion of the vascular bed was attenuated in the hypertensives, this effect was due to a more rapid urinary excretion and a more rapid shift of the fluid in the extravascular space.
4. Excess sodium excretion was dependent on the values of PRA and MAP before the start of the infusion.
5. It is concluded, that the capacity of the kidney to excrete sodium is not affected in essential hypertension.

References

Birchall R, Tuthill SW, Jacobs WS, Trautmann jr WJ, Finlay T (1953) Renal excretion of water, sodium and chloride. Comparison of the responses of hypertensive patients with these of normal subjects primed with various hormones. Circulation 7 : 258

Cushny AR (1917) The secretion of urine, Longmans, Green, London

Farnsworth EB (1946) Renal reabsorption of chloride and phosphate in normal subjects and in patients with essential arterial hypertension. J Clin Invest 25 : 896-905

Guyton AC, Coleman TG (1969) Quantitative analysis of the pathophysiology of hypertension. Circ Res Suppl 1 24/25 : 1-14

Hanenson IB, Tamsky HH, Polasky N, Ranschoff W, Miller BF (1959) Renal excretion of sodium in arterial hypertension. Circulation 20 : 498

Kiil F (1975) Pressure diuresis and hypertension. Scand J Clin Invest 35 : 289-293

Messmer K, Sunder-Plassmann L, Klövekorn WP, Holper K (1972) Circulatory significance of hemodilution: Rheological changes and limitations. Adv Microcirc 4 : 1-77

Raeder MG, Ombik jr P, Kiil F (1974) Effect of acute hypertension on the natriuretic response to saline loading. Am J Physiol 226 : 989

Schalekamp MADH, Krauss XH, Schalekamp-Kuyken MPA, Kolsters G, Birkenhäger WH (1971) Studies on the mechanism of hypernatriuresis in essential hypertension in relation to measurements of plasma renin concentration, body fluid compartments and renal function. Clin Sci 41 : 219-231

Ulrych M, Hofman J, Hejl Z (1964) Cardiac and renal hyperresponsiveness to acute plasma volume expansion in hypertension. Am Heart J 68 : 193-203

Winton FR (1951/52) Hydrostatic pressure affecting the flow of urine and blood in the kidney. Harvey Lecture 47 : 21

Hypertension and Public Health

An Overview of the National High Blood Pressure Education Program in the United States

G. W. WARD

Hypertension is one of the most prevalent chronic disease conditions in the United States.

Approximately 35 million Americans, about one in six, have high blood pressure warranting some form of treatment. An additional 25 million are estimated to have borderline high blood pressure requiring medical surveillance. Untreated hypertension is the largest single contributor to stroke, and a major contributor to heart disease and kidney failure. It is the complications caused by hypertension rather than hypertension that generally results in hospitalization. Hypertension is more common among blacks than whites-about one out of four blacks has definite high blood pressure, contrasted to one in six in the general population.

In addition to being a major accelerating factor in the 500.000 strokes (175.000 stroke deaths) and 1.250.000 heart attacks (650.000 heart attack deaths) each year, hypertensive heart disease, hypertension, and ischemic heart disease with hypertension accounted for more than 90.000 deaths in the U.S. in 1976. While direct hypertension deaths are a gross underestimate of the effect of hypertension on overall cardiovascular disease mortality, they clearly indicate its significance.

Actuarial, epidemiologic and clinical data confirm that the risk of subsequent illness and/or death increases with blood pressure. Even within the normal blood pressure ranges the relationship persists: a person with a blood pressure of 130/80 is at greater risk of premature mortality or morbidity from heart failure, heart attack, stroke and renal failure than an individual with a blood pressure of 110/70. These risks begin to accelerate at about a level of 140/90; a level now accepted as the arbitrary threshold of borderline hypertension.

The specific causes of 90 to 95 percent of hypertension remain unknown. We do not yet know enough about the fundamental processes involved to prevent or cure it. Thus, short term emphasis must be placed on optimizing control of existing hypertension. Studies indicate that chemotherapeutic lowering of blood pressure can be accomplished on a sustained basis with concomitant lowering of morbidity and mortality. In some individuals nutritional changes such as salt and weight control may lesson the degree of or even obviate the need for drug therapy.

In 1972, the nation faced a contradictory situation vis-a-vis hypertension control. On the one hand, therapies proved to lower blood pressure and its dreadful complications were available. On the other hand, within the large population of hypertensive patients, many were not aware of their condition, some were receiving treatment, but only a few were successfully controlling their blood pressure.

The reasons for this proved to be many. Public and professionals alike tended to regard anything but severe hypertension in a ho-hum fashion, not clearly recognizing the health hazard represented by even mild hypertension. Among professionals, confusion existed in selecting among a multitude of drugs, each with a differing mode of action. Most professional publications on hypertension focused on the diagnosis of the few cases of secondary hypertension and neglected the management of essential hypertension — the ultimate diagnosis in more than 90 percent of our nation's 35 million hypertensive patients. Regimen adherence issues were poorly addressed by both physicians and patients.

Physicians must turn their attention to the potential of preventive cardiology rather than the current crisis care cardiology. Problems of regimen adherence must be met. Comprehensive efforts at high blood pressure control require a multidisciplinary team approach. There exist both professional reluctance to make full use of allied health personnel and legal barriers to their use. In addition, such comprehensive efforts require sophisticated planning and management skills long used by industry, but still new to the health care delivery system.

The existing health care system contains inadequate mechanisms both for accomplishing and for financing detection and treatment of high blood pressure for large segments of the population. Existing means for continuing education of health professionals are often poorly organized and rarely relate to a demonstrated education need. Lacking at times are resources and mechanisms to accomplish long term (chronic) patient education and follow-up any significant amount of consumer education. Currently a large and sometimes disproportionate reliance must be placed on voluntary activity to accomplish these tasks often leading to extreme variance in quality and considerable discontinuity of effort.

Thus, although the nation is progressing in its capability to control hypertension, it is still realistic to expect further gains.

The National High Blood Pressure Education Program

The National High Blood Pressure Education Program (NHBPEP), inaugurated in 1972, is a coalition of about 15 federal agencies, some 150 major national organizations, 50 state health departments, some 2.000 organized community control programs and a variety of other facilitating groups which is coordinated by the National Heart, Lung, and Blood Institute (NHLBI).

Although the NHLBI role is authorized by public law and its continued role
consistenly endorsed in Congressional reports, the Program itself is mandated
by a jointly expressed need among the participants, not by law. It is this common agreement, this broad consensus — not an executive or legislative fiat —
which fuels the NHBPEP. The Program is one of few true, participative part-
nerships among federal government, local government and private interests
which makes the most of the unique resources and capabilities each sector can
offer. As such, it represents an apparently successful experiment to determine
whether such a cooperative, multidisciplinary effort is possible and whether it
can achieve lasting change to meet a clear social need — reduction of excess
illness, disability and death from uncontrolled hypertension.

Program Scope

The National High Blood Pressure Education Program was organized in 1972.
The National Heart, Lung, and Blood Institute was designated as the coordinating agency. Begun as a Secretary's initiative, this Program was quickly given
additional impetus by passage the same year of legislation authorizing NHLBI
activity in prevention, education and control.

Program is a complex, multi-faceted effort having extraordinary depth and
breadth. Its scope includes a multitude of organizations, a wide range of interrelated issues and a host of activities.

Organizations

It was clear from the outset of the Program that the National Heart, Lung, and
Blood Institute could not alone identify and define all the issues which had to
be addressed, provide all the educational materials that were required, nor de-
liver the necessary services to some 60 million Americans requiring blood pressure surveillance or treatment. Only by developing a coordinated network involving many organizations could any progress be made. Thus, the organizations participating in the Program serve not only as the Program backbone, but
also provide much of its brains and muscle.

The scope of participating organisations who have willingly entered into a
partnership with the Federal government to achieve hypertension control is
broad and varied. Over 150 major national organizations — professional, voluntary, and representing components of industry — have participated regularly
in the Program, many of them since its inception. Professional groups include
virtually every type of provider in a position to provide assistance to the hypertensive patient: physicians, nurses, pharmacists, dentists, health educators,
pediatrists, optometrists, and nutritionists. Both majority and minority organizations among these professions have contributed significantly to both planning and implementation of the Programm effort.

National voluntary organizations are also well represented in Program acitivites. Among these are the American Heart Association, American Red Cross, National Kidney Foundation, and Citizens for the Treatment of High Blood Pressure. These groups have participated both in a planning and advisory function at the national level and as key action leaders in local communities.

The National High Blood Pressure Education Program has been uniquely successful among public health programs in eliciting assistance from the private, industrial sector. Pharmaceutical companies, insurance companies, equipment manufacturers, and a wide array of industrial firms, many having no direct relationship to health care have generously and continuously lent their expertise and resources to hypertension control.

Nor has local government been remiss in assuming responsbility and investing resources. Virtually every state health department has a specifically labeled component to deal with hypertension control; a few of which are nationally recognized as pioneers in this regard, having been engaged in hypertension control activities of major size even before the National High Blood Pressure Education Program was begun. Many county and community health departments have been actively involved as well; Milwaukee and Savannah serve as excellent models which can be cited as exemplars of this kind of effort.

Many federal agencies have been involved on both a continuing and intermittent basis. In addition to the National Heart, Lung, and Blood Institute, many agencies within HEW have been significant participants. The Health Services Administration, Bureau of Community Health Services supports not only special service programs aimed specifically at hypertension, but also has made significant effort to increase attention to hypertension among its many other service delivery programs such as neighborhood health centers, migrant health programs, rural health initiatives, and the Indian Health Sercive. The National Center for Health Statistics has provided invaluable help to the Program through its data base and willing staff assistance. The Health Resources Administration overviews the health planning organizations of the nation and has accepted Program guidance regarding incorporation of issues relevant to hypertension control planning in its advisory documents.

The Food and Drug Administration, in addition to serving as a data base for certain specific issues, used its own resources to asisist the Program in conducting a national probability sample survey to help assess physician knowledge and actions regarding hypertension. A partial list of other cooperating HEW agencies includes the National Cancer Institute, the Office of Health Information and Health Promotion, the Bureau of Health Manpower, the Bureau of Health Education, and the Office of the Assistant Secretary for Planning and Evaluation.

The Veterans Administration, the largest health agency outside HEW and the largest single organized health care delivery system in the nation, operates a series of hypertension clinics treating thousands of patients each year. The VA also regularly provides the Program with valuable counsel.

234

Among other federal agencies is the Office of Personnel Management
the Civil Service Commission) whose Occupational Health Divisions has actively
assisted the Program in development of hypertension education and control
programs for the three million civilian employees of the federal government.
The U.S. Department of Agriculture has assisted through its extension program
efforts. The Department of Defense has distributed many Program materials
among the health personnel of its branches and adopted many of the treatment
recommendations developed by the Program.

Program Emphasis Areas

Another at least partially unique characteristic of the National High Blood Pressure Education Program has been its intent and ability to modify the direction
of Program focus to reflect the constantly changing status of hypertension control in the nation. Initial Program focus concentrated upon increasing awareness
among the public, patients and health professionals of the health risk presented by uncontrolled hypertension. As data became available suggesting that this
awareness was increasing, the Program shifted and now operates in a mode which
emphasizes maintenance of therapy and long-term control of blood pressure.
Within these broader focuses, however, are a large number of more specific
issues which must be addressed.

Medical Guidelines Development and Adoption: A major Program emphasis
area is seeking the updating through consensus of developed medical guidelines
for the identification, evaluation, treatment, and counseling of hypertensive
patients. Guidance has been developed which addresses not only the technical
and clinical aspects of these issues, but also how they may be implemented
within the roles of a variety of health professionals.

Therapy maintenance is not only a major Program focus at this time but also a
topic with a technology of its own which must be translated to practitioners. It
is also the focus of most Institute produced massmedia materials. If regimen
adherence and long-term control is not attained, then all the preceding steps of
detection, referral and care, and selction of therapy have been fruitless.

The worksetting represents a major focus area for the Program. The health care
services provided by many small companies and large corporations across the
country as well as the comprehensive union organization which exists in many
industries serve as resources for delivery of services and communicating the
message of the Program.

Interdisciplinary Roles: The Program is concerned not only with the independent actions of a variety of health professionals, but also with development of
effective interaction among these professionals. Thus, a significant effort has
been expended to identify and promote interactive roles for health professionals
with particular interest devoted to decreasing barriers and constraints to effective use of non-physician personnel.

Minority Populations: A singularly important Program emphasis area deals with the unique problems of hypertension control among the nation's various minority populations. Both low income and low education appear to be risk factors for hypertension and these risk factors are much more prevalent among many minority groups. Minority populations frequently have greater difficulty gaining access to the necessary care. Educational materials, to be most effective, must be sensitive to the unique cultural aspects of these populations.

Blood Pressure Measurement: Because accurate determination of blood pressure is the ultimate measure of the hypertension problem and its resolution, the Program has an ongoing interest in both the training of personnel to perform this function well and the development of standards to help insure both the accuracy and precision of blood pressure measurement devices.

Rural areas do not appear to have experienced the same rate of progress in achieving hypertension control as have major metropolitan areas. For this reason, the National High Blood Pressure Education Program contains a priority emphasis area to explore the unique characteristics of rural populations and rural health care delivery with the intent of increasing among the nation's non-metropolitan regions development of needed capacities for hypertension control.

Dietary Management: Although drug therapy is the mainstay of hypertension control and is likely to remain so for the forseeable future, it is not the only useful modality. A long considered and recently implemented program emphasis area deals with dietary management of hypertension and its utility as an alternative or adjunct to drugs.

Elderly and Youth Populations: Two additional special population groups constitute Program emphasis areas. These are the pediatric and elderly populations of the nation. As research continues, it has become evident that the precursors of fixed adult hypertension may begin quite early in life. In addition, appreciable numbers of young people, although we cannot currently label them as hypertensive, have blood pressures well above those of their age and sex peers. The Program is pursuing both research and consensus on establishing normal blood pressure ranges by age and sex in young people and in better refining the need for and the effects of therapies in this age group.

The elderly have unique problems of their own. In addition to limited resources, social isolation and other factors which may serve as care access barriers to the elderly, the benefits of intervention for some forms of hypertension in the elderly (isolated systolic hypertension) are not yet well established. Side effects and other risks of therapy may be more severe among older persons. The National High Blood Pressure Education Program, thus, has a Program emphasis area to examine, and hopefully, to resolve questions of this nature.

International Acitivities: Interest in hypertension control is not solely an American phenomenon. The US-USSR cardiovascular research exchange program incorporated a hypertension component about two years ago. Recently signed agreements with the Federal Republic of Germany and with Italy also include this interest. In addition, many education documents have been widely

circulated abroad. The Joint National Committee Report has been translated
into Japanese, French and Flemish. International visitors to NIH frequently
inquire about the NHBPEP. Program activities and results have been presented
to such diverse nations as Saudi Arabia, Finland, Canada, England, Yugoslavia,
Tanzania, China, Japan, England and Israel. Although international activities
are small in relation to the overall effort, they represent an important aspect of
the Program by disseminating the United States experience as well as allowing
the U.S. an opportunity to learn from parallel activities in other nations.

Program Activities

Given the large number of participating organizations and the broad range of
issues described in the proceeding sections, it is difficult to compress the totality of activity for the entire program into a readable document. And, in truth,
the Institute does not have complete data on all the activities of the participating organizations.

The Program, early on, chose to work with many organizations in a cooperative manner. These working relationships created a network — a National High
Blood Pressure Education network — through which to transmit and receive
ideas and information. The dissemination of this information and ideas went
primarily to the major participating organizations. These primary contacts in
turn relay, translate and disseminate information out to their following and
constituents. At times this relaying of information may exchange organizatio-
nal hands four and five times — eventually reaching the grass roots for implementation. Without omniscience and microscopic vision it is difficult to ascertain the totality of implementation at these grass roots levels. In addition, the
diffusion of any innovation requires an unpredictable quantity of time. After
concepts or ideas are planted with the primary contacts, the ideas may take
several weeks, months, or even years to trickle down and be implemented at
the local level. It is not surprising, then, that we hear of some innovations that
we hear of some innovations that are finally being implemented after an apparent two or three year time lag. Thus, we anticipate that many innovations that
are eventually adopted are done so without the knowledge of the Program.

High Blood Pressure Information Center: A key focal point within the Program
and the Program's primary interface with the general public and health professionals is the High Blood Pressure Information Center. The Center answers public inquiries about high blood pressure and distributes free educational materials,
short reports, bibliographies and studies, posters, radio and television materials,
reprints and other items. The Information Center also acts as a clearingshouse
for similar materials prepared by non-government sources, for relevant articles
in the professional literature, and for community and state programmatic activity. It schedules educational exhibits for both professional and lay group
meetings and conventions. A speaker's roster provides lecturers knowledgeable
about high blood pressure or helps organiuations find qualified speakers in their
own localities. The Center annually receives approximately one-hundred and

twenty-five thousand individual inquiries and distributes well over one million pieces of informational material.

Community Program Development: On request, the Community Program Development Service offers technical assistance to help community organisations to develop plans for improved efforts to control high blood pressure. The service draws on federal government experts and experienced practioners from successful community programs. Periodically, the service sponsors special invitational workshops: it also helps communities to develop their own workshops. For the past several years, activities of this component have been managed and coordinated using states as working units primarily because Institute resources available to the program are indidequate to reach all community programs on an individual basis. Some two-thousand active community programs have been identified. In addition, Institute and Contractor Program staff work closely with the HSA's Bureau of Community Health Services personnel to coordinate hypertension control activity supported by that Bureau.

Educational Materials Assessment: The Program reviews and endorses, on request, public and professional educational materials being developed by any source. The Program "logo" and the phrase "prepared in cooperation with the National High Blood Pressure Education Program" can be included on these materials if they meet these criteria: the items must not be sold for profit, must contain no product endorsement, and must be technically accurate.

Professional Education: Recommendations for detection, treatment, and patient education have been developed for the Program by nationally recognized experts. These recommendations are the basis for both content of a variety of professional education materials developed by the Program and for those developed by many other sources. This activity relates closely to and maintains liaison with a variety of groups including major professional organizations such as the American and National Medical Associations, American and National Dental Associations, American and National Nurses Associations, American and National Pharmaceutical Associations, American Association of Medical Colleges, National Board of Medical Examiners, American Academy of Family Physicians, American College of Cardiology, American Heart Association, pharmaceutical companies and others. A considerable array of educational materials have been developed.

Public Education: The Program coordinates a cooperative public education effort involving both local and national organizations and the media. The primary function of this component is to develop and coordinate distribution of mass media materials. In past years, the Institute, through its contract with the Advertising Council, has acquired between $3 to 5 million annually in free advertising space. When the success of other participating groups is added to this figure it is not unreasonable to estimate that as much as $20 million worth of free advertising space and time on radio and television and in print materials is garnered each year. This estimate does not include value impact of blooklets, leaflets, flyers, and posters distributed by the Institute's High Blood Pressure Information Center and the many other participant organizations each year.

238

Patient Education: The Program has taken the posture that patient education is a requisite component of therapy and that control of high blood pressure eventually involves to an irreducible two member team of the patient and provider. The concept that the patient is a member of the health care team is considered vital. Many organizations participating within the Program have developed and distributed patient education materials. The Institute has been involved in developing effective methods for pretesting these materials prior to their distribution. In addition, the Institute and several other participating groups are actively and effetively in patient education activities. Toward this end, a recent major activity of the Institute has been to support curriculum and materials development — in collaboration with the American Academy of Family Practitioners and The Society of Teachers of Family Medicine — to assist improved training of family practive residents in patient education.

Minority Populations: The Program has long recognized the unique needs of the variety of minority populations in the United States. In 1975, the Program held its first National Forum on Hypertension Among Minority Communities and plans a second National Forum in 1980. An outcome of the first forum was establishment of an ongoing Ad Hoc Committee on Hypertension in Minority Populations which has directed the conduct of workshops for many minority groups including Native Americans, Asian Americans, Hispanic origin groups including Puerto Ricans, Cubans and Mexican Americans, and Blacks. In addition, for two years the Institute has supported the Black Health Providers Task Force whose recommendations recently presented at a White House Conference may have considerable impact on the delivery of hypertension care services to Black populations.

School Health Education: School health education is a new planning effort to be developed during the coming years. Studies have shown that the adult population is frequently ill-informed about the health care system, the functions of the body an the nature of health risk factors. Although life-long reinforcement of health messages can never be eliminated, this activity can be substantially reduced if all children learn in their basic primary and secondary education the essentials of these topic. The function of this program area is not to directly engage in school education activities, but rather to work with persons in the field of education toward improving health curricula and positioning the NHLBI and other organizations participating in the Program as a resource to school health education.

Educational Research Grants Program: The scientific base for developing effective educational programs for the public, patients and health professionals is still developing. A major interest of the Program is the conduct of educational research and the exploration of innovative, cost effective ways of using education as a primary tool to gain greater control of high blood pressure. The Institute has, since 1974, provided continuing support to a variety of grants performing such research.

Demonstration Projects: The NHLBI has developed three major demonstration areas. These are: 1) Statewide Coordination of High Blood Pressure Control;

2) High Blood Pressure Control at the Worksetting; and 3) Community High Blood Pressure Control Demonstration Projects. The Statewide projects are intended to assess the impact of resource/activity coordination upon hypertension control status of patients and upon selected morbidity and mortality outcomes. Worksetting demonstrations will assist the ability of industry to mount and evaluate programs to detect hypertension, educate empolyees, and maintain hypertension control as well as to ascertain costs of such efforts. An additional project, operated through the Health Education Branch (HEB), is exploring the role of health insurers in stimulating and assisting development of work site based hypertension education and control programs. The Community Demonstration Program is examining models for implementation at the local level and measuring outcomes of both health care status and operational costs. Model sites have been chosen in both urban and rural areas.

Special Studies and Evaluation: To provide baseline evaluation data and to acquire planning information, the Institute has supported a variety of special studies of varying scope and depth and has made an active effort to secure data from other sources for this purpose. Examples of major studies supported include a national sample of the general public to determine existing knowledge, attitudes and behavior related to high blood pressure. This study, initially conducted in 1973, is currently being replicated. Under the auspices of the Food and Drug Administration, a similar study was conducted among physicians in 1978. Other studies include examination of the relationship between high blood pressure and life insurance, charateristics of automated blood pressure measuring devices, emplyment policies related to high blood pressure and state health department high blood pressure activities. A key study concerns the cost/benefits of high blood pressure therapy; it is contemplated that this study will be revised and refined on a continuing basis as a tool for assisting national and community program planning.

Program Progress

Since the inception of the National High Blood Pressure Education Program, few would deny that there has been substantial measurable progress in hypertension control in the United States. This progress has been achieved only by the willing participation of many individuals and organizations, a willingness derived from presentation of convincing arguments based on sound data that:
1. a real problem exists,
2. practical solutions exist,
3. that benefits are likely if the solutions are implemented, and
4. provision of feedback that progress was made which was commensurate with the implementation investment.

Such a response does not happen by accident nor does it happen frequently by fiat. To achieve this response, the NHBPEP leadership has pioneered — at least within the National Institutes of Health, if not within much of government — the use of consensus development to define the problems, solutions and benefits of hypertension control and to ascertain the degree or rate of progress.

One success of the Program, then, has been establishing the wide-spread acceptability of using the consensus process. Its utility is seemingly high. The necessity for using broad participation with the subsequent commitment to consensus outcomes by participants has undoubtedly been advantageous in advancing Program goals. At the same time, one must recognize that the consensus process has limits, it does not necessarily produce an optimum recommendation in terms of desirable goals, but rather, produces an outcome to which most people will agree. Decisive action comes, but it comes in small increments over time.

Another major area of Program success lies in development of a coordination mechanism to increase the level of concerted action among many disparate groups having varying interest in health, health care, and hypertension control. (It is important to note, at this point, that neither coordination nor consensus necessarily means selling "the Program", but rather our objective is to stimulate interest in and action upon high blood pressure control irrespective of whether an individual or group chooses to ally itself with the organization now known as the National High Blood Pressure Education Program.) A primary coordinating mechanism has been the National High Blood Pressure Education Coordinating Committee previously mentioned in the section describing Program organization. This committee, initially comprised of eight participating organizations, has grown in five short years to include over twenty professional, voluntary and other private organizations which regularly send representatives to a recognized forum for debate and resolution of issues in hypertension control.

Many of the consensus documents disseminated by the Program have arisen from needs identified and clarified within the Coordinating Committee. A few examples include: the Report of the Joint National Committee on High Blood Pressure, Detection, Evaluation and Treatment; a statement of the benefits and hazards of consumer operated blood pressure measurement devices; a position statement on the utility of dietary management of hypertension; and a statement of issues related to hypertension control among the elderly.

To achieve maximum from these position papers it has been necessary to use many redundant channels, each fine tuned to a specific audience or community of interest. The NHBPEP has succesfully developed such a structure using the coordinated resources and communications capabilities of many of its participating organizations. For example: the NHLBI has directly supported the operation of a community program develment service which provides on-site, tailored technical assistance to both regional and community levels. The Institute supports the High Blood Pressure Information Center which provides a variety of services to individuals. Under the aegis of the Coordinating Committee, the Program sponsors each year National High Blood Pressure Month which is designed to draw concentrated attention to the hypertension control problem and serve as a catalyst for year round activity among many organizations. The Committee also sponsors an annual National Conference on High Blood Pressure Control which provides for exchange of practical nuts and bolts implementation experience among an ever increasing variety of health and related professionals.

These and a variety of other nationwide efforts to bring high blood pressure under control have been under way for the past seven years. Various statistical indicators show that definite progress is being made. The public is developing a more accurate understanding of high blood pressure; patients are learning the importance of treating the problem and are living healthier lives as a result; health professionals have accepted the Program's recommended approach for managing the disease. Most significantly, progress in controlling high blood pressure is apparently contributing to a dramatic decline in death rates from cardiovascular disease.

The Change in Public Knowledge of High Blood Pressure

From the beginning it has been clear that there was, among the general public, both a lack of information and the existence of misinformation regarding high blood pressure and its control. An early survey in 1973, documented many of these deficiencies. In 1976, following additional research, the Program identified some specific widely held misconceptions regarding high blood pressure. Combating these misconceptions became the purpose of public and patient education efforts. Two national surveys although not readily comparable, indicate, for example, that only 39 percent of the public in 1973, versus 57 percent of the public in 1978, understood that hypertension usually has no symptoms. The misconception that dizziness was a symptom of high blood pressure was held by 86 percent in 1973 and by only 51 percent in 1978. Headaches as a condition associated with hypertension was cited by 75 percent in 1973 and by only 48 percent in 1978. Thus, belief in these misconceptions appears to be declining.

Treatment Practices by Health-Care Practitioners

When the National High Blood Pressure Education Program was formed, there was no general agreement by physicians on the most effective treatment methods for hypertension. The Program formed a task force to address the issue of treatment and a few years later convened a second group to revise treatment recommendations. These recommendations have been widely disseminated and adopted. The Food and Drug Adminstration in 1977 conducted a nationwide survey of physician's knowledge, attitudes and reported behavior regarding hypertension. Results of the survey indicate that physician's practices generally concur with national treatment recommendations in the areas of screening, blood pressure confirmation, and management goals. Physicians seem to be initiating drug therapy at slightly lower blood pressure levels than those suggested by the guidelines. There is a lower but still substantial concurrence concerning use of certain evaluation tools, non-drug therapies and the use of the recommended stepped-care approach. Additional data from the *National Disease and Therapeutic Index* strongly suggests a time associated increase between physician prescribing patterns for anti-hypertensive medications and the continuing efforts of the Program.

There is little hard data available to assess the practices of other health practitioners, however, an observed increase in articles within the professional literature for nurses, pharmacists and dentists during the course of the Program, as well as anecdotal field observations, strongly suggests that these professionals as well are contributing more often, more aggressively, and more appropriately to achieving hypertension control.

Patient Visits

Another changing indicator which reflects the actions of practitioners and patients is patient visits for hypertension. Data from the *National Disease and Therapeutic Index* indicates that the number of visits for hypertension has increased 20.7 percent from 1971 to 1978, while visits to physicians for all other causes decreased by 14.2 percent during the same period.

Death Rate Changes

Age-adjusted cardiovascular mortality rates have declined almost 32 percent over the last 30 years. In the last 10 years, however, the decline has accelerated precipitously and accounts for over two-thirds of the total 30 year decline. This decline is seen in both sexes, in the white and non-white and in every age decade band from the 2nd to beyond the 8th. Not only have death rates declined but despite an aging and ever increasing population the total number of cardiovascular deaths fell below one million in 1975 for the first time in almost a decade and the estimated 960 000 cardiovascular deaths in 1977 represent the lowest level since 1963. During the nine years since 1968, coronary heart disease mortality rates (the leading cause of death in the U.S.) declined 23 percent. For stroke the decline was even greater, 32 percent.

Stroke still ranks as the third most common cause of death in the United States (an estimated 182.840 in 1977). It is also the cause of disability for an estimated one million Americans. A downward trend in stroke mortality has been apparent for more than 50 years. Of importance is the fact that the downward trend in stroke death rate appears to have accelerated. In recent years, death rates for stroke have declined more rapidly than for any other component of cardiovascular motality. In the 1940's and 1950's stroke mortality declined less than 1 percent per year, in the 1960's 1.7 percent per year and, since 1972, by over 5 percent per year. Though sizable geographic differences have been noted in the past in stroke death rates in the United States, rates in all regions have fallen in the last 15 years with rates tending to converge with less variation from region to region.

All four major age-sex-color groups have shared in the stroke decline but the decline by sex for non-whites (primarily blacks) is relatively and absolutely greater than for the comparable white population. In fact the 48.5 percent decline in non-white females age 35-74 over the period 1960-1975 represents a fundamental change in the pattern of this disease.

In addition to observing national data on stroke death rates, the Program has made a preliminary analysis of similar trends in communities. Ten communities having known high rates of hypertension, education, and control activity were compared with two similar sets of ten communities not known to have well-organized efforts. The group of high activity communities experienced a 24 percent decline in crude stroke deaths from 1972 to 1976. The groups of presumed low activity communities each experienced a decline of only about 19 percent in the same period. Although these data clearly do not confirm a causal relationship, they do add weight to the association of increased hypertension control activity and declining stroke death rates.

Obviously, hypertension control is not the sole factor in these declining death rates. Both improved medical care and declines in other risk factors (smoking, blood lipids, lack of exercise and weight) have, doubtless, had their impact as well. However, the persistantly strong association between hypertension and cardiovascular death and documented progress in hypertension control produce a highly suggestive temporal relationship supporting the notion that blood pressure control has been a major contributor to these mortality declines.

Campaigns Against High Blood Pressure in Switzerland and the National Research Program 1 "Methodology of Primary Prevention of Cardiovascular Diseases"[1]

F. GUTZWILLER[2]

Introduction

This article attempts, in a first part, to describe the hypertension detection campaigns and their evaluations so far undertaken in Switzerland, and, in a second part, to discuss the National Research Program 1 "Primary Prevention of Cardiovascular Diseases in Switzerland". This latter program is a community-based life-style intervention trial [1, 2].

Epidemiology, Detection and Treatment Status of High Blood Pressure in Switzerland

In this framework, it is not possible to enumerate every activity regarding detection and long-term control of hypertension in Switzerland. A recent report of the Swiss Association against high blood pressure summarized these activities succinctly [3].

Basically, detection activities of different types have been, and are, undertaken at factories, during blood denation campaigns, and in the military service. Most important among those activities is the so-called "incidental" screening, i.e. blood pressure measurements taken by practising physicians during patient consultations for reasons not related to hypertension. It is estimated that through this incidental screening, some 35% of the adult Swiss population benefit yearly from a blood pressure measurement [4].

Furthermore, there is a whole range of continuing education activities sponsored by academic institutions, physician associations, or the pharmaceutical in-

---

1 Grant Nr. 4.077.0.76.01, Swiss National Science Foundation
2 National Research Program Collaborative Group
Project Directors: F. Gutzwiller, B. Junod; Scientific Expert: F.H. Epstein;
Local Coordinators: A. Crisinel, K. Röthlisberger; Scientific Committee:
Th. Abelin. M. Bassand, L. Billand, H.R. Brunner, W. Büri, A. Delachaux,
H. Howald, O. Jeanneret, H. Micheli, T. Moccetti, O. Oetliker, O. Ritter,
G. Ritzel, J.L. Rivier, M. Schär, H.B. Stähelin, W. Vetter, L.K. Widmer;
Statistical Analysis: M. Lejeune; Program Director: W. Schweizer

dustry. Finally, large scale trials based on physician offices, such as the Swiss Hypertension Treatment Program involving some 400 practitioners certainly contribute considerable to this process of continuing education [5].

The following section describes the two largest detection campaigns undertaken so far in Switzerland. They also illustrate two common approaches to mass screening: one uses events with massive gatherings of people, the other combines the system of mass-radiography existing in most Swiss cantons. Finally, both of these campaigns were evaluated.

Blood pressure measurements (Physiometrics SRI) were performed on 21.589 persons visiting the Swiss Trade Fair in Basel in 1974. Diastolic pressures were found to be $\geq$ 95 mm Hg in 12% of the screened population. Including those under antihypertensive treatment, the prevalence of high blood pressure (diastolic pressures were found to be $\geq$ 110 mm Hg in 3%, $\geq$100 mm Hg in 7% and $>$ 95 mm Hg in 12% of the screened population. Including those under antihypertensive treatment, the prevalence of high blood pressure (diastolic pressure $\geq$ 95 mm Hg) amounted to 19% of the adult population [6].

The combination of mass radiophotography and blood pressure measurement was started in the canton of Berne (population approx. one million) in 1974. An average of 80% of the personnel from various enterprises attended mass radiophotography on a voluntary basis and 97-100% participated in the blood pressure measurement. The costs were low because a well-established service could be utilized. In this way, it was possible to examine 90.000 persons within three years, or 45% of the population (age 30 to 65 years) [7].

For the following results, a total of 17.112 persons aged 30 years and more and belonging to the working population were examined: 14.6% of the screened population had a blood pressure of $\geq$ 160 and/or $\geq$ 95 mm Hg. Diastolic pressure was found to be $\geq$ 100 mm Hg in 5.9% and $\geq$ 110 mm Hg in 1.8%.

Table 1 summarizes the data regarding treatment status from these two studies and from the representative population samples of the National Research Program, that will be discussed later.

Thus, according to the population under study, a third to half of the population were unaware of their high blood pressure. Only 13% to 35% are under satisfactory control, with marked differences according to the different linguistic regions of the country.

Thus, the situation in Switzerland seems not very different compared to recent data from the National High Blood Pressure Education Program in the United States [8].

An evaluation of both these studies showed, that four to six months after the screening and the recommendation to see a practising physician, only one third of hypertensives were still under regular care, another third were not confirmed as hypertensive or were lost to follow-up, and one third did not even seek care (Swiss Trade Fair) [9]. The figures in Berne were somewhat, but not decisively, better: 58% were still under care, 17% were not called back for a further appointment, and 25% did not even see their physician [7].

246

Table 1. High blood pressure and treatment status in three Swiss studies

study	all hypertensives		unaware	without treatment	treated but not controlled ($\geq$ 160/95 mm Hg)	controlled ($\leq$ 160/95 mm Hg)
	N	%				
swiss trade fair, 1974 (6)	3.042	100%	32%	19%	14%	35%
mass radiophoto-graphy, bern, 1977 (7)	2.419	100%	51%	14%	14%	21%
national research program 1 (1977/1978)						
— swiss german part	472	100%	40%	15%	21%	25%
— swiss french part	370	100%	53%	17%	17%	13%

In contrast to the campaigns just described, high blood pressure is only one of several risk factors included in the National Research Program 1 which attempts to modify the whole range of known risk factors for cardiovascular disease in a comprehensive fashion, thus intregrating screening and follow-up activities.

The National Research Program 1

Objectives

The main objectives of the National Research Program are 1) the evaluation of possible ways to reduce known cardiovascular risk factors among the local populations of two intervention communities compared to two "regular care" communities and 2) the provision of tested cost-effective methods for nationwide use in the future control of cardiovascular disease. To this extent, comparable communities between 10.000 and 20.000 inhabitants were selected (one pair in the French-speaking part, one pair in the German-speaking part of the country). For the purpose of epidemiological comparisons, a fifth community in the Italien speaking part of the country was also included.

Study Design

This five-year program started in 1977 after the planning phase, with baseline assessment including comparable random samples in all four communities and additional volunteers in the two intervention communities. Baseline assessment is followed by 2 1/2 years of intervention in two of the four communities, including intermediate assessment. At the end of 1980, there will be a final assessment, including all those screened at the first examination and a further random sample of those not screened at the beginning of the program. Thus, a specific effect of the examination particularly on the behavior of members of the random samples in the control communities can be assessed.

Baseline Assessment

Baseline screening in the four cities is now completed, covering roughly 10.000 persons. This includes a questionnaire covering the following main areas: family history, dietary habits, smoking behavior, physical activity, psychosocial assessment (Bortner-scale), general health status, including Rose questionnaire for chest pain, knowledge and attitudes. In addition, the following measures were obtained: blood pressure, cholesterol, glucose, ergometry, height and weight for all screenes; high-density-lipoproteins, Thiocyanates in the blood to validate the questionnaire answers for smokers and non-smokers for sub-samples. Participation rates for Swiss citizens in the stratified random population samples average roughly 70%; with documented information on the reasons for non-participation from the rest. Baseline assessment is not only a necessary part of the

248

evaluation scheme, but also the beginning of the intervention: in the two intervention communities, results were transmitted to participants, using a "health passport" which also included an assessment of the individual health score, using a information on tobacco consumption, blood pressure, index of obesity, blood cholesterol and physical activity.

The Intervention

Three main principles of health education guide all local intervention techniques:
— active *participation* of the population
— *mobilization* of all personal and community resources
— *integration* of the new program into existing local health and social servies

The local action committee, with its coordinator, assumes responsibility for these three functions. The main tasks include the conceptualization, planning and implementation of the various compenents of the intervention program in the community as a whole as well as in specified high risk groups.

Specific Intervention Activities Regarding High Blood Pressure

The "health passport" already reffered to included information regarding high blood pressure. An individual follow-up system for hypertensives was instituted through control-cards mailed back by the physicians as soon as the hypertensives identified during the screening had visited their offices. In contrast to the studies discussed before, 95% of all hypertensives followed the advice to seek care with their practicing physicians.

To raise awareness regarding high blood pressure and its problems, there is a continuous range of activities, such as newspaper information, exhibitions, film shows, screening campaigns at different sites, and promoting incidental screening by the locally practising physicians. There is, particularly in mass-media campaigns, an integrated approach to health information: thus, information regarding modern dietary habits includes guidelines on salt intake and similar issues.

Besides raising awareness, and enhancing detection activities, long-term control presents a major problem. In this domain, a series of activities is undertaken, including continuing physician education (addressing questions such as patient complicance). Furthermore, the development of self-help groups of hypertensives, assisted by trained nurses is promoted. This type of patient counselling includes also the promotion of self-measurement. Finally, courses on relaxation training for hypertensives are offered.

Evaluation

Instruments for the evaluation of feasibility and effectiveness include random sample surverys covering risk factors, socioeconomic and psychological data as well as knowledge, attitude and practice, administered at baseline screening, at intermediate tests, and repeated at the end of the program. Each individual action during the program is monitored in addition: with those actions, where the name of the participating individual is known, follow-up questionnaires at 6, 12 and 24 months' interval are used.

For mass-media action, where individual participants are not known, random sample procedures are used. Furthermore, a sociological analysis will investigate factors determining preventive health behavior and finally, a cost-benefit analysis of all aspects of the program will be carried through.

Conclusion

The activities just described attempt to discover the most effective methods of reducing risk factor levels in the population at large. Thus, it was for instance demonstrated that screening activities have to be embeded in a referral system to result in a meaningful long-term follow-up. These activities are based on the assumption that it is important to initiate model community programs and act now, rather than to wait for an uncertain period of time.

A final report integrating all the data from the National Research Program 1 will hopefully give Swiss decision makers the oppotunity to determine whether future country-wide use of such intervention activities is warranted.

References

1. National Research Program Collaborative Group (1978) National Research Program 1: Planning and organisation. Sozial- und Präventivmedizin 23 : 280-281
2. Gutzwiller F, Junod B, Schweizer W (eds) (1979) Prévention des maladies cardio-vasculaires. Le programme national suisse de recherche No. 1 A. Cahiers Médico-Sociaux
3. Fabre J (1979) Rapport d'activité de la commission sociale et préventive de l'association Suisse contre l'hypertension artérielle, Genève
4. Gutzwiller F (1977) Präventivmedizin im Kanton Basel-Stadt. Basler Statistik 2
5. Bühler FR (1978) Schweizer Hypertonie-Behandlungsprogramm: SHBP. Schweiz Aerztezeitung 23
6. Bühler FR, Lèche AS de, Schüler G, Gutzwiller F, Baumann F, Schweizer W (1976) Das Hypertonieproblem in der Schweiz. Analyse einer Blutdruckuntersuchung an 21.589 Personen. Schweiz Med Wochenschr 106 : 99-107

7. Stephan E (1979) Kombination Schirmbild-Blutdruckmessung. Erfahrungen und Ergebnisse im Kanton Bern. Schweiz Med Wochenschr 109 : 234-243
8. National Institutes for Health (1976) National High Blood Pressure Education Program. DHEW Publication No. (NIH) 76-632, Washington, DC
9. Gutzwiller F, Bühler FR, Kamm M (1976) Oeffentliche Hypertonie-Erfassung und Problematik der individuellen Langzeitkontrolle. Schweiz Med Wochenschr 106 : 1687-1692

Rundtisch-Gespräch:
Möglichkeiten der Hypertonieintervention in Deutschland

Moderator: K.D. Bock, Essen
Teilnehmer: K.D. Haehn, Hannover; J. Jahnecke, Bonn; U. Laaser, Köln;
Th. Philipp, Mainz; F.W. Schwartz, Köln

Bock: Meine Damen und Herren, wir kommen jetzt zum abschließenden Rundtisch-Gespräch mit dem Thema: „Möglichkeiten der Hypertonieintervention in
Deutschland". Der Begriff Intervention bedeutet Eingriff und in diesem Zusammenhang das Eingreifen in den Verlauf, die Entstehung oder die Behandlung
einer Erkrankung. Die große gesundheitspolitische Bedeutung des hohen Blutdruckes ist einerseits auf seine Häufigkeit zurückzuführen, andererseits darauf,
daß bei dieser Erkrankung, im Gegensatz zu vielen anderen Krankheiten, die
Möglichkeiten einer Intervention besonders erfolgversprechend erscheinen. Wir
verfügen heute über Behandlungsverfahren, die die Krankheit zumindest partiell
reversibel machen und die Patienten vermutlich vor Komplikationen bewahren.
Die Intervention läßt sich in eine Reihe von Schritten gliedern. Weitgefaßt
kann man sogar die Praevention als erste Maßnahme einer Intervention betrachten. Bei der Praevention unterscheiden wir wiederum zwischen primärer und
sekundärer Praevention. Unter primärer Praevention verstehen wir Maßnahmen,
die die Entstehung der Krankheit überhaupt verhindern, unter sekundärer
Praevention sind prophylaktische Maßnahmen zu verstehen, die zur frühzeitigen Erfassung der Erkrankung führen, um hierdurch rechtzeitig weitere
Interventionsmaßnahmen einzusetzen. Dadurch sollen Komplikationen verhütet und die Mortalität reduziert werden.

Im Rahmen dieses Rundtisch-Gespräches wollen wir uns im wesentlichen mit
der sekundären Praevention beschäftigen. Abschließend werden wir dann noch
auf einige Aspekte der primären Praevention eingehen. Ich darf zunächst die
Teilnehmer des Rundtisch-Gespräches vorstellen: von links nach rechts: Herr
Professor Philipp von der I. Medizinischen Universitätsklinik Mainz, daneben
Herr Professor Jahnecke, Chefarzt des St. Johannes-Hospitals in Bonn, weiterhin Herr Dr. Schwartz als Geschäftsführer des Zentralinstituts für die kassenärztliche Versorgung in Deutschland, Herr Professor Haehn, als Inhaber des
Lehrstuhl für Allgemeinmedizin an der Medizinischen Hochschule Hannover
und gleichzeitig niedergelassener Allgemeinarzt und abschließend Herr Dr.
Laaser, der als Epidemiologe am Institut zur Bekämpfung des hohen Blutdruckes in Heidelberg tätig ist.

Beginnen wir mit der sekundären Praevention. Der erste Schritt betrifft die Erfassung der betroffenen Patientengruppen, also der Hypertoniker, wobei uns
die allgemein akzeptierte Vorstellung leiten sollte, daß eine möglichst frühzeitige Erfassung der Kranken besonders gute Chancen bietet, die Krankheit auch

erfolgreich behandeln zu können. Diese Erfassungsaktionen werden als
„Screening''-Verfahren bezeichnet. Hier gibt es unterschiedliche technische
Verfahren, die schon vieler Orts angewendet worden sind. Wir müssen aber davon ausgehen, daß wir nicht einfach die Verfahren anderer Länder kopieren
können, weil Screening ebenso wie andere Interventionsverfahren entscheidend
von der Struktur eines Gesundheitssystemes abhängen. Man sollte hierbei immer berücksichtigen, daß unser Gesundheitssystem im wesentlichen auf 60.000
praktizierenden Ärzten basiert.

Haehn: Ich darf über die Maßnahmen im Bereich der kassenärztlichen Tätigkeit
berichten, wo heute der Blutdruck eigentlich routinemäßig gemessen wird. Ich
will nicht davon sprechen, daß bei jedem Patienten jedesmal der Blutdruck gemessen wird, aber wir sehen unsere Kranken, die wir über Jahre oder Jahrzehn-
te verfolgen, sehr häufig zu Untersuchungen, bei denen die Blutdruckmessung
ohnehin durchgeführt werden muß. Zunächst haben wir die sportmedizinischen
Untersuchungen, die schon bei den Zehnjährigen durchgeführt werden und
dann alle zwei Jahre wiederholt werden, so lange die Jugendlichen sich mit dem
Sport auseinandersetzen. Nahezu alle Personen werden blutdruckmäßig erfaßt,
wenn sie die Schule verlassen und ihre Lehre oder Berufsausbildung beginnen,
da sie zu diesem Zeitpunkt in der Regel noch keine 18 Jahre alt sind und nach
dem Jugendarbeitsschutzgesetz untersucht werden müssen. Im Rahmen dieser
Untersuchung ist die Blutdruckmessung ebenfalls vorgeschrieben. Im weiteren
Verlauf ihres Lebens werden die Menschen in den Betrieben durch betriebsärzt-
liche Zentren blutdruckmäßig erfaßt. Bekannt ist auch die Blutdruckmessung
im Rahmen der Krebs-Früherkennung, zu der sich die Kassenärzte verpflichtet
haben. Einen Sonderfall stellt das Blutdruckmessen im Rahmen der Blutspendeaktionen dar, die bei ländlicher Bevölkerung eine große Rolle spielen. Hierbei
werden recht häufig Hochdruck-Patienten entdeckt. Bekanntlich wird auch bei
Wehrtauglichkeitsuntersuchungen eine Blutdruckmessung durchgeführt.

Ich darf darauf hinweisen, daß gut 90% aller Bürger sozialversichert sind und
daß von diesen Versicherten wiederum 80% in der Regel einmal jährlich den
Arzt aufsuchen. Auch hierbei ergibt sich jeweils die Möglichkeit einer Blut-
druckkontrolle.

Bock: Was Sie beschrieben haben, Herr Haehn, ist das, was wir als „incidental screening'' bezeichnen, d.h. die Blutdruckmessung bei jeder Gelegenheit,
bei der ein Arztkontakt erfolgt. Hierbei hat die Kassenarztpraxis natürlich einen
besonderen Stellenwert. Neben dieser besten Methode gibt es auch einige alternative Möglichkeiten, die wir kurz erörtern sollten. So ist in den USA hinsichtlich der Effizienz das „door to door''-Screening untersucht worden. Hierbei
werden die Leute in den Wohnungen aufgesucht und somit naturgemäß um-
fassend erreicht. Eine andere Möglichkeit besteht in dem Einsatz mobiler Un-
tersuchungseinheiten, wobei beispielsweise die Bevölkerung aufgefordert wird,
in einer Schule, in einem Gemeindezentrum, in einem Krankenhaus oder in
einer anderen ärztlichen Versorgungseinrichtung den Blutdruck messen zu lassen. Ich möchte bei dieser Gelegenheit Herrn Philipp fragen, ob er noch etwas
zu diesen alternativen Möglichkeiten beitragen kann.

Philipp: Unabhängig voneinander haben Herr Jahnecke und ich ein Zentrum-Screening mit dem Einsatz einer mobilen Einheit über einige Jahre durchgeführt. Ich darf über meine Ergebnisse und somit über die Effektivität dieses Screening-Verfahrens einige Zahlen beitragen. In Zusammenarbeit mit der Barmer Ersatz-kasse und der Landeszentrale für Gesundheitsvorsorge in Rheinland-Pfalz wurde über 18 Monate ein Hochdruck-Screening durchgeführt, wobei zwei Nichtmediziner im Umgang mit einem halbautomatischen Blutdruckmeßgerät und der Blutdruckmeßtechnik geschult worden sind. Nach Vorankündigung in der regionalen Presse wurden an besonderen Plätzen Blutdruckmeßaktionen angeboten. Hierbei wurden Großveranstaltungen wie Messen und Landesausstellungen gewählt, aber auch frequentierte Kaufhäuser und öffentliche Plätze mit eingeschlossen. Als Blutdruckgrenzen wurden die von der Deutschen Liga zur Bekämpfung des hohen Blutdruckes zugrundegelegten oberen Normgrenzen gewählt. Die Blutdruckmessung erfolgte einmalig nach einer Minute Sitzen am rechten Arm. Insgesamt zeigten 61.100 der 218.000 untersuchten Personen über die Norm erhöhte Blutdruckwerte und konnten somit als Hypertoniker identifiziert werden. Von den 61.100 gaben nur 20.600 an, zu wissen, daß sie einen hohen Blutdruck hätten. Auch von diesen 20.600 gab nur die Hälfte an, daß sie unter einer antihypertensiven Therapie ständen. Diese Zahlen übersteigen die bekannten Zahlen über die Praevalenz der Hypertonie, was teilweise auf die besonderen Umstände der Untersuchung zurückzuführen ist. Einerseits wurde nur eine einmalige Messung durchgeführt, wobei bekannt ist, daß durch Wiederholungsmessungen der Prozentsatz an verbleibenden Hypertonikern abnimmt. Andererseits war der Altersdurchschnitt der untersuchten Population mit über 37 Jahren recht hoch. Somit können diese Daten nicht Anspruch auf eine epidemiologisch relevante Aussage erheben.

Einen Punkt möchte ich jedoch hervorheben, der bislang nicht angesprochen wurde. Wir haben versucht, eine sogenannte Kosten-Nutzen-Analyse durchzuführen. Die Aktion kostete insgesamt 177.000 DM einschließlich ihrer statistischen Auswertung. Demzufolge betrugen die Screening-Kosten und somit das Blutdruckmessen für die einzelne Person 0.84 DM. Die Entdeckung eines Hypertonikers, der bislang noch nicht wußte, daß er einen Hochdruck hatte, betrug 4.35 DM. Somit scheint dieses Screening-Verfahren ein sehr preiswertes Verfahren zu sein, um unbekannte Risikofaktoren-Träger zu finden.

Jahnecke: Ich kann natürlich nicht mit solchen Zahlen wie Herr Philipp glänzen. Wir haben ein Hochdruck-Screening mit einer etwas anderen Fragestellung durchgeführt, das ich kurz skizzieren will. In 21 Städten, die über das Gebiet der Bundesrepublik verteilt lagen, wurde jeweils für einen Tag mit einer mobilen Blutdruckmeßeinheit, die mit zwei Medizinstudenten besetzt war, Blutdruckmessungen angeboten. Unsere Frage war, ob man durch örtliche Aktionen kostenlos in die Presse einsteigen und somit die Botschaft „Hochdruck ist eine gefährliche Krankheit, die behandelt werden muß" praktisch kostenlos verbreiten kann. Das Echo, das wir erfuhren, ließ diese Frage ganz klar mit ja beantworten. In einer Gesamtauflage von über 22 Millionen wurde unsere „Botschaft" in die Zeitung und somit in die Öffentlichkeit gebracht. Wir haben bei über 32.000 Menschen den Blutdruck messen können, wobei die Ergebnisse im einzelnen nicht so interessant sind. Die Zahlen lagen etwas tiefer, als die, die Herr Philipp nannte, da wir jeweils die einzelnen Altersstufen auf die tatsächliche Stärke des entsprechenden Jahrganges in der Bundesrepublik umgerechnet haben. Rechnet man aber unsere Zahlen hoch, so muß die Angabe, daß 6 Millionen Hochdruckkranke in der Bundesrepublik existieren, angezweifelt werden. Vielmehr scheint die Zahl bei 10-12 Millionen zu liegen. Hierbei sind die Menschen gemeint, die bei einer einmaligen Messung einen eindeutig erhöhten Blutdruck aufweisen.

Wichtig für mich an dieser Aktion war, daß die Menschen derartige Aktionen annehmen. Überall war der Wunsch, den Blutdruck gemessen zu bekommen, größer als er technisch verkraftet werden konnte. Die Leute standen häufig in langen Schlangen vor dem Blutdruckmeßplatz und warteten nicht nur Minuten.

Bock: Bei der Einrichtung solcher Programme muß natürlich bedacht werden, daß jedes Screening-Verfahren die Forderung erfüllen muß, daß es immer und immer wiederholt wird, um neu auftretende Hypertoniker erfassen zu können. Mit einmaligen Aktionen kann man Querschnitte aufzeigen, aber es bedarf dann der Institutionalisierung auf Dauer. Ein anderer kritischer Punkt liegt darin, daß sie natürlich eine Selektion der Bevölkerung erreicht haben und eines der Kriterien für Screening-Prozeduren ist natürlich der Prozentsatz der Bevölkerung, der erfaßt werden konnte. Können Sie hierzu etwas sagen?

Haehn: Ich wollte noch fragen, ob bei diesen eindrucksvollen Zahlen bekannt wurde, welche der kontrollierten Patienten wirklich nachhaltig Hypertoniker waren. Wir haben ja bei der gynäkologischen Vorsorge und auch bei Blutspendeaktionen erkennen müssen, daß immer wieder zu hohe Blutdruckwerte gemessen wurden, die sich bei späteren Kontrollen nicht bestätigen ließen.

Philipp. Das eben Gesagte zeigt natürlich, daß derartige Untersuchungen sehr kritisch analysiert werden müssen. Diese Zahlen können nicht als repräsentativ im epidemiologischen Sinne angesehen werden. Nachuntersuchungen sind in unserem Falle bei dem hier gezeigten Kollektiv nicht durchgeführt worden.

Bock: Ich darf noch einmal auf meine Frage zurückkommen. Wieviel Prozent der Bevölkerung werden durch derartige Screening-Verfahren erfaßt, wieviel könnte man regelmäßig erfassen, wenn man derartige Aktionen wiederholt?

Philipp: Für die dargestellte Blutdruckmeßaktion kann diese Frage nicht beantwortet werden. Eine ähnliche Aktion in Cochem an der Mosel, auf die ich später noch eingehen möchte, zeigte aber, daß innerhalb einer Woche an einem Ort mit entsprechendem publizistischem Aufwand nahezu 40% der Bevölkerung über dem 16. Lebensjahr durch ein derartiges Screening erfaßt werden konnte.

Jahnecke: Unser Screening ist natürlich von der Kapazität aus begrenzt gewesen. Insgesamt haben wir 0.7% der erwachsenen Bevölkerung erfaßt, was natürlich eine sehr geringe Zahl ist und Hochrechnungen nicht zuläßt. Möglicherweise hätte man mit mehr Meßplätzen an einem Ort auch mehr erreichen können.

Bock: Diese Zahlen sind insofern von Bedeutung, als in Amerika die unterschiedlichen Screening-Verfahren speziell unter dem Gesichtspunkt der Effi-

zienz getestet wurden. Beim „door to door"-Screening wurden meines Wissens
50-70% der Bevölkerung erfaßt. Von Herrn Haehn haben wir erfahren, daß bei
unserer Art der kassenärztlichen Versorgung, die ja 90% der Bevölkerung um-
faßt, 80% der Leute innerhalb von zwei Jahren Arztkontakte haben. Somit wäre die Form des incidental-screening die vermutlich effektivste Form. Würden
Sie dem zustimmen, Herr Laaser?

Laaser: Ja, ich glaube, daß die Frage der Beteiligung nicht so entscheidend ist, wenn
man Screening als Maßnahme der gesundheitlichen Versorgung und des gesundheitlichen Angebots sieht, als wenn man Screening im Rahmen wissenschaftli-
cher Untersuchungen beurteilt. Ich denke, daß ein Screening-Verfahren gut ist,
wenn es sinnvoll ist. In diesem Falle reichen auch 30% der erfaßten Bevölkerung,
denen dann ja geholfen werden kann. Eine andere Frage ist natürlich, ob derartige Prozentzahlen, Prävalenzzahlen im eigentlichen Sinne, bei einer selektierten
Beteiligung ein völlig verzerrtes Bild geben können. Es kann durchaus sein und
ich möchte es fast unterstellen, daß gerade die Hypertoniker seltener an einer
Untersuchung teilgenommen haben, und sich dadurch der Bekanntheitsgrad
bzw. das Ausmaß an Unbekanntheit mindestens so deutlich darstellt, wie es
von Herrn Philipp genannt worden. ist.

Bock: Unsere Frage ist, welche Screening-Prozedur als langfristige Erfassungs-
möglichkeit der Hypertoniker empfehlenswert ist. Ich kann nicht zustimmen,
wenn Sie sagen, wenn nur 30% erfaßt werden, dann ist das in Ordnung. Wir sollten so viel wie möglich von der Bevölkerung erfassen. Was mit den erfaßten
Hypertonikern geschehen soll, ist ein weiteres Problem, das wir anschließend
besprechen wollen.

Laaser: Natürlich soll der Prozentsatz der erfaßten Hypertoniker so hoch wie
möglich sein. Man darf aber nicht den Kostengesichtspunkt aus dem Auge ver-
lieren. Es ist durchaus denkbar, daß die Kosten in der Arztpraxis viel höher wären, als die Kosten eines öffentlichen Screenings. Unter diesem Gesichtspunkt
kann kostenbezogen die Erfassung von 30% der Bevölkerung durch öffentliches
Screening besser sein als die Erfassung von 80% durch Maßnahmen der Praxis.

Bock: Es ist zweifellos richtig, wenngleich man auch sagen könnte, man soll
nicht soviel Krebserkrankungen früh erfassen, weil das eine Menge Geld kostet.
Ich bin nicht dieser Meinung, aber grundsätzlich haben sie recht. Die Kosten
müßten unbedingt verglichen werden.

Schwartz: Ich glaube, daß die Einführung von Früherkennungsmaßnahmen oder
Screening-Maßnahmen in Deutschland kein organisatorisches Problem darstellt,
weil wir ein Land sind, das eine sehr hohe ärztliche Versorgungsdichte hat. Insbesondere gibt es bei uns außerordentlich viel Primär-Ärzte wie Praktiker, Internisten, Kinderärzte und mit Einschränkung auch Gynäkologen. Richtig ist, daß
80% unserer versicherten Bevölkerung unmittelbar oder mittelbar einen dieser
eben genannten Primär-Ärzte pro Jahr aufsucht, d.h. Ärzte, in deren Aufgabenbereich die Blutdruckmessung liegt. Interessant hierbei ist, wie der Anteil der
Bevölkerung sich auf die einzelnen Arztgruppen verteilt. 68% dieser Gruppe
suchen unmittelbar einen Allgemeinarzt auf, 10% einen Internisten, 12% einen

Frauenarzt und 6% den Kinderarzt. Soweit zur oraganisatorischen Seite. Nun zu den Kosten: Die Propagierung eines Screenings im Rahmen der bestehenden kassenärztlichen Versorgung würde gebührentechnisch meßbare Kosten auf der Screening-Stufe zunächst kaum verursachen. Es gibt keine Gebührenziffer für die Blutdruckmessung und es ist derzeit auch nicht beabsichtigt, eine Blutdruck-meßziffer einzuführen, wie wiederholt mit den Gremien der Krankenkassen besprochen. Vielmehr ist es so, daß die sogenannte „Beratung" oder auch die „eingehende Untersuchung", d.h. die beiden Grundleistungsziffern der ärztlichen Honorierung, die Blutdruckmessung im Bedarfsfalle mit einschließen. Auch bei der Empfehlung, die Blutdruckmessung im Rahmen der Krebsfrüher-kennungsmaßnahmen durchzuführen, sind auf der Screening-Stufe keine zusätzlichen Kosten angefallen. Hierbei werden jährlich immerhin 5 Millionen Erwachsene untersucht. Selbstverständlich ist eine solche Methode dennoch nicht kostenlos, weil die Folgekosten erheblich sind, die bei der Aufklärung entdeckter Verdachtsfälle entstehen. Von der Kostenseite wie auch von der organisatorischen Seite her würde sich ein Screening auf hohen Blutdruck vordergründig problemlos propagieren lassen. Offen bleibt neben der Frage der Folgekosten die nach jener Bevölkerungsgruppe, die nicht zu diesen 80% gehört, die in Kontakt mit einem Arzt steht. Es scheint mir von besonderem Interesse zu sein, wie diese Problemgruppe aussieht und wieviel Hypertoniker in ihr enthalten sein werden, anders gefragt: erfassen wir mit den Patienten, die ohnehin zum Arzt gehen, die richtige Zielgruppe.

Bock: Ich glaube, daß darüber niemand Bescheid weiß. Es gibt ja chronische Nicht-Patienten, die niemals einen Arzt aufsuchen. Kostenlos ist sicher nicht nur, was keine Folgekosten verursacht. Die Blutdruckmessung wird ja nicht dadurch kostenlos, weil sie nicht in der Gebührenordnung erscheint. Herr Haehn wird dem sicher widersprechen, denn auch wenn das Blutdruckmessen nicht abzurechnen ist, kostet ihn das eine Menge Geld.

Haehn: Zur Kostenfrage sind zwei Dinge zu sagen. Hierbei sollten die Patienten in zwei getrennten Gruppen betrachtet werden. Die Patienten der einen Gruppe kommen mit einer Befindensstörung, wobei im Rahmen der Abklärung auch der Blutdruck gemessen wird. Hierbei entstehen naturgemäß keine Sonderkosten. Wird man aber der gesamten Bevölkerung mitteilen, sie möchte jährlich einmal den Blutdruck messen lassen, dann kommt natürlich die zweite weitaus größere Gruppe der Patienten ohne subjektive Erkrankung. So lange aber dieses Screening nicht durch die RVO abgedeckt ist, dürften wir formell gesehen, diese Tätigkeit überhaupt nicht durchführen. Denn unser Aufgabenbereich erstreckt sich auf das Behandeln von Krankheiten bzw. auf das Durchführen von Früherkennungsuntersuchungen bei Erkrankungen. Natürlich ist die Kostenfrage nicht einfach zur Seite zu legen. Wenn man in seiner Praxis bemüht ist, derartige Messungen durchzuführen, dann kostet dieses eine Menge Arbeitszeit für Arzt und Arzthelferin, die im Grunde nicht finanziell abgedeckt ist. Sie sagen zwar, daß die Blutdruckmessung im Prinzip immer dazu gehört, aber der Arzt, der dieser Aufforderung nicht folgt, bekommt dafür natürlich dasselbe Honorar für seinen Patienten, als wenn er zusätzlich noch den Blutdruck mißt. Insofern spielen finanzielle Dinge natürlich eine gewisse Rolle. Ich hoffe aber, daß der einzelne

Arzt, insbesondere bei der zunehmenden Anzahl von Ärzten, die in der Zukunft praktizieren werden, nicht mehr so kleinlich sein wird und sich etwa solchen Maßnahmen verschließt. Hierzu sollte die heutige Diskussion positiv beitragen.

Laaser: Wir sollten noch einmal darauf zurückkommen, daß man bei der vollständigen Erfassung der Hypertoniker von den Konsequenzen her argumentieren sollte. In jedem Fall werden wir unterscheiden müssen zwischen denen, bei denen gegenwärtig eine pharmakologische Behandlung indiziert sein könnte und den anderen Hypertonikern, bei denen gesundheitserzieherisch im Sinne der allgemeinen Lebensstil- bzw. Verhaltensveränderung interveniert werden sollte. Meines Wissens existiert bislang nur eine einzige Untersuchung, die uns eine Begründung für die Indikation zur pharmakologischen Behandlung gibt, nämlich die Veterans Administration Studie, die in einer sehr eng umgrenzten männlichen Bevölkerung gezeigt hat, daß bei diastolischen Werten von 105 mm Hg und höher die pharmakologische Behandlung eine Reduktion der Mortalität erbringt. Gehen wir hiervon aus, dann werden nur sehr wenige, vermutlich kaum 10% aller Hypertoniker, pharmakologisch behandlungsbedürftig sein. Wenn aber eine pharmakologische Behandlung für einen großen Teil der Hypertoniker nicht zur Debatte steht, d.h. lediglich Gesundheitserziehung, Lebensstilveränderung, Gewichtsreduktion empfohlen werden können, dann wird ein Screening nicht gebraucht. Diese Maßnahmen sind an sich jedem zu empfehlen, auch einer ganzen Reihe von Gesunden, die keinen hohen Blutdruck haben. Nur für die pharmakologische Indikation ist ein Screening begründet, und diese Indikation bezieht sich vorläufig auf 10% der Hypertoniker. Wenn wir davon ausgehen, daß 20% der Bevölkerung einen hohen Blutdruck hat und von diesen wiederum die Hälfte nicht darüber Bescheid weiß, dann bezieht sich eine denkbare pharmakologische Konsequenz auf weniger als 1% der durch Screening erfaßbaren Bevölkerung. Wir müssen also damit rechnen, daß bei 100 untersuchten Probanden lediglich ein bis zwei Hypertoniker gefunden werden, bei denen eine pharmakologische Therapie begründet wäre und neu begonnen werden müßte. Diese Zahl reduziert sich sogar noch weiter, wenn man in Betracht zieht, daß die medikamentöse Behandlung wahrscheinlich nur bei einem Teil der neu aufgefundenen Hypertoniker beibehalten wird und tatsächlich zu einer dauerhaften Blutdrucksenkung führt.

Schwartz: Es ist sicher notwendig, derartige Rechnungen zu Beginn jeder Screening-Maßnahme anzustellen, aber wir müssen diese Kosten relativ werten: Im Rahmen der Krebsfrüherkennungs-Untersuchungen beliefen sich 1977 die Entdeckungskosten je nach Krebsart auf ca. 42.000 bis 100.000 DM pro entdecktem Fall. Bei dem von Herrn Laaser zugrunde gelegten Aufwand-Nutzen-Relationen würden sich die Entdeckungskosten eines behandlungsbedürftigen Hypertonikers auf nur 80 bis 100 DM belaufen, wenn man die einzelne Blutdruckmessung so niedrig wie Herr Philipp kalkuliert und ohne Berücksichtigung der Folgekosten. Diese Zahl ist relativ gesehen sehr niedrig.

Philipp: Wir sind von der Gegenüberstellung des incidental Screenings und dem Zentrums-Screening ausgegangen. Wichtig für uns scheint zu sein, was aus den Patienten wird, die im Rahmen eines Zentrums-Screenings gefunden werden und die dann zum behandelnden Arzt geschickt werden. Wir haben ähnlich deprimierende Daten gefunden, wie sie Herr Gutzwiller in seinem vorangegangenen Vortrag angedeutet hat. Ich beziehe mich jetzt auf die Untersuchung, die wir in Cochem an der Mosel über zwei Jahre durchführten. Hierbei wurden 2.800 Einwohner von Cochem auf freiwilliger Basis innerhalb einer Woche untersucht. Das entspricht ca. 40% der Einwohner von Cochem über dem 14. Lebensjahr. Wir fanden bei Zugrundelegung der Blutdrucknormgrenzen der Deutschen Liga zur Bekämpfung des hohen Blutdruckes 546 Hypertoniker. Lediglich 262 hiervon wußten, daß sie einen erhöhten Blutdruck hatten. Mit jedem Hochdruckpatienten wurde ein eingehendes Gespräch geführt, sie erhielten Aufklärungsmaterial und Broschüren, sowie die mündlich und später auch schriftlich ausgesprochene Aufforderung, ihren Hausarzt aufzusuchen. Mit den in Cochem ansässigen Hausärzten war die ganze Aktion wiederholt und ausführlich besprochen worden. Von den 546 Hypertonikern gingen jedoch nur 422 zu ihrem Arzt. 124 folgten auch späteren schriftlichen Aufforderungen nicht. Durch die Hausärzte wurde nur bei 302 Patienten das Vorliegen einer Hypertonie bestätigt. Diesen Punkt muß man vermutlich akzeptieren, da bei Wiederholungsmessungen, wie bereits mehrfach angeklungen, eine abnehmende Anzahl von manifesten Hypertonikern festzustellen ist. Verabredungsgemäß sollten alle Hypertoniker in 3-monatigen Abständen zu Kontrolluntersuchungen bei ihren Hausärzten sich vorstellen. Nach 6 Monaten waren aufgrund der von den Hausärzten dokumentierten Bögen nur noch 242 in Behandlung, nach 18 Monaten lediglich noch 178. Von diesen 178 waren 100 normotensiv eingestellt. Zusammenfassend wurden also von 546 als hyperton erkannten Personen nach 18 Monaten lediglich 100 effektiv kontrolliert. Diese Zahlen zeigen, daß ein Screening, so gut es auch gemeint sein mag, nur der Anfang einer Reihe von Aktivitäten sein kann.

Bock: Richtig, aus diesem Grunde haben wir ja auch die einzelnen Schritte der Intervention angefangen vom Screening, in kleine Teilschritte aufgegliedert. Der Gesamteffekt eines Screening ist sicher wesentlich von den weiteren Schritten abhängig. Es gibt verschiedene Möglichkeiten: So wurden wiederholt Hochdruckpatienten bei Screening-Maßnahmen ausgedruckte Meßzettel in die Hand gedrückt mit dem Inhalt: Gehen Sie zu Ihrem Arzt, Ihr Blutdruckwert liegt etwas zu hoch. Bei extrem hohen Werten sollte man sicher anders handeln als bei Patienten, deren Wert im Grenzbereich liegt. Im Rahmen des incidental Screening kommt es ja vor, daß der Arzt, der den erhöhten Blutdruck mißt, nicht mit dem sonst behandelnden Arzt identisch ist. Die Weiterleitung des Patienten und die Benachrichtigung des behandelnden Arztes müßten sicher rationalisiert werden. Herr Haehn, wie sehen Sie diesen Punkt?

Haehn: Für mich wäre der Schritt nicht so schwierig, weil ich davon ausgehe, daß die Screening-Stelle vorwiegend eben die Arztpraxis ist. Wenn der Betroffene erst einmal in der Praxis ist und eine geeignete Anleitung erhält, dann entfällt der Schritt einer Weiterleitung.

Bock: Gehen wir doch aber davon aus, daß der erhöhte Blutdruck nicht durch den Arzt selber, sondern in einem Kaufhaus, einer Apotheke, bei einem Den-

tisten oder eben einem anderen Fachkollegen gemessen worden ist. Was soll
dann geschehen?

Haehn: Dieser Punkt ist sicherlich von Bedeutung, hier haben wir überall schon
über unerfreuliche Ergebnisse gehört. Aus diesem Grunde bin ich auch so sehr
dafür, daß das Screening möglichst in den Arztpraxen stattfindet. Nehmen wir
an, mein Kollege in der Nachbarschaft stellt für mich bei einem Patienten eine
Hypertonie fest, so bin ich sicher, daß er die Hypertoniebehandlung einleitet
oder den Patienten zu dem eigentlich behandelnden Arzt überweist. Anders
könnte die Situation bei sehr fachspezialisierten Kollegen, wie Augenarzt oder
HNO-Arzt sein.

Bock: Wenn wir die Angaben von Herrn Philipp als repräsentativ ansehen, dann
müßten wir schlußfolgern, daß alle zusätzlichen Aktionen dieser Art über ihren
,,public relation''-Wert hinaus nichts bringen.

Laaser: Es könnte eine mögliche Schlußfolgerung unserer Diskussion darstellen,
daß man feststellt, daß diese Schwerpunktaktionen überflüssig sind, da 80%
aller Versicherten ja ohnehin pro Jahr beim niedergelassenen praktischen Arzt
auftreten.

Bock: Unsere Empfehlung wäre demnach, das incidental screening in der Arztpraxis zu forcieren. Eine solche Empfehlung an unsere Ärzteorganisationen soll
zwar schwerpunktmäßige Einzelaktionen nicht verhindern, jedoch ist darauf
hinzuweisen, daß damit im wesentlichen nur ein ,,public relation''-Effekt erzielt
wird. Würden Sie dem zustimmen?

Haehn: Ja, das erfordert nur, daß die Ärzte das incidental Screening als Bewäh-
rungsprobe bestehen. Ich bin vielleicht vorhin von Herrn Philipp etwas mißver-
standen worden. Tatsächlich gehen 80% der Versicherten jährlich zum Arzt,
aber bislang wird bei ihnen noch nicht in ausreichendem Maße der Blutdruck
gemessen.

Bock: Herr Schwartz scheint dem nicht ganz zustimmen zu wollen.

Schwartz: Tatsächlich. Ich finde solche Untersuchungen, wie sie Herr Philipp
gemacht hat, sehr wichtig. Hierbei sollte besonders Wert darauf gelegt werden,
wieviel der bekannten und auch der unbekannten Hypertoniker in der letzten
Zeit in Arztkontakt standen und wieviel in der Regel überhaupt nicht zum Arzt
gehen. Möglicherweise kann hierdurch festgestellt werden, ob gerade diejenigen,
die zu diesen Schwerpunktmessungen gehen, die im Rahmen anderer großer
Aktionen stattfinden, gerade zu dem Personenkreis zählen, der auch regelmäßig
zum Arzt geht. Es wäre interessant zu wissen, ob durch derartige Schwerpunktaktionen neue Bevölkerungsgruppen erschlossen werden können, die sonst
nicht zum Arzt gehen. Wird diese Frage verneint, so werden diese Aktionen
nicht sehr sinnvoll sein.

Bock: Das würde sich aber lediglich um die 10-20% Nicht-Patienten handeln.

Laaser: Ich glaube, Herr Schwartz, die Problematik reicht noch weiter. Sicher,
wenn man tatsächlich neue Bevölkerungsgruppen dadurch erschließen kann,

dann muß man das noch einmal überdenken. Nur, das weitergehende Problem bleibt trotzdem ungelöst: Wie erreiche ich bei den durch Screening-Maßnahmen neu entdeckten Hypertonikern eine erfolgreiche, dauerhafte Behandlung. Darüberhinaus ist es auch nicht angemessen, die Kosten für das Screening bei Hypertonie mit den Kosten für das Krebs-Screening in Beziehung zu setzen. Beim Krebs-Screening diskutiert man ja auch die Nützlichkeit im Sinne der Kosten-Nutzen-Analyse. Darüberhinaus sind aber bei meiner Hochrechnung zwei entscheidende Schnittstellen zu berücksichtigen, an denen wesentliches verbessert werden kann.

1. Von Bedeutung ist, ob der Prozentsatz der adäquat behandelten Hypertoniker angehoben werden kann von beispielsweise z.Zt. 12.5 auf 25% oder noch höher.

2. Es ist denkbar, daß nach Abschluß und bei Vorliegen der Ergebnisse der jetzt laufenden Interventionsstudien zur milden Hypertonie es zu einer Ausweitung der pharmakologischen Behandlungsindikationen kommen wird, wie z.B. auf Hochdruckpatienten, die lediglich eine Grenzwerthypertonie haben.

Philipp: Wenn wir von der Kosten-Nutzen-Analyse sprechen, sollten wir auf der einen Seite immer wissen, daß die Behandlung des hohen Blutdruckes generell sehr teuer ist und sollten gleichermaßen wissen, daß wir tatsächlich über den Langzeiteffekt einer Therapie noch sehr wenig wissen. Falls wir uns für die allgemeine Intensivierung des incidental-Screening aussprechen — und die Deutsche Liga zur Bekämpfung des hohen Blutdruckes hat diese Maßnahme ja schon lange progagiert — so müßten wir unbedingt eine Effektivitätskontrolle dieser Maßnahme herbeiführen. Hiermit meine ich, daß festgestellt werden muß, in welchem Ausmaße und ob überhaupt das incidental-Screening durchgeführt wird. Wir gehen davon aus, daß 80% aller Versicherten im Jahr einmal den Arzt aufsuchen. Aufgrund der Krankenschein-Kontrollen kann sicher festgestellt werden, ob ein Patient bei einem Arzt gewesen ist und man müßte relativ einfach feststellen können, ob bei diesen in Kontrolle befindlichen Patienten in der Tat der Blutdruck gemessen worden ist.

Bock: Sie sprachen wieder von Effektivität. Wir müssen jedoch streng zwischen der Effizienz der gesamten Intervention, die sich ja darin ausdrücken wird, ob am Schluß weniger Todesfälle oder Komplikationen zu finden sind und der Effektivität jedes Teilschrittes, also hier des Screenings, unterscheiden. Hierbei kommt es darauf an, bei wieviel der den Arzt aufsuchenden Personen der Blutdruck tatsächlich gemessen wird und natürlich, was der Arzt mit dem Patienten macht, der eine Grenzwerthypertonie oder eine manifeste Hypertonie hat. Nachdem was Sie vorher gezeigt haben, Herr Philipp, scheint dies ein weiterer Schwachpunkt zu sein.

Philipp: Ich hatte nicht die Absicht, diesen Eindruck zu erwecken. Wir haben gesehen, daß 25% der als Hochdruckpatienten zum Arzt geschickten Personen vom Hausarzt nicht als solche eingestuft wurden. Zweit- und Drittmessungen haben wiederholt gezeigt, daß die Hochdruckhäufigkeit mit der Anzahl der Wiederholungsmessungen abnimmt. Daneben gibt es sicherlich ein großes Kollektiv von Patienten mit erhöhtem Blutdruck, bei denen es fraglich ist, ob die

pharmakologische Behandlung sinnvoll ist. Ich möchte hier insbesondere auf
die Grenzwerthypertonie und die Hypertonie im Alter abzielen.

Bock: Natürlich ist es notwendig — nicht nur um Kosten zu sparen, sondern um
die Patienten zu schützen — daß durch den behandelnden Arzt die Behandlungs-
indikation kritisch bedacht wird. Diesen Punkt sollten wir aus Zeitgründen nur
grob besprechen. Was tut der Arzt, um festzustellen, ob der Betreffende tatsächlich eine Hypertonie hat, ob dieser Hochdruck eine behandlungsbedüftige
Erkrankung ist und ob in diesem Fall Allgemeinmaßnahmen ausreichen oder
pharmakologische Maßnahmen indiziert sind. Alle diese Überlegungen müssen
in der Allgemeinpraxis getroffen werden, wobei die Patienten mit erhöhtem
Blutdruck, die lediglich mit Allgemeinmaßnahmen behandelt werden sollten,
vermutlich die größte Gruppe in der Allgemeinpraxis sein werden.

Haehn: Es ist atsächlich eine schwierige Frage, wann ein Hypertonus behandlungsbedürftig ist und noch schwieriger wie. Lassen Sie mich kurz auf die viel-
zitierte Diät abheben mit all der Problematik, die in der Motivation der Kranken liegt. Nur in Ausnahmefällen gelingt es, eine Gewichtsreduktion zu erreichen und auch die Kochsalzreduktion wird nur unbefriedigend eingehalten.
Aus diesen Überlegungen heraus stellt sich leider für den behandelnden Arzt
selten die Frage, ob pharmakologisch oder mit Allgemeinmaßnahmen behandelt werden muß, sondern lediglich die Frage, ob pharmakologisch behandelt
werden muß oder nicht.

Bock: Das ist sicherlich richtig. Einzelne Kliniken in Amerika lehnen einen Versuch mit Allgemeinbehandlung einschließlich Gewichtsreduktion ab, da sie sagen, es hat keinen Sinn, die Patienten zu frustieren und ihnen ihre Lebensge-
wohnheiten zu manipulieren. Besser ist es, ihnen gleich einen β-Blocker oder
ein Diuretikum zu geben. Diese Alternative muß man als Realist durchaus mit
einbeziehen.

Laaser: Ich habe noch einmal eine Frage an Herrn Philipp bezüglich der 322
behandelten Hypertoniker in Cochem. Gesichert ist bisher ja nur die Behand-
lungsnotwendigkeit für Blutdruckerhöhungen von diastolisch 105 mm Hg und
höher. Demzufolge sind in Cochem sicherlich mehr Hypertoniker als, strengge-
nommen, notwendig behandelt worden. Die nicht-pharmakologischen Bemü-
hungen der Ärzte sind sicher weiterhin in ihren Erfolgen sehr begrenzt. Aus diesem Grunde scheint, das möchte ich noch einmal betonen, das Screening für die
nicht-pharmakologisch indizierten Hypertoniker nicht sinnvoll zu sein. Die
Konsequenzen, nämlich die Allgemeinmaßnahmen wie Gewichtsreduktion und
Salzreduktion, werden nicht durchgesetzt werden können. Sinnvoll ist eine Umstellung des Hypertonikers vermutlich nur, wenn die Nachbarschaft, die Umge-
bung und besonders die Familie des Hypertonikers den Patienten gleichgerich-
tet mit unterstützt. Eine isolierte Behandlung in der Praxis scheint mir nicht
möglich zu sein.

Bock: Screening bedeutet für mich, daß erst einmal alle untersucht werden müssen. In welche Gruppe ein Hypertoniker dann gehört, muß später festgestellt
werden.

Schwartz: Aus meinen ersten Bemerkungen ließe sich vielleicht herauslesen, daß ich eindeutig für ein solches Screening bin. Jetzt aber, wo wir über die Therapiemöglichkeiten sprechen, möchte ich pointiert sagen, daß eine bloße Frühentdeckung ohne gleichzeitige Sicherstellung weiterer standardisierter Diagnostik und Therapie, und zwar kontinuierlicher Therapie mit nachweisbarem Erfolg, ganz sinnlos ist. Falls nicht wenigstens gezeigt werden kann, daß das Problembewußtsein der Bevölkerung und auch bei den Ärzten durch deratige Screening-Maßnahmen nachhaltig angehoben wird, möchte ich mich gegen diese Maßnahmen aussprechen. In der derzeitigen Situation mit der therapeutischen Vielfalt und gewissen Uneinigkeiten über die Behandlungsmedikationen, insbesondere bei Grenzwerten und im Alter, wird sich die Kassenärzteschaft auch nur schwer zu einem bundesweiten umfassenden Screening-Programm entschließen. Nicht die Entdeckung neuer Fälle ist das Problem, sondern die sinnvolle und richtige Dauerbehandlung derjenigen, die diese am meisten benötigen. Sinnvoll scheint hier ein mehrstufiges Vorgehen: Zunächst durch die vermehrte Propagierung der Blutdruckmessung als „case-finding", ebenso durch öffentliche Aktionen das Problembewußtsein bei Ärzten und Patienten zu stärken und zugleich für die Verbreitung akzeptabler und gerechtfertigter Indikations- und Therapieschemata zu sorgen. Dann erst ist umfassendes Screening diskutabel.

Bock: Hier muß ich widersprechen. Es gibt bei uns Empfehlungen sowohl für die Diagnostik als auch für die Art der Therapie, für ihre Überwachung, für ihre Indikationen. Diese kurzgefaßten und übersichtlichen Merkblätter der Hochdruck-Liga entsprechen inhaltlich im wesentlichen den Empfehlungen in anderen Ländern, z.B. in der Schweiz und in den USA und auch dem jüngsten WHO-Report. Es sind Leitlinien für den niedergelassenen Arzt, mit Hilfe derer er sehrwohl in der Lage ist, jeden Hypertoniker diagnostisch und therapeutisch individuell zu betreuen. Wenn das bis heute nicht ausreichend geschieht, so liegt das nicht am Fehlen von Richtlinien oder an irgendeinem wissenschaftlichen Dissens, sondern daran, daß diese Empfehlungen der Ärzteschaft nicht genügend nahegebracht worden sind, d.h. es handelt sich um eine Frage der ärztlichen Fortbildung. Die Tatsache, daß eine wirksame Diättherapie mit Kochsalzrestriktion oder Gewichtsreduktion auf erhebliche praktische Schwierigkeiten stößt, ist meines Erachtens kein Argument gegen ihre grundsätzliche Empfehlung. Hier wären Forschungsprogramme in Gang zu setzen mit dem Ziel, für den praktischen Arzt Behandlungsmethoden zu entwickeln, die diesem eine wirksame Diättherapie ermöglichen. Aus den vorhandenen praktischen Schwierigkeiten, die z.T. nur Umsetzungsprobleme darstellen, aber zu folgern, daß man am besten gar nichts tut, halte ich für verfehlt.

Haehn: Es gibt natürlich schon Ansätze, allgemeine Maßnahmen besser durchzusetzen. Wir haben in Hannover eine kleine Studie mit dem Ziel gemacht, ob man durch verhaltenstherapeutische Maßnahmen Gewichtsreduktion und später auch Blutdruckbeeinflussung erzielen kann und insbesondere ob diese Maßnahmen unter Praxisbedingungen eingesetzt werden können. Hierzu haben wir 70 Hypertoniker in meiner eigenen Landpraxis mit einem großen Aufwand gruppentherapeutisch behandelt mit einem verhaltenstherapeutischen Programm, das von Psychologen durchgeführt wurde. Im Einzelfall haben wir tatsächlich

innerhalb von zwölf Wochen eine Gewichtsreduktion um 18 Pfund erreicht.
Aber bei allen wurde das Gewicht insgesamt reduziert und bei allen konnte der
Blutdruck gesenkt werden. Mich hat das gute Durchhaltevermögen der Patienten in der Gruppe beeindruckt und ich denke, daß derartige gruppendynami-
schen und basistherapeutischen Methoden eingeführt werden sollten. Hierbei
ist allerdings ein großer Aufwand und eine große Organisation erforderlich. Dieser Ansatz ist aber sicherlich nicht nur für Patienten mit Hochdruck anwendbar,
sondern auch für andere Erkrankungen.

Bock : Wir sollten jetzt in der Diskussion weitergehen. Nehmen wir an, der neu
entdeckte Hypertoniker ist diagnostisch abgeklärt und nach der Schwere seiner
Erkrankung eingestuft worden und wird jetzt behandelt. Herr Schwartz, sehen
Sie eine Möglichkeit, daß man in regelmäßigen Abständen Stichproben aus der
Bevölkerung untersucht und überprüft, wieviele der neu entdeckten Hypertoni-
ker behandelt werden oder nicht? Gibt es eine Möglichkeit, dieses über die
Krankenscheine oder auf anderem Wege zu überprüfen?

Schwartz: In Niedersachsen ist eine Studie mit unserer finanziellen Unterstützung durchgeführt worden. Hierbei hat Professor Pflanz an Mitgliedern der Be-
triebskrankenkasse Volkswagen AG und Salzgitter AG versucht, die Frage der
Behandlungskontinuität zu überprüfen. Bei allen wurden Früherkennungsmaßnahmen, die auf Herz-Kreislauf-Krankheiten zielten, durchgeführt. Von den
dort entdeckten Hypertonikern standen nach einem Jahr noch 27% unter me-
dikamentöser Therapie. Die angeblich leichte Messung über die Krankenscheine
ist vielen Irrtumsmöglichkeiten ausgesetzt. Insbesondere sind die Diagnosen auf
den Krankenscheinen nicht klar und verbindlich. In der Regel steht einfach Hypertonie darauf, ohne daß etwa Form und Schweregrad erkennbar wären. Hinsichtlich antihypertoner Behandlungen sind die Gebührenziffern zu unpräzise,
wie etwa die unscharfe Definition der häufigsten Ziffer 1, der „Beratung", zeigt.
In Niedersachsen wurden deswegen spezielle Fragebögen eingesetzt.

Bock: Es wäre sicher nötig, einmal eine Effizienzmessung bei diesem Schritt
der Intervention durchzuführen.

Laaser: Ich möchte an dieser Stelle kurz versuchen, den Begriff der Effizienz
und der Effektivität voneinander abzusetzen. Effektivität würde bedeuten zu
prüfen, ob eine Maßnahme einen Effekt hat, also ob Gruppentherapie einen
Effekt auf die Gewichtsreduktion hat. Das läßt sich vermutlich mit wenigen
Mitteln leicht klarstellen, und hierzu ist die Praxis ein idealer Studienplatz.
Schwieriger ist die Frage nach der relativen Effizienz, nämlich, welche Maßnahme am kostengünstigsten ist in Beziehung auf den gewünschten Effekt. Der ge-
wünschte Effekt kann nur in der Reduktion der Herz-Kreislauf-Erkrankungen
liegen. Dieser Effekt kann nur in großen Studien geprüft werden.

Bock: Vielen Dank für die Klarstellung. Wir kommen nun zum nächsten Schritt.
Das ist die Problematik der Dauerbehandlung und Dauerbetreuung der Hypertoniker, die als solche identifiziert wurden. Wir wissen alle, daß ein Teil der Patienten sich im Laufe der Zeit der Behandlung entzieht und es sind in den letzten Jahren eine Reihe von Möglichkeiten geprüft worden, die Gruppe dieser

„drop outs" zu verkleinern. Vielleicht können Sie, Herr Haehn, hierzu eine stichwortartige Bemerkung machen.

Haehn: Ich habe vorhin schon auf die Grundtherapie als Methode hingewiesen, die Patienten zu motivieren, bei der Stange zu bleiben. Im Rahmen einer Dissertation wurde in meiner Praxis untersucht, wie sich das Verhalten der „drop outs" entwickelt, wenn man ein Einbestellsystem einführt. Bei aller Fragwürdigkeit des methodischen Ansatzes, da wir ja ein Teil retrospektiv analysieren mußten, zeigte sich folgendes: Nach unserer Definition war ein „drop out" bzw. ein Therapieabbrecher ein Patient, der länger als 12 Wochen nicht mehr in der Praxis erschienen war. Nach Einführung unseres Patienten-Terminierungssystems mit terminlicher Einbestellung konnte die Zahl der Therapieabbrecher um über 1/3 reduziert werden. Weitere Vorteile des Einbestellungssystems sind eine bessere Organisation des Praxisablaufes, die es dem Kranken ermöglicht, einen festen Termin zu haben, er braucht nicht zu warten und er ist entsprechend engagierter. Den Wiedereinbestellungstermin kann sich unser Patient z.T. selber aussuchen, was seine Motivation sicher auch fördert. Dieses Einbestellungssystem ist für die Behandlung aller chronischer Erkrankungen unbedingt zu fordern.

Bock: Was machen Sie aber, wenn der Patient nicht wiederkommt?

Haehn: Dann steht man in einem Gewissenskonflikt. Normalerweise ist der Arzt gehalten, dem Patienten, der nicht wiederkommt, nicht nachzulaufen, weil er ja möglicherweise den Arzt gewechselt hat. Von Seiten der Bundeskassenärztlichen Vereinigung wird zum Glück aber jetzt der Versuch unternommen, die Ärzte zu animieren, im Rahmen der Vorsorgeuntersuchungen ruhig auf die Patienten zuzugehen und sie aufzufordern. Ich persönlich laufe dem Hypertoniker nicht nach, im Gegensatz etwa zu dem Diabetiker, der insulinpflichtig ist und einer größeren aktuellen Gefahr ausgesetzt ist.

Bock: Es gibt auch noch andere Möglichkeiten zur Verbesserung der Patienten-Compliance, z.B. ein möglichst einfaches Behandlungsregime mit nur einer Tablette pro Tag, insgesamt nur wenige Verordnungen, diese aber ganz klar mündlich durch den Arzt und unterstützt durch schriftliche Unterlagen, die Vermittlung von Erfolgserlebnissen, etwa bei der Selbstmessung des Blutdrucks durch den Abfall auf Normwerte.

Philipp: Das was Herr Haehn ausführte, möchte ich voll unterstreichen. Meiner Überzeugung nach dürfen Hypertoniepatienten nur mit Festsetzung eines neuen Vorstellungstermins entlassen werden. Von Seiten einer Klinikambulanz ist dieses Vorgehen natürlich leichter, da es uns nicht sehr trifft, wenn der Patient zu einem anderen Arzt gegangen ist. Wir registrieren jedoch genau, wenn ein Patient nicht gekommen ist und schicken ausnahmslos bei Nichterscheinen eine sachliche Einbestellungskarte. Genaue Zahlen über die Effektivität dieses Einbestellungs- und Kontrollsystems kann ich noch nicht vorlegen; aber es ist sicher so, daß mehr als 70% der Patienten, die eine Einbestellungskarte erhalten, sich anschließend sofort wieder melden. Lassen Sie mich auf einen zweiten Punkt eingehen, der sicher die Patienten-Compliance deutlich verbessern kann,

die Blutdruckselbstmessung. Wir haben versucht, beide Systeme, die Blutdruckselbstmessung und das Einbestellsystem miteinander zu verknüpfen. Zu diesem
Zweck wurde ein Abkommen mit den RVO-Kassen in Rheinhessen getroffen.
Alle Patienten, die eine medikamentös behandlungsbedürftige Hypertonie haben, erhalten von uns ein Blutdruckgerät verordnet. Dieses Blutdruckgerät steht
ihnen jedoch nicht als Eigentum zur Verfügung, sondern es wird von der Krankenkasse prinzipiell nur verliehen. Das hat zunächst den simplen Vorteil, daß
die Krankenkasse sich die Geräte im großen Stil einkaufen kann und dadurch
weniger finanziell belastet wird. Der zweite Vorteil liegt darin, daß die Auslei-
hungszeit jeweils auf zwölf Monate begrenzt ist. Nach zwölf Monaten erhalten
die Patienten automatisch von der Krankenkasse eine schriftliche Aufforderung,
das Gerät zurückzubringen, oder aber alternativ von ihrem Arzt eine Bescheini-
gung vorzulegen, nach der sie 1. in Behandlung stehen, 2. den Blutdruck auch
regelmäßig messen, 3. den Blutdruck messen können und 4. die Weiterverord-
nung für das nächste Jahr ärztlich angezeigt ist. Der Vorteil ist offensichtlich:
Die Kassen zahlen weniger für das Blutdruckmeßgerät, die Patienten messen
ihren Blutdruck regelmäßig selber, die Patienten-Compliance wird durch das
Selbstmessen erhöht, da die Patienten den Erfolg der antihypertensiven Therapie
beobachten und insbesondere den Erfolg eines Absetzens registrieren können
und schließlich der entscheidende Erfolg dieses Systems: Die ,,drop outs'' der
Hochdruckpatienten werden nach zwölf Monaten durch diese Aufforderung
dem behandelnden Arzt wieder zugeführt und können erneut behandelt werden.

Schwartz: Ich finde diesen Gedanken ausgezeichnet und habe ihn mir sofort
notiert. Seit langem gibt es schon die Diskussion auf Bundesebene mit den
Krankenkassen, wie die Modalität des Blutdruckselbstmessens zu handhaben
ist. Verordnung eines Blutdruckmeßgerätes auf Rezept hat zu deutlichen Wi-
derständen bei den Krankenkassen geführt. Ich sehe hierin jedoch einen sehr
guten Weg. Vielen Dank.

Haehn: Lassen Sie mich als weiteren Grund für die hohe Non-Compliance der
Patienten als letztes noch die Nebenwirkung von Medikamenten anführen. Die
Normotonie ist zwar erstrebenswertes Therapieziel, aber keinesfalls immer ein
erreichbares Ziel und wenn, dann nur unter Einkaufen von Nebenwirkungen, die
dann wiederum zur Verstärkung der Non-Compliance führen können.

Jahnecke: Ich glaube, die Formulierung scheint überspitzt zu sein, Herr Haehn.
Das ist sicher wieder ein graduelles Problem, womit ich Normotonie erreichen
kann oder muß. Ein juveniler Grenzwerthypertoniker wird durch seine Medikamente kaum Nebenwirkungen verspüren. Es gibt jedoch genügend Hochdruckkranke, die Nebenwirkungen in Kauf nehmen müssen, und das umso mehr, umso schwerer ihr Hochdruck ist. Hier ergibt sich dann ein großes zeitliches Problem in den Praxen, die für die Erhöhung der Compliance erforderliche Kon-
taktzeit mit dem Patienten zu erbringen. Ich bewundere immer wieder die niedergelassenen Kollegen, die in kürzester Zeit zahlreiche Patienten durchschleu-
sen können. Ich brauche eine halbe Stunde bei einer Erstvorstellung für einen
Hochdruckpatienten, bis der Patient einigermaßen begreift, worauf es ankommt,
warum ich ihn behandle und daß er einen Wechsel für seine Zukunft unter-

schreiben muß, daß ich ihn vor einem Herzinfarkt beschützen will, der in 15 Jahren oder später kommt, wenn er nicht behandelt wird. Es ist nicht durch eine in die Hand gedrückte Broschüre getan. Vielleicht kann man durch Gruppenbildung und Gruppentherapie den Kontakt vertiefen und Zeit sparen. Hierbei könnten uns auch die Massenmedien sehr helfen. Im letzten Hugenpoet-Symposion 1977 wurde sachkundig mit den Herren diskutiert, die im Fernsehen die bekannte Sendung „Der 7. Sinn" kreiert hatten. Durch diese Sendung, die über Jahre lang konsequent gesendet wurde, ist es tatsächlich gelungen, verkehrserzieherisch auf die Bevölkerung einzuwirken. Ich glaube es wäre wichtig, über einen ähnlichen Zugang gesundheitserzieherisch auf die Bevölkerung einzuwirken.

Bock: Die Massenmedien sind ein Kapitel für sich. Ich habe auf diesem Symposion durch Kontakt mit Medizinjournalisten, Rundfunk- und Fernsehleuten lernen müssen, daß wir Ärzte uns eine falsche Vorstellung über das machen, was über Massenmedien ankommt und was nicht. Unsere Artikel, Broschüren und Nachrichten, so schön sie im einzelnen auch immer sein mögen, werden von der Bevölkerung nicht akzeptiert. Die Sensation, der Aufhänger ist es, der mit der Nachricht verbunden werden muß. Brustkrebs ist schlimm, diese Aussage wirkt aber nicht. Aber wenn Betty Ford Brustkrebs hat, dann ist dies eine Nachricht, die Wirkung zeigt. Insgesamt möchte ich warnen, daß wir uns als Amateure auf das Gebiet der Werbung und der Massenmedien begeben. Hierbei muß man sich professionellen Rates versichern.

Die Nebenwirkung von Medikamenten, um das kurz zu streifen, sind ein recht wichtiges Problem. Ein Patient mit schwerster Hypertonie wird Nebenwirkungen in Kauf nehmen müssen, ein Grenzwerthypertoniker kaum. In der Regel sollten wir bei dem umfangreichen Medikamentenangebot durchaus die Alternative finden, mit der wir relativ nebenwirkungsfrei behandeln können.

Schwartz: Wir haben in Deutschland einen Arzneimittelmarkt mit einem sehr hohen Anteil von Kombinationspräparaten. Dies gilt vermutlich auch für die blutdrucksenkenden Medikamente. Es sind nun Bestrebungen im Gange, im Rahmen von Transparenzlisten die Kombinationspräparte einer Bewertung zuzuführen, wie sie beispielsweise auch von der amerikanischen Arzneimittelbehörde angewandt wird. Die vorliegenden Kriterien sehen das Stichwort Compliance nicht vor. Meine Frage an diejenigen, die in der Hypertonietherapie Bescheid wissen: Wie ernst ist das Argument zu nehmen, daß Kombinationspräparate unter dem Gesichtspunkt der Compliance einen ernsthaften Stellenwert haben?

Philipp: Nach den bislang nur wenigen vorliegenden Untersuchungen scheint es recht sicher zu sein, daß die Verringerung der Tablettenzahl die Patientencompliance verbessern kann. Um die tägliche Tablettenzahl aber verringern zu können, sind natürlich Kombinationspräparate insbesondere in der Hochdrucktherapie geeignet und zu propagieren.

Bock: Es ist auch international akzeptiert, daß die Hochdruck-Kombinationspräparate eine echte Bereicherung darstellen. Von den 80-100 Kombinationspräparaten sind jedoch nur etwa 20-25 sinnvoll zusammengesetzt. Wir haben im Merkblatt der Liga zur Therapie diese Kombinationspräparate aufgeführt. In der Hochdrucktherapie sind wir also von unseren puristischen Empfehlungen einer grundsätzlich freien Kombination zu Gunsten einer besseren Compliance abgegangen und haben, wie auch die FDA, Kombinationspräparate propagiert. Voraussetzung ist aber eine zweckentsprechende Zusammensetzung.

Jahnecke: Nur ein kleiner Einwand. Zunächst sollte geprüft werden, ob eine Monotherapie nicht ausreicht. Von Monat zu Monat erfahren wir, daß die potentiellen, waschzettelbedingten Nebenwirkungen sehr zur Non-Compliance beitragen. Und die Kombinationspräparate mit Dreierkombinationen haben natürlich die größte Liste an sogenannten potentiellen Nebenwirkungen. Aus diesem Grunde trotz meiner Zuneigung zu Kombinationspräparaten zunächst die Bitte, eine einfache Monotherapie zu versuchen.

Bock: Diese Klarstellung war nötig. Ich möchte jetzt Herrn Laaser noch einmal bitten, bevor wir zum letzten Teil, der Primärpraevention kommen, in ein paar Stichworten uns zu sagen, welche Möglichkeiten er sieht, die Effizienz oder zunächst einmal die Effektivität eines Praeventionsprogrammes zu demonstrieren, Möglichkeiten, die bei uns realisierbar sind.

Laaser: Wenn man die Blutdrucksenkung als Maß für die Effektivität eines Interventionsprogrammes ansieht, so ist dieses sicher nur ein intermediäres Kriterium, das man allerdings auch in großen Bevölkerungen einfach messen kann. Ein Interventionsprogramm kann durchaus im Rahmen einer Aktion, wie sie Herr Philipp durchgeführt hat, auf seine Effektivität überprüft werden. Wir haben eine ähnliche Screening-Untersuchung, wenn auch unter schwierigeren Voraussetzungen, in Köln durchgeführt, wobei wir an den dortigen Schulen insgesamt 6.300 Schüler, das entsprach einer Beteiligung von 76%, mit einem Primär-Screening fassen konnten. Ein Jahr später wurden von den ersterfaßten Schülern noch einmal 80% nachuntersucht. Bei solchen Beteiligungsraten kann man — vor allem, wenn man zusätzlich auch noch eine Analyse der Nichtteilnehmer durchführt — Selektionsphänomene nachweisen und so zu einer Aussage über die Bezugsbevölkerung kommen. Wenn die Populationsbasis in diesem Sinne ausreichend genau definiert wird, dann kann die Effektivität des Interventionsprogrammes unter Einschluß von Diagnostik, Therapie und Compliance durch das Ausmaß der erreichten Blutdrucksenkung bewertet werden. Eine nationale Studie ist hierzu nicht notwendig, andererseits wird eine Praxis wiederum für solche Untersuchungen zu klein sein. Eine mittlere Stadt als Ausgangsgröße wäre sicherlich für derartige Untersuchungen ausreichend. Die Senkung des Blutdruckes an sich aber nachzuweisen, reicht noch nicht aus. Denn wenn er keine Beschwerden macht, schadet er eigentlich nicht, und wir wollen ihn ja nur senken, um seine Folgen, d.h. Herzinfarkt, Schlaganfall bzw. arteriosklerotische Komplikationen, zu verhindern. Die nun zu erfassen und in Beziehung zu Anfangsmaßnahmen wie Screening und zu den nachfolgenden Maßnahmen der Behandlung und auch zur Compliance zu setzen, hierzu braucht man ein Register, wie es z.Zt. nur in Heidelberg in Form des Herzinfarkt-Registers von Professor Nüssel existiert. Dieses Register wurde durch die WHO angeregt und derartige

Register müßten meiner Ansicht nach in mehreren Städten, regional wiederum
begrenzt, eingerichtet werden. Wenn die arteriosklerotischen Komplikationen
über mehrere Jahre hinweg kontinuierlich, ausreichend vollständig und definiert erfaßt werden, dann erlauben diese Daten eine Effizienzanalyse von Screening und Behandlungsmaßnahmen.

Bock: Um es für unsere Zuhörer klarzustellen, Register heißt in diesem Zusammenhang nicht, daß Sie alle Hypertoniker erfassen, sondern daß Sie lediglich
bestimmte Komplikationen vollständig erfassen wollen, ist das richtig?

Laaser: Es kommt auf die Enddefinition an. Es gibt auch Register, die sich auf
die Enddefinition Hypertonie beziehen. Von größerer Bedeutung sind aber die
Register, die sich auf die harten Daten wie Herzinfarkt und Schlaganfall beziehen.

Bock: Die Krebsregister erfassen meines Wissens ja alle Fälle von bestimmten
Krebserkrankungen, auch unabhängig davon, ob die Personen hieran sterben
oder nicht.

Laaser: Es ist hiermit auch nicht gesagt, daß nur die an einem Herzinfarkt Ge-
storbenen registriert werden sollen. Uns interessiert die Morbidität und die
Mortalität der Komplikationen.

Bock: Wie sehen Sie, Herr Laaser, die institutionellen Möglichkeiten, so etwas
durchzuführen? Können Sie uns das beispielsweise erklären, wie Sie eine Region
geographisch abgrenzen wollen und wie Sie an alle Herzinfarkte herankommen
wollen, z.B. auch die, die plötzlich zu Hause tot umfallen.

Laaser: Ich kann mich hierbei auf das bereits bekannte konkrete Beispiel in
Heidelberg beziehen. Hier werden alle Herzinfarkte erfaßt, und hier existieren
umfangreiche Erfahrungen und detaillierte Techniken. Man braucht natürlich
viel Detailkenntnisse, um allen Quellen nachzugehen, um die Informationen
aus Krankenhäusern, aus Praxen, aus Instituionen und auch den einzelnen Dorf-
gemeinschaften zu gewinnen. Man muß ganz besonders die Melde- und die Stan-
desämter durchforsten, und hierzu gehört ein erheblicher Personalaufwand.
Aber schließlich wird eine sinnvolle Kosten-Nutzen-Analyse nur dann durchzuführen sein, wenn die Endkriterien betrachtet werden. Ich glaube persönlich
nicht, daß eine einzelne Forschergruppe oder gar ein einzelner Wissenschaftler
sich mit Erfolg diesem Forschungsgebiet zuwenden kann. Diese umfangreichen
Studien müssen multizentrisch mit einer personalintensiven großen Gesamtan-
strengung durchgeführt werden. Aus diesem Grunde sollen derartige Studien
auch über die WHO laufen und von ihr koordiniert werden. Herr Ward hat uns
ja heute über ähnliche Aktivitäten in den Vereinigten Staaten berichtet, insbesondere über das National High Blood Pressure Education-Program, in dem solche Maßnahmen multizentrisch entwickelt und auch koordiniert werden. Ein
analoges Programm ist für die Bundesrepublik im Sinne eines Bluthochdruck-
Aufklärungs- und Fortbildungsprogrammes (BAF) geplant.

Schwartz: Meine Anmerkung zielt fast schon auf den nächsten Punkt hin, wie
ein derartiges Programm zu organisieren ist. Besonders wichtig, Herr Laaser, ist

m.E., daß eine solche Registrierungsstudie nur dann gelingen kann, wenn die
mitarbeitenden Epidemiologen sich in ihrem Umfeld wie die Fische im Wasser
bewegen, was bedeutet, daß sie einen ausgezeichneten Kontakt zu den niedergelassenen Ärzten wie auch zu den in der Klinik arbeitenden Kollegen haben müssen. Ein wesentliches Zwischenziel muß es sein, die Motivation aller mitarbeitenden Gesundheitsberufe dauerhaft aufrecht zu erhalten, alle Ereignisse tatsächlich zu melden. Analog gilt dies natürlich auch für alle späteren Interven-
tionsschritte.

Jahnecke: Ich habe leichte Schwierigkeiten mit dem Verständnis einer Kontrollregion. In einer umgrenzten Region würde bei diesem Modell, Herr Laaser, alles
medizinisch notwendige und denkbare durchgeführt werden. Wo wollen Sie
dann die Kontrollregionen ansiedeln? Ich könnte mir kaum vorstellen, in einer
Kontrollregion mitarbeiten zu wollen. Sie können vermutlich ihre Interven-
tionsregion nur mit historischen Daten vergleichen und dann wird die Vergleich-
barkeit ziemlich schwierig.

Laaser: Vermutlich wissen Sie, Herr Jahnecke, gar nicht, daß sie Kontrollregion sind. Zur Zeit werden einige derartige Studien geplant, wobei vergleichbare
Einheiten, beispielsweise zwei Dörfer oder zwei mittlere Städte in gleicher
Größe miteinander verglichen werden. In der einen Region wird mit den her-
kömmlichen Methoden der Gesundheitszustand erhalten oder gebessert. In der
Vergleichsregion werden nun gleichzeitig ausgedehnte gesundheitserzieherische
und Aufklärungsprogramme laufen müssen.

Jahnecke: Nun wird es etwas klarer, aber kann man wirklich aus ethischen Er-
wägungen heraus sagen, ich forciere in einer Region alle denkbaren Aktivitäten
und bremse die Aktvitäten in der anderen?

Laaser: Lassen Sie mich dazu direkt antworten: Die Kontrollregion für eine
epidemiologische Studie ist ein offensichtliches Problem. Als Kontrollregion ist
jedoch im allgemeinen das reguläre normale Gesundheitssystem mit allen seinen
bereits existierenden Versorgungsmöglichkeiten vorgesehen. Für das Krankheits-
bild der Hypertonie sind allerdings tatsächlich die epidemiologisch orientierten
Kollegen im Zweifel, ob es unter ethischen Gesichtspunkten zu rechtfertigen
ist, der Kontrollregion nur das zu bieten, was „normalerweise" angeboten wird.
Als Alternative könnten wir das Interventionsprogramm gestuft in drei Städten
durchführen, wobei wir zwar auf eine Kontrollregion im engeren Sinne verzich-
ten, aber zu den bereits existierenden gesundheitlichen Versorgungsmöglichkeiten in der einen Stadt nur zusätzliche minimale Anstrengungen aufwenden.
Falls wir nun nach fünf Jahren keine entscheidenden Unterschiede zwischen
minimalen und maximalen Interventionsbemühungen sehen, so ist dieses
natürlich auch ein entscheidendes Endergebnis.

Bock: Könnten Sie nicht eine Region ganz sich selbst überlassen?

Laaser: Ja, indem wir das normal existierende Gesundheitssystem zugrundele-
gen. Aber es entsteht tatsächlich die Frage, ob ein derartiges Programm noch
ethisch zu vertreten ist.

Bock: Ich hoffe, daß wir das noch vertreten können!

Schwartz: Vor diesem Forum, Herr Laaser, sollten wir ehrlich genug sein, auszusprechen, daß man möglicherweise die Effektivität gar nicht feststellen kann. Jede Kampagne, auch wenn sie nur in einer Gemeinde durchgeführt wird, wirkt wie eine Infektion. Es gibt auch eine geistige und soziale Infektionsausbreitung, so daß Vergleichsgruppen nie ganz unbeeinflußt gesehen werden können und alle Vermutungen und Schlußfolgerungen nur relativ sein werden. Es gibt auch bekanntermaßen säkulare Trends, die die Entwicklung überlagern. Es besteht also durchaus die Möglichkeit, daß wir große Anstrengungen unternehmen, viel Geld investieren und zum Schluß keinen Beweis führen können. Ich befürchte aber, daß wir mit dieser Möglichkeit einfach leben müssen.

Bock: Wir kommen jetzt zu unserem letzten Thema, der Primär-Praevention. Ihr Ziel ist es zu verhindern, daß eine Hypertonie überhaupt erst entsteht. Hier ist das tierexperimentelle Modell der genetischen Hypertonie zu erwähnen. Freis hat genetisch hypertensiven Ratten in der Phase, bevor sie hyperton wurden, Antihypertensiva verabreicht mit dem Ergebnis, daß kein Hochdruck auftrat. Ein analoges Verfahren beim Menschen, d.h. die prophylaktische Verabreichung von Antihypertensiva an Normotoniker, kommt natürlich nicht ernsthaft in Betracht. Was könnten wir sonst tun?

Soweit ich sehe, gibt es eigentlich nur zwei Ansatzpunkte. Einer ist die Gewichtsreduktion. Man würde damit allerdings nur 40-50% aller potentiellen Hypertoniker erfassen, nämlich die, die deutlich übergewichtig sind. Der zweite Ansatzpunkt betrifft die Reduktion des Kochsalzkonsums. In den Vereinigten Staaten ist von der Regierung ein gesundheitspolitisches Programm, die ,,dietary goals'', veröffentlicht worden. Darin werden recht detaillierte Empfehlungen für die Ernährung der Bevölkerung gegeben, u.a. für die Kohlenhydrate, die Fette und vor allem das Kochsalz. Es hat viele Einwände von ärztlicher Seite gegen dieses Programm gegeben, die sich vielfach darauf bezogen, daß für manche der empfohlenen Maßnahmen der Wirksamkeitsnachweis ausstehe. Es wurde ferner darauf verwiesen, daß sich manche ältere Empfehlungen später als unrichtig herausgestellt haben und daß durch eine Revision von Empfehlungen das Vertrauen der Bevölkerung erschüttert werde, so daß dann auch neue Empfehlungen nicht mehr ernst genommen werden.

Was das Kochsalz betrifft, so wissen wir, daß der Mensch bei uns nur 1-2 g pro Tag benötigt, der Durchschnittsverbrauch aber etwa bei 13 g pro Tag liegt. In der ersten Fassung der ,,dietary goals'' wurde empfohlen, den Kochsalzkonsum der Bevölkerung auf 3 g pro Tag zu reduzieren. Die Gegner haben das Argument vorgebracht, daß man dann auch empfehlen müßte, den Eiweißkonsum auf 40 g pro Tag zu beschränken, weil der Mensch ja mit etwa 35 g pro Tag auskommen könne. In der zweiten Fassung der ,,dietary goals'' wurde dann eine Reduktion des Kochsalzkonsums auf 5 g pro Tag empfohlen. Auch eine solche Reduktion beinhaltet eine beträchliche Umstellung von Ernährungsgewohnheiten. Von der Säuglingsnahrung angefangen über Brot, sonstige Backwaren und sämtliche Konserven, müßte der Kochsalzgehalt überprüft und gegebenenfalls reduziert werden. Man muß berücksichtigen, daß Kochsalz ein uraltes Konservierungsmittel ist und außerdem zahlreiche Back- und Treibmittel Natrium enthalten. Ein brauchbarer Kochsalzersatz ist nicht in Sicht. Potentielle Ersatzstoffe bei den Backmitteln und bei der Lebensmittelkonservierung müßten auch hinsichtlich ihrer Langzeittoxizität beurteilt werden. Die Erfahrung mit Rohrzuckerersatz durch Süßstoffe oder Ersatzzucker sollten eine Warnung sein.

Darf ich die Teilnehmer fragen, ob sie eine Empfehlung, den Kochsalzkonsum der Gesamtbevölkerung zu reduzieren, für gerechtfertigt halten, oder eine andersartige oder gar keine Empfehlung vorzuziehen?

Philipp: Meiner Meinung nach sollte man zunächst überprüfen, was in unseren Breitengraden machbar und erreichbar ist, bevor wir Dinge fordern, die letztlich nicht durchsetzbar sind. Wie möglicherweise bekannt ist, führen wir an der Mainzer Universitätsklinik in Verbindung mit den Kliniken Zürich und Münster eine mehrjährige Untersuchung mit dem Ziel der Kochsalzrestriktion durch. Hierbei wird der Einfluß einer eingehenden diätetischen Beratung auf die Inzidenz der Hypertonie untersucht. Untersuchungskollektiv sind Angehörige von Patienten mit essentieller Hypertonie, die noch keinen hohen Blutdruck haben. Untersuchungsziel ist es, festzustellen, ob wir durch solche intensiven diätetischen Maßnahmen die Häufigkeit der Hypertonieentstehung überhaupt reduzieren können. Und dieses Kollektiv von Kindern von Hypertonikern hat sicher ein gesteigertes Risiko in sich, einmal eine Hypertonie zu bekommen.

Bock: Sie würden also sagen: Generelle Empfehlung nicht, aber prüfen ja?

Philipp: Prüfen auf jeden Fall ja.

Jahnecke: Eine generelle Empfehlung würde ich vom Praktischen aus für gar nicht durchführbar halten. Lassen Sie mich es an einem Beispiel ausführen: Wir wissen, daß 10% aller Menschen fett werden, wenn sie mehr als 1.500 Kalorien am Tag essen. Vermutlich gehöre ich auch selbst dazu. Aber kann man einer Patientengruppe sagen, alle Menschen dürfen bloß 1.500 Kalorien essen, damit keiner fett wird? Ich denke, ein derartiges Vorgehen ist nicht durchführbar. Kein Mensch würde sich daran halten. Wie sollte man überhaupt organisatorisch den Salzkonsum per Dekret reduzieren können? Und dann stellt sich erst die Frage, ob es sinnvoll ist. Bei Hochdruckkranken wissen wir, daß durch Salzreduktion der Blutdruck gesenkt werden kann. Aber bislang ist meines Wissen noch nicht gesichert, daß die Hochdruckentstehung durch Salzreduktion verhindert werden kann.

Bock: Das ist keineswegs gesichert, aber natürlich auch nicht ganz unwahrscheinlich. Sie haben aber ein Problem angeschnitten, das sich bei allen derartigen Maßnahmen stellt, nämlich das Verhältnis der von einer solchen Empfehlung profitierenden Menschen zur Zahl derer, die keinerlei Vorteil davon haben. Wenn wir davon ausgehen, daß 20% der Bevölkerung potentielle Hypertoniker sind, würden wir 80 von 100 Menschen einer Population mit einer Kochsalzrestriktion belästigen, ohne daß sie davon den geringsten Nutzen hätten. Bei den übrigen 20 wäre zunächst einmal gar nicht sicher, ob es gerade die wären, die sich an die Empfehlung halten würden, und wenn, ob dann bei ihnen ein Hochdruck verhindert, vielleicht auch nur hinausgeschoben würde. Dann gibt es natürlich, noch den etwas theoretischen Einwand, daß möglicherweise bei einer generellen Kochsalzrestriktion eine neue Morbidität entstehen würde, z.B. die Zahl der Hypotoniker zunimmt oder vermehrt Salzmangelzustände auftreten.

Schwartz: Ich halte grundsätzlich Dinge, gegen die der einzelne sich selber schützen kann, in diesem Fall durch Wahl seiner Nahrung, für Angelegenheiten des einzelnen und nicht des Staates. Der Staat ist dafür da, allgemeine Gefahrenabwehr durchzuführen und nicht dem Individuum diese Entscheidung abzunehmen, es sei denn, es wäre in den Grundnahrungsmitteln, etwa wie Brot, ein außerordentlich überhöhter Salzanteil festzustellen.

Haehn: Meiner Meinung nach gibt es überhaupt keine Möglichkeit, eine derartige Kochsalzrestriktion zu erreichen. Obendrein, wie wir schon gehört haben, ist der Effekt überhaupt nicht gesichert. Somit wäre ich gegen derartige Maßnahmen.

Laaser: Nachdem offenbar alle Teilnehmer gegen eine Empfehlung sind, möchte ich doch versuchen, eine Art Gegenposition darzulegen. Ich meine, daß Brot ein schlechtes Beispiel ist. Wie ist es aber mit der künstlichen Flaschenmilch für Säuglinge? In diesem Nahrungsmittel ist der Salzgehalt häufig wesentlich höher, als in der normalen Muttermilch, und es gibt Untersuchungen, speziell bei der spontan hypertensiven Ratte, die zeigen, daß gerade in der frühkindlichen Phase eine erhöhte Sensibilität für eine später zu entwickelnde Hypertonie erzeugt wird, wenn man in dieser Phase mit erhöhtem Salzgehalt ernährt. Ich könnte mir schon vorstellen, daß man sich nicht ohne weiteres auf den Standpunkt zurückziehen kann, das sei Sache des einzelnen, sondern daß man sagen müßte, der einzelne braucht zwar nicht die Verordnung, nicht das Dekret, aber die Unterstützung, die Beratung auch im Sinne einer allgemeinen Empfehlung; die geben wir für die Hypertoniebehandlung ja auch. Andererseits muß ich mich trotz allem der vorherrschenden Meinung anschließen: Zwar gibt es für die individuelle Beratung genügend Hinweise, daß eine Reduktion der Salzaufnahme sinnvoll ist, vor allgemeinen Empfehlungen ist jedoch die Prüfung in einer Bevölkerungsstudie notwendig. Bei Empfehlungen für die Gesamtbevölkerung sollten wir daran denken, daß es nicht darauf ankommt, daß nun kein Mensch mehr Salz ißt, sondern darauf, daß jeder etwas weniger ißt und die Salzaufnahme im Bevölkerungsdurchschnitt gesenkt werden kann.

Bock: Wir müssen uns darüber im klaren sein, daß die Teilnehmer dieses Gespräches eine recht konservative Meinung vertreten. Unsere Auffassung deckt sich mit der der Kritiker an den schon erwähnten „dietary goals" in den Vereinigten Staaten, aber man darf auch nicht vergessen, daß dieses gesundheitspolitische Programm von namhaften Fachleuten auf diesem Gebiet erarbeitet und empfohlen worden ist, und daß für seine Durchsetzung viel Geld aufgewendet wird. Wenn wir aber mit guten Gründen der Meinung sind, daß eine Empfehlung an die Gesamtbevölkerung, die Kochsalzaufnahme auf 5 g zu reduzieren, nicht vertretbar, nicht durchsetzbar oder zumindest verfrüht erscheint, so sollten wir auch mögliche Alternativen erwägen. Eine Alternative könnte es sein, daß man diätetische Praeventionsmaßnahmen auf die Risikopopulation beschränkt. Diese Risikopopulation, die potentiellen Hypertoniker, beträgt zahlenmäßig nur ein Fünftel der Gesamtbevölkerung und wäre, als unmittelbar Betroffene, wahrscheinlich leichter zu Präventivmaßnahmen zu motivieren. Das entscheidende Problem ist nur, die Risikopopulation zu definieren und zu erfassen. Das gelingt heute nur auf recht unzulängliche Weise, in dem man z.B. alle Menschen, deren Blutdruck in der obersten Quintile des Normalbereichs liegt und/oder diejenigen, bei denen zwei nahe Verwandte einen Hochdruck haben, als Risikopopulation ansieht. Die so definierte Gruppe enthält aber einerseits Menschen, die dennoch keinen Hochdruck bekommen und erfaßt andererseits auch nicht alle Risikoträger. Es wäre sicher ein ganz wichtiges Forschungsvorhaben, Methoden zu entwickeln, die es ermöglichen, die potentiellen Hochdruckkranken zu erfassen, bevor sie hyperton werden. Vielleicht sind die von Herrn Losse und seinen Mitarbeitern gefundenen Abweichungen im Natriumgehalt der Erythrozyten ein Weg in dieser Richtung.

Meine Damen und Herren, ich darf in wenigen Worten zusammenfassen: Wir haben versucht, einen Überblick über die Möglichkeiten der primären und sekundären Praevention des Hochdrucks zu geben. Die Interventionsmaßnahmen zur sekundären Praevention reichen vom Screening der Bevölkerung auf unerkannte Hypertonien über eine Basisdiagnostik bis hin zu einer wirksamen blutdrucksenkenden Therapie bei möglichst allen erfaßten Hypertonikern. Die einzelnen Schritte der Intervention sollten in Zukunft in bezug auf ihre Effektivität, das gesamte Programm einer sekundären Praevention in bezug auf seine Effizienz laufend kontrolliert werden. Die Möglichkeiten zur Primär-Praevention des Hochdrucks sind begrenzt und bedürfen dringend der weiteren Ausarbeitung.

Ich danke dem Auditorium für seine Aufmerksamkeit und unserer Tischrunde für die lebhafte Diskussion.

Subject Index

spironolactone, 212
spontaneously hypertensive rats,
   cAMP in   86 ff.
   —, pathophysiology of hypertension
   in 76
SQ 14.225 see captopril
sympathetic nervous system, activity
   of   3 ff., 11 ff., 15 ff.
   —, activity of, in mineralocorticoid-
   hypertension   18 ff.
   — and haemodynamics   50, 60 ff.

—, see also noradrenaline
stress, emotional   102

teprotide   114, 130
tiamenidine (HOE 440), therapy with
   4, 7, 9

valsalva manoeuvre   101
vasodilatory drugs (L 6150), noradrenaline and renin   52 ff.

Adaptability of Vascular Wall

Proceedings of the XIth International Congress
of Angiology – Prague 1978
Editors: Z. Reiniš, J. Pokorný, J. Linhart, R. Hild, A. Schirger
1980. 486 figures, 205 tables. XIX, 755 pages
ISBN 3-540-09907-7
Distribution rights for all socialist countries:
Avicenum, Czechoslovak Medical Press, Prague

Antihypertensive Agents

Editor: F. Gross
With contributions by numerous experts
1977. 120 figures. XV, 779 pages
(Handbuch der experimentellen Pharmakologie, Band 39)
ISBN 3-540-07594-1

The Arterial System

Dynamics, Control Theory and Regulation

Editors: R. D. Bauer, R. Busse
1978. 132 figures, 18 tables. X, 310 pages
ISBN 3-540-08897-0

Assisted Circulation

Editor: F. Unger
With contributions by numerous experts
1979. 322 figures, 73 tables. XXIII, 653 pages
ISBN 3-540-09308-7

Atherosclerosis V

Proceedings of the Fifth International Symposium
Editors: A. M. Gotto Jr., L. C. Smith, B. Allen
1980. 250 figures, 183 tables. XXXIX, 843 pages
ISBN 3-540-90473-5

Brain and Heart Infarct II

Editors: K. J. Zülch, W. Kaufmann, K.-A. Hossmann,
V. Hossmann
With contributions by numerous experts
1979. 114 figures, 22 tables. XII, 330 pages
ISBN 3-540-09401-6

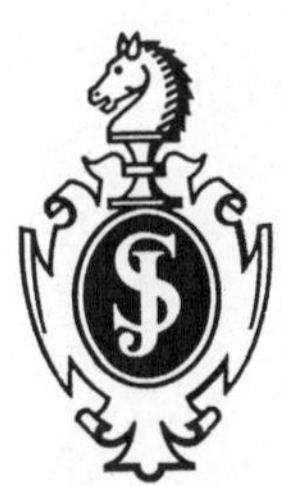

Springer-Verlag
Berlin
Heidelberg
New York

Cardiac Nuclear Medicine

Editors: B. L. Holman, H. L. Abrams, E. Zeitler
With contributions by numerous experts
1979. 47 figures, 22 tables. V, 88 pages
ISBN 3-540-09803-8

Coronary-Prone Behavior

Editors: T. M. Dembroski, S. M. Weiss, J. L. Shields,
S. G. Haynes, M. Feinleib
1978. 6 figures, 13 tables. XVI, 244 pages
ISBN 3-540-08876-8

Evaluation of Cardiac Function by Echocardiography

Editors: W. Bleifeld, P. Hanrath, D. Mathey, S. Effert
1980. 145 figures, 13 tables. Approx. 210 pages
ISBN 3-540-10045-8

B. J. Harlan, A. Starr, F. M. Harwin
Manual of Cardiac Surgery

Volume 1

1980. 193 figures. XV, 204 pages
(Comprehensive Manuals of Surgical Specialties)
ISBN 3-540-90393-3

Hypertension and the Kidney

Proceedings of a Symposium on 'Hypertension and the
Kidney', Milan, Italy, September 28-29, 1974
Guest Editors: B. Kincaid-Smith, M. H. Maxwell
1975. 26 tables. I, 140 pages
(Kidney International Supplement 5 to Volume 8)
ISBN 3-540-90146-9

B. E. Strauer
Hypertensive Heart Disease

Translated from the German
1980. 65 figures, 19 tables. VII, 105 pages
ISBN 3-540-10041-5

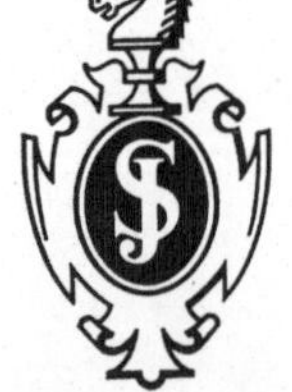

Springer-Verlag
Berlin
Heidelberg
New York